U0308155

教育部人文社会科学研究青年基金项目（18YJCZH017）资助成果

《黄帝内经素问》
隐喻英译对比研究

主　编　陈　战

全国百佳图书出版单位
中国中医药出版社
·北　京·

图书在版编目（CIP）数据

《黄帝内经素问》隐喻英译对比研究/陈战主编.—北京：中国中医药出版社，2022.12

ISBN 978－7－5132－7812－6

Ⅰ.①黄…　Ⅱ.①陈…　Ⅲ.①《素问》—英语—翻译—研究

Ⅳ.① R221.1 ② H315.9

中国版本图书馆 CIP 数据核字（2022）第 172355 号

中国中医药出版社出版

北京经济技术开发区科创十三街 31 号院二区 8 号楼

邮政编码　100176

传真　010-64405721

三河市同力彩印有限公司印刷

各地新华书店经销

开本 710×1000　1/16　印张 21.5　字数 525 千字

2022 年 12 月第 1 版　2022 年 12 月第 1 次印刷

书号　ISBN 978－7－5132－7812－6

定价　148.00 元

网址　www.cptcm.com

服 务 热 线　010-64405510

购 书 热 线　010-89535836

维 权 打 假　010-64405753

微信服务号　zgzyycbs

微商城网址　https://kdt.im/LIdUGr

官 方 微 博　http://e.weibo.com/cptcm

天猫旗舰店网址　https://zgzyycbs.tmall.com

如有印装质量问题请与本社出版部联系（010-64405510）
版权专有　侵权必究

《〈黄帝内经素问〉隐喻英译对比研究》
编委会

主　审　刘桂荣

主　编　陈　战

副主编　李茂峰　徐　丽　姚秋慧　曲　悃
　　　　宋红波　孔冉冉　刘晓杰

编　者　（以姓氏笔画为序）
　　　　王　莹　文世芳　孔冉冉　曲　悃
　　　　刘晓杰　刘晓燕　李茂峰　李淑燕
　　　　宋红波　陈　战　陈学习　赵文竹
　　　　姚秋慧　徐　丽

编写说明

　　认知语言学认为，隐喻无处不在。它不仅是一种语言现象，更是一种认知现象，是人们认识周围世界的重要工具。长期以来，中医学因其晦涩的语言和独特的思维方式而不为国际科技界理解和接受。从隐喻的角度研究中医学的奠基之作《黄帝内经》可以了解语言背后古人的思维和认知方式，为研究其他中医典籍提供有益的参考。从英译的角度研究《黄帝内经》中的隐喻现象，总结和归纳隐喻的英译策略和方法，更是可以在中医学古奥的语言和独特的思维方式与现代语言之间搭建一座桥梁。这不仅有助于从更深层次理解和阐释中医学的语言，而且能为深入研究和准确翻译其他中医典籍提供相似的途径和方法，从而推动中医典籍英译事业和中医药跨文化传播事业的发展。

　　本书从翻译理论和隐喻英译的基本知识出发，聚焦《素问》中不同类型的隐喻，对比四个英译本对隐喻的不同译法，总结不同译者的翻译风格及认知隐喻观指导下《素问》隐喻的英译策略和方法。全书分上、中、下篇。上篇首先介绍翻译的基本概念、原则和标准、方法和技巧及翻译的过程，然后从认知角度探讨影响隐喻翻译的因素并提出具体可行的隐喻翻译策略。中篇以自建的汉英双语平行语料库为工具，结合中医学、语言学和翻译学等学科理论，从语言与内容等角度对四个英译本中的空间隐喻、本体隐喻、结构隐喻、社会关系隐喻等四类隐喻译文进行对比分析，尤其注重隐喻跨文化交际效果的实现。下篇首先从语言风格、翻译策略和目标实现等方面描述四位译者的翻译风格，从原文解读和文化意识等角度分析出现不同翻译风格的原因。

在此基础上，总结出对等策略、本体补偿策略、舍喻体译喻底策略和隐喻显化策略等翻译策略以及相对应的直译法、意译法、直译意译结合法和音译（加注）法等翻译方法。

　　本书选择《素问》的四个典型英译本进行英译对比研究，分别为：①中国学者李照国：*Yellow Emperor's Cannon of Medicine·Plain Conversation*（世界图书出版西安有限公司，2005），简称李本；②美国人威斯（Ilza Veith）：*The Yellow Emperor's Classic of Internal Medicine*（台湾南天书局有限公司，1982），简称威本；③德国汉学家文树德（Paul U. Unschuld）、美国学者田和曼（Hermann Tessenow）和中国学者郑金生：*Huang Di Nei Jing Su Wen: An Annotated Translation of Huang Di's Inner Classic — Basic Questions*（University of California Press，2011），简称文本；④旅美华人中医师吴连胜、吴奇：*The Yellow Emperor's Canon of Internal Medicine*（中国科学技术出版社，1997），简称吴本。需要说明的是，对于以上译本中出现的少许错误，本着"尊重原作，不做改动"的原则，如实呈现译文原貌，以便读者全面了解和把握译者特点和译文质量。李本译文 [ ] 中的内容是译者因为语法结构或者语义表达的需要而补充增加的词语。文本译文 { } 里的内容是译者对其认为的衍文而作的标记。中文释义主要参考：①张灿岬：《黄帝内经素问语释》（山东科技出版社，2017）；②郭霭春：《黄帝内经素问语译》（人民卫生出版社，2013）。从二者中选择更为合理的释义，作为衡量英译本质量的参照。

　　本书具体撰写分工如下：陈战撰写第一章第一、二、三节，第三章第一、二节；李茂峰撰写第一章第四节；刘晓杰撰写第三章第三节；姚秋慧撰写第四章，第九章第一节；曲恤撰写第五章第一节前半部分，第八章第一、二节；文世芳撰写第五章第一节后半部分；孔冉冉撰写第五章第二、三节，第八章第三、四节；刘晓燕撰写第二章第一节，第五章第四节，第六章第一节；宋红波撰写第二章第二、三节，第六章第二节；李淑燕撰写第六章第三节，第七章；徐丽撰写第六章第四节前半部分，第九章第二节；王莹撰写第六章第四节后半部分；陈学习负责第一至五章审校工作；赵文竹负责第六至九章审校工作。

　　本书是在教育部人文社会科学研究青年基金项目"基于语料库的《黄帝内经素问》隐喻英译对比研究"（18YJCZH017）的资助下完成，部分内容曾以论文的形式发表于《中国中医基础医学杂志》《时珍国医国药》《环球中医药》《西部中医药》《海外英语》等学术期刊，并引用参考了我们以前的研究成果，在此特别说明。

由于时间仓促，加之水平有限，书中难免存在疏漏甚至错误之处，恳请读者和专家批评指正，以便再版时修订完善。

《〈黄帝内经素问〉隐喻英译对比研究》编委会

2022 年 4 月

编写说明

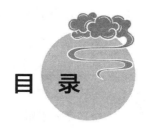

目 录

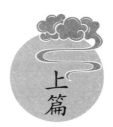

上篇

翻译与隐喻的翻译

第一章　翻译基本知识

第一节　翻译的概念

翻译活动与社会变化密切相关。自人类沟通交流伊始，翻译活动就相伴相随。据现有的文字记载，中国的翻译历史已达三千余年[1]。《礼记·王制》提到"五方之民，言语不通"，为了"达其志，通其欲"，各方都有专人，而"北方曰译"。《周礼》中的"象胥"，即为四方译官之总称。我国历史上出现最早的、较大规模的文字翻译活动是佛经翻译。佛经译者在"译"字前加"翻"，成为"翻译"一词，一直流传到今天。

在漫长的翻译历史长河中，古今中外从不同角度对"翻译"进行了界定和阐释，反映出人们对翻译实践活动的认识。我国《辞海》把"翻译"定义为"把一种语言文字的意义用另一种语言文字表达出来"。英国《牛津英语词典》给"翻译"下的定义是：to turn from one language into another（从一种语言转换成另一种语言）。美国《新编韦氏国际词典（第三版）》定义为：to turn into one's own or another language（转换成本族语或另一种语言）。美国翻译理论家尤金·奈达（Eugene Nida）在给翻译下定义时，把翻译中的"意义"概括成"语义"和"文体"。他说：Translating consists in reproducing in the receptor language the equivalent of the source-language message, first in terms of meaning and secondly in terms of style.（所谓翻译，是指在译语中用最切近而又自然的对等语再现源语的信息，首先在语义上，其次是文体上。）

由此可见，翻译是把一种语言/语言变体（即译语，target language）表

---

[1]　马祖毅.中国翻译简史[M].北京：中国对外翻译出版公司，2004：1.

达的意义用另一种语言/语言变体（即源语，source language）传达出来，以达到沟通思想情感、传播文化知识、促进社会文明的目的。"翻"是指两种语言的转换，而"译"是指两种语言转换的过程。二者构成一般意义上的翻译，让更多人了解其他语言的含义。

翻译属于交叉学科，与语言学、符号学、修辞学、心理学、人类学等有着密切关系。它是一种跨语言、跨文化、跨时间、跨空间的复杂言语交际活动，使原作者的思想与读者的思想得以沟通。翻译过程不仅涉及两种语言，而且还涉及两种文化，因为语言是文化的载体。翻译是一种创造性实践活动，形成于社会、文化和语言现实中，同时又为促进社会、文化和语言发展服务。

第二节　翻译的原则和标准

翻译原则与翻译标准，实际上是同一事物的两个方面。翻译原则是就译者而言的，即译者在翻译时应遵循的原则；而翻译标准是就读者或评论家来说的，是评价译文优劣的标准。翻译原则和标准是指导翻译实践的准绳，也是衡量译文好坏的尺度。

唐代翻译大师玄奘主张"既需求真，又需喻俗"的翻译标准。"求真"即忠实原文，"喻俗"即译文应合乎译语的表达习惯，让读者感觉译文通俗易懂。玄奘的"求真喻俗"总结了翻译的核心标准，与现代翻译标准较为契合。

18世纪末，爱丁堡大学教授亚历山大·F·泰特勒（Alexander Fraser Tytler）在《论翻译的原则》（*Essay on the Principles of Translation*）一书中系统地提出了翻译和评价译文的三条基本原则：

1. A translation should give a complete transcript of the ideas of the original work.（译文应完全传达原文的思想。）

2. The style and manner of writing should be of the same character as that of the original.（译文的风格和笔调应与原文一致。）

3. A translation should have all the ease of the original composition.（译文应与原文一样流畅。）

19 世纪末，翻译家严复在《天演论·译例言》中提出了"信、达、雅"（Faithfulness, Expressiveness and Elegance）的三字标准。"信"即译文应表现作者的真实意图；"达"表示译文应与原文表达同一个意思；"雅"指译文要有文采。"信""达""雅"之间是相互关联的递进关系，"信"为基础，"达"为核心，"信达而外，求其尔雅"。

无论泰特勒的三原则，还是严复的三字标准，都对翻译界产生了很大的影响。特别是后者的提法简明扼要、层次分明、主次突出，虽争议颇多，却一直在翻译界占有一席之地。

后人批判性地继承并发展了严复的三字标准，总结出"忠实、通顺"（Faithfulness and Smoothness）的四字标准。"忠实"首先指译文内容应该忠实于原作。译者必须把原作内容完整而准确地表达出来，不得有任何篡改、歪曲、遗漏或增删现象。"忠实"还指译文要保持原作风格，包括民族风格、时代风格、语体风格、作者个人风格等。所谓"通顺"，指译文语言必须通顺易懂，符合规范。译文必须明白流畅，没有佶屈聱牙、文理不通、晦涩难懂等现象。忠实和通顺相辅相成。忠实而不通顺，读者无法看明白，失去了翻译的意义；通顺而不忠实，脱离了原文的内容和风格，翻译便成了无益之举。

翻译是一种创造性的交流活动，译者需要坚持翻译的标准和原则。然而在翻译实践中，不同体裁、不同题材、不同读者和不同工作方式，对翻译的要求不尽相同。这就要求译者在坚持翻译标准和原则的前提下，相应地采取灵活机动的方法，满足各类翻译工作的需要，而不是将翻译标准视为一成不变的教条，生搬硬套。译者的任务是在翻译中将原则性和灵活性有机结合在一起，实现奈达提出的"动态对等"（dynamic equivalence）。

第三节　翻译的方法和技巧

翻译是一种涉及两种文化之间信息转换的跨文化活动。两种文化在风俗习惯、历史、地理和宗教等方面以及两种语言的结构本身都存在很多差异，这就要求好的译文需要综合运用多种翻译方法。翻译方法是翻译得以实现的具体途径。不同的方法会使译文风格千差万别,也会直接影响译文质量的优劣。一般而言,翻译界大都认为翻译方法有直译和意译之分。

不过,翻译时到底应该采取直译或意译,还是直译和意译相结合的方法,这不仅取决于翻译目的、读者对象和语篇类型,还取决于译者的理解能力和写作水平。通常来说,当原文与译文在形式和意义上基本一致时,一般选择直译;当原文的形式或意义在译语中难以找到对应的表达时,就需要灵活运用直译或意译。

一、直译方法及技巧

直译是指译文的语言表达形式,在译语规范容许的范围内,基本上遵循源语的表达形式且忠实于原文意思。简而言之,直译就是按照原文的字面意思直接翻译为译语的翻译方法。

直译最大的优势在于能在译文中保留源语的文化观念和价值观,特别是保留原文的比喻、形象和民族地方色彩等。鲁迅十分尊重原作,坚持"宁信而不顺"的翻译原则,主张直译,不仅强调忠实于原作思想,而且力图不随便改动原文句式,以保存原作风貌并输入新的表达方法,但这绝不是主张逐字"死译"或"硬译"。

交际语言所包含的意思可以细分为三个方面:字面意义、形象意义和隐含意义,即真实含义。人类在感情、社会经历及对客观事物的感受等方面会有相似之处,因此不同语言中通常会有少量相同或相似的表达方式。这些语言的字面意义、形象意义相同或相似,隐含意义也十分接近,即所传达的文化信息是相同的。采取直译的方法直接套用相同的表达方式,既可保留原文的字面意义、形象意义和隐含意义,又可保留源语的风格,使译文易于理解和接受。

由于中西方在文化背景和思维方式上存在很大不同,人们对周围环境做出的反应及表达方式也各异。翻译时,如果源语形象所承载的比喻意义无法在译语中再现,根据上下文,可以选用译语读者所熟知的形象替换源语形象。虽然这样会导致译语和源语的形象意义不同,但是传达了真实含义,可达到相同的语用效应,使读者产生相同或相近的感觉。例如,spring up like mushrooms 如果译为"雨后蘑菇"也可以接受,但汉语中读者更熟悉的形象为"雨后春笋"，因此译成"雨后春笋"更符合中国文化意象，也更贴切。

另外，汉语中存在大量的俗语和习语。它们不仅形象直观，说服力强，而且隐含着中华民族特定的历史、经济、文化信息。翻译时应该尽可能保持原文的文化价值和形象比喻，同时也应考虑到读者的接受能力。换言之，只要译语读者可以理解，最好进行直译。例如，中医学的"肝""心""脾""肺""肾"等概念在西医中存在对应词。虽然这些概念在两大体系中的内涵不尽相同，但为了便于西方读者接受，一般将这些概念直译为 liver、heart、spleen、lung、kidney[1]。

直译也是有条件的，前提是必须达意，要在译语能力所及的情况下，尽可能保留原文的风格，表达源语的意义。否则，因为缺乏相应的知识，望文生义，将一些不相干的词语堆砌在一起，太过于直译就可能成为"死译"或"硬译"，导致译文令人费解，甚至成为笑柄。例如，有人把"带下医"译成 doctor under the skirt。实际上，"带下"指的是妇科疾病，从语言的角度来看，使用了借代的修辞格。"带下医"实际上是指妇科大夫，正确译法应为 gynecologist[2]。

二、意译方法及技巧

意译是指在忠实原文内容的前提下，不拘泥于原文的语言形式，摆脱原文结构的束缚，使译文的表达完全遵循并符合译语语言规范的翻译方法。

汉语和英语属于不同语系，两者的语言文化及思维方式不同，词汇、句法结构及表达方法差异较大，两种语言的字面意义、形象意义和隐含意义也不尽相符，某些意义甚至完全缺失。在这种情况下，直译无法兼顾原文的意义和文化内涵，甚至会影响对语言的理解或相互之间的交流。为了再现源语的语义效果，传达原文的语用目的，译者只能舍弃原文语言形式或字面形象的对等，采用意译法，在译语中寻找能够表达源语真正含义的表达形式，必要时调整、甚至改变源语的句式结构，或直接译出语言的隐含意义，使译语和源语达到意义上的对等。

例如，"龙"在中西方文化中代表的寓意完全不同。在汉语中，"龙"

---

[1] 陈战 . 中医药术语文化因素英译浅析 [J]. 西部中医药，2014，27（3）：145.

[2] 陈战 . 中医文献英译中的文化缺省与补偿 [J]. 西部中医药，2014，27（5）：143–144.

象征着吉祥如意，很多具有积极意义的成语都与"龙"有关，如"卧虎藏龙""龙马精神"等。然而在西方传统文化中，龙是邪恶、毁灭与贪婪的象征。经典方剂"青龙白虎汤"如果直译为 Blue Dragon and White Tiger Decoction，可能会使西方读者产生误解，认为此药以青龙和白虎为原料。他们会感到纳闷："中国人太奇怪了，怎么吃龙这样的怪物？白虎是濒危动物，应该妥善保护，怎么能入药呢？"[1] 其实，橄榄是治喉病的"青龙"，萝卜是治喉病的"白虎"。橄榄与萝卜一同煎汤，谓之"青龙白虎汤"。对于这类方剂名称，可以采用"原料 + 制作方法"的译法，译成 Olive and Turnip Decoction。

一些词句源于典故或国家经济、文化领域的大事，往往难以在译语中找到对应语，翻译时一般采用意译，译出其隐含意义。例如，英语典故 Achilles' heel 出自荷马史诗《伊利亚特》，若直译为"阿喀斯的脚后跟"或"阿喀斯之踵"，不了解希腊神话故事的读者就会感到费解，因此应该采用意译，译出其隐含意义——"致命弱点"。再如，"天有不测风云"出自北宋吕蒙正的《破窑赋》，比喻有些灾祸是无法预料的。由于英语中的 wind 和 cloud 无法表达出这种含义，所以，翻译时就无法保留"天"和"风云"的字面意义和形象意义，而是意译出其中的隐含意义——Something unexpected may happen anytime。

另外，有些语句既可以进行直译，也可以进行意译，同一文本可能有多种不同译文。好的译文应以能够较为圆满地再现原作的人物形象和写作风格为标准。例如，kill two birds with one stone 可以译成"一石二鸟""一箭双雕"或"一举两得"等。译文的确定必须根据具体文本的类型和主题，以及翻译的目的、译者的取舍、译语的容许度和读者的接受能力来决定。

总之，直译与意译各有所长。无论是直译还是意译，均应首先忠实于原文内容。如果忽略内容，只追求与原文形式一致，则是硬译、死译；如果偏离原文内容，只依据语言的表层意义，片面追求译文形式，随意编造句子，则是滥译和乱译。真正的意译是在正确理解原文内容的基础上，灵活运用翻译技巧，适当调整原文结构，采用恰当、规范的译语形式表达源语。成功的翻译无论采取何种翻译方法，即使改变语言形式，也能准确表达其隐含意义，

[1] 陈战 . 中医文献英译中的文化缺省与补偿 [J]. 西部中医药，2014，27（5）：143–144.

做到思想内容正确而又表达贴切。

第四节　翻译的过程

　　翻译的心理过程由两部分组成：第一，必须掌握原文作者的思想；第二，必须用译文的语言把原文作者的思想表达出来。译者只有透彻理解原作思想之后，才能着手翻译。翻译犹如把一座房子拆掉，然后用原有的这些材料在另一个地方建造起一座同样的房子。也就是说，翻译要经过两个过程：第一个过程是"拆房子"，把语言结构分解开来，这是一个分析的过程；第二个过程是"重建房子"，把语言内容重新建构起来，这是一个表达的过程。

　　具体而言，翻译的过程包括理解、表达和校核三个阶段。

　　1. 理解　目的是全面领会原文作者所要表达的思想内容，不仅要弄清原文的字面意思和主要思想，还要透彻理解原文字里行间的深刻含义。本阶段关注的焦点是原文的内容和形式，明确原文的文本结构、词汇和修辞等各方面的意义。本阶段主要包含两个步骤：①通读源语全文，宏观把握整篇文章的内容，真正读懂原文，以便正确理解句子间的逻辑关系，弄清代词的指代内容，为正确翻译原文内容做好铺垫。②分析句式结构，透彻理解原文语句，这是正确翻译的关键。首先应该找出句子的主干结构，确定句子的主语、谓语和宾语；同时，关注句子成分是否有省略、主句和从句之间的关系是否明确等语法问题。准确把握句式结构及其关系是保证译文语法正确、语言得当的重要环节。

　　2. 表达　是译者在译语中寻找恰当的词语，运用合适的方法和技巧，将自己理解的原文内容加以转换的过程。表达是将源语转换成译语的核心阶段，译者应注意语义和结构的调整。表达的好坏取决于译者对原文的理解程度及其译语的素养和水平。理解是表达的基础，表达是理解的结果。译者把分析过程中所理解的深层结构及意义转换成译语的表层结构，帮助译文读者获得与原文读者相近的感受。同时，由于两种语言代表两种完全不同的文化，其表达习惯也不尽相同，正确的理解并不一定会有正确的表达。因此，表达时需要灵活运用各种翻译方法和技巧。

3. 校核　是复读原文及译文，进一步校对、核实、推敲、修改原文理解及译语表达的阶段，是前两个阶段的深化。校核内容主要包括审查词语、句式及文本内容的翻译是否精准或存在错漏，是否有笔误、拼写错误等问题。校核是翻译过程中相当重要的一个阶段。通过校核，对比原文和译文，检查两者在文字及语法上的对应，并根据原文检测译文的准确性、可理解性以及词汇、句法、篇章和文体等方面的对等情况，使译语准确再现源语的文化内涵，满足译语读者的阅读审美。

在这三个阶段中，理解和表达是两个关键环节，需要译者具备一定的能力和技巧。理解是表达的基础和前提，表达是对源语理解及向译语转换的体现，没有准确的理解就没有顺畅的表达，二者不可分割。理解与表达是相互关联、往返反复的过程，表达的过程中需要更进一步地理解原文。因此，英汉互译时，译者往往需要经历从英语到汉语，再从汉语到英语反复推敲的过程。

小　结

本章介绍了翻译的基本概念、翻译的原则和标准、翻译方法以及翻译的过程。翻译是一种跨语言、跨文化、跨时间和跨空间的复杂言语交际活动，翻译过程不仅涉及两种语言，而且涉及两种文化，因为语言是文化的载体。翻译原则和标准是指导翻译实践的准绳，也是衡量译文好坏的尺度。译者需要坚持翻译的标准和原则，翻译时将原则性和灵活性有机结合起来，实现源语与译语的"动态对等"。在翻译方法上，翻译界大都认为有直译和意译之分。采用哪种方法不仅取决于翻译目的、读者对象和语篇类型，还取决于译者的理解能力和写作水平。翻译的过程包括理解、表达和校核三个阶段。理解是表达的基础和前提，表达是对源语理解及向译语转换的体现。校核有助于检测译文的准确性、可理解性，使译语准确再现源语内容，提高译文的可读性。

第二章　隐喻的翻译策略与方法

美国学者乔治·莱考夫（George Lakoff）与马克·约翰逊（Mark Johnson）出版《我们赖以生存的隐喻》（*Metaphors We Live By*）标志着隐喻认知研究的开始。他们认为，隐喻普遍存在于我们的日常生活中，不仅存在于语言中，而且存在于我们的思想与行动中；我们赖以思考和行为的日常概念系统在本质上是隐喻性的；隐喻是一种思维方法，是人类将某一领域经验用来说明和理解另一领域经验的一种认知和思考的基本方式；作为一种重要的认知手段，它使我们能够通过具体熟悉的事物来理解相对抽象生疏的事物；隐喻作为构建和表达新概念的一种重要的思维认知方式，普遍存在于人的概念系统中[1]。

美国语言学家爱德华·萨丕尔（Edward Sapir）在《语言论：言语研究导论》（*Language: An Introduction to the Study of Speech*）中指出，语言有一个环境，不能脱离文化而存在[2]。文化可以解释为"社会所做的和所想的"，而语言则是"思想的表达方式"。概括地讲，语言是文化不可分割的一部分，是文化的载体；文化则是语言的"底座"或环境。不同民族的人会根据不同的原因创造出不同的比喻，产生这些差异的主要因素就是语言的"底座"[3]。时代背景、文化与地理环境、社会生活、伦理价值观念等无不对喻体的选用产生影响。

从认知角度讲，翻译是从始源域到目标域的映射，翻译过程本质上也是认知过程。隐喻翻译是双重认知建构，包括译者认知重构和读者再认知重构

---

[1]　Lakoff, G. & Johnson, M. *Metaphors We Live By*[M]. Chicago: University of Chicago Press, 1980：3.

[2]　Edward Sapir. *Language: An Introduction to the Study of Speech*[M]. 北京：外语教学与研究出版社，2002：221.

[3]　束定芳，庄智象. 现代外语教学——理论、实践与方法（修订版）[M]. 上海：上海外语教育出版社，2008：129.

两方面。不同语言中的隐喻往往打上原生文化的烙印，翻译既要充分考虑保留或重构源语隐喻的必要性，又要适当兼顾译语读者的认知接受能力，才能最大限度地实现认知建构价值上的对等，从而让译语读者获得与源语读者相同或相近的反应。由于受多种因素制约，译者往往会采用不同的翻译策略和方法以达到有效交流的目的。

第一节　隐喻翻译的影响因素

　　正确翻译隐喻并非易事，要求译者在翻译时要特别注意两种语言之间的差异以及语言背后的文化差异。文化差异和心理差异会直接影响到隐喻由源语向译语映射的准确性。

一、文化差异

　　隐喻翻译不是把两种语言进行简单的语义对应输出，而是在关注两种语言背后文化差异的同时，进行语言转换。汉语与英语分属于汉藏和印欧两个语系，由于中英文化差别较大，导致两种语言的语法和使用习惯差别很大。这些差别往往造成译作与原作在语言上的鸿沟，甚至无法译出。著名翻译家许渊冲指出："根据计算机统计，西方文字之间的对等词达到90%，因此西方译论家提出了对等的理论；但中文和英语之间的对等词只有40%左右，因此西方的对等译论只能解决其中一小部分中英互译问题，而大部分问题都不能解决。"[1] 由此可见，汉英两种语言的差别的确非常大，即使貌似对等，实际上也不完全对等，可以说完全对等的词语极少。面对这些差异，既要充分认识，认真处理，又不能随意夸大或缩小。毕竟，两种语言之间既有个性又有共性。

　　文化，作为一个民族的根基，包罗万象、涉及面广，并且与翻译之间总是存在着千丝万缕的联系。无论使用何种方法进行翻译，文化规约及社会历

---

[1]　张光明 . 认知隐喻翻译研究 [M]. 北京：国防工业出版社，2010：116.

史语境总是在一定程度上制约着译者的翻译活动。正是因为文化与翻译之间存在这种无法割裂的纽带关系，才使得翻译研究能够从文化因素中寻找解释，而文化研究需要以翻译研究为辅助。

总之，文化是人类独有的精神财富。生活在不同地区的人们，因生活环境、风俗习惯和文化背景不同，价值观和人生观也必然存在一定差异，这种差异在翻译时表现得尤为明显。由于中西方的习俗和价值观、语言结构和思维习惯、生活习惯存在差异，译者在翻译策略和喻体选用上也会不同。文化差异是翻译的一大障碍，只有全面理解文化差异并进行适当处理，才能进行准确的翻译。

二、心理差异

在日常翻译实践中，由于受到自身的文化立场、社会身份和自我定位等诸多因素的影响，译者要想分毫不差地译出与原文一致的作品几乎不可能[1]。正是这些个体差异导致风格迥异的翻译流派产生。此外，译者的语言能力也会直接影响翻译策略的选择。同样，对于作为语言现象和思维方式的隐喻，译者在进行翻译时，必然也会受到个体认知和心理差异的影响。

隐喻作为一种思维方式，具有普遍性和共通性。在翻译时，译者对喻体的选择往往会基于相似的构造、心理基础和共同的经验，这使得不同语言之间存在一致的隐喻表达成为可能。同样，不同的思维方式、价值观念等也会导致人们对客观世界的认知不尽相同，译者对喻体的翻译也存在差别。因此，翻译隐喻要求译者基于客观实际，用符合译语表达习惯的喻体进行代替。在一定程度上，译者的喻体转换能力体现出译者对两种语言文化的驾驭能力，而成功的隐喻是译者将源语中的隐喻，通过喻体或调整结构来转译目标域中的隐喻，使其具备形象特征[2]。

在翻译隐喻时，译者对隐喻的转换力是隐喻能否成功实现从源语到译语"映射"的关键。译者对隐喻的转换失当或失误，会影响译语读者对原文的理解，因此也就无法有效传递信息，甚至可能造成误导。考量原文与译文的喻体是否能够做到喻意对应，关键看两者"映射"出来的特性对译语读者来说

---

[1] 许芳琼. 论译者因素对翻译策略的影响 [J]. 开封教育学院学报，2019，39（10）：53.

[2] 黄金德. 认知语言学视域下的英汉翻译策略研究 [M]. 沈阳：东北大学出版社，2019：135.

是否在概念上一致，这也体现了译者在翻译时的喻体转换能力。

第二节　隐喻的翻译策略

认知语言学认为，隐喻的产生既有生理基础，也有心理上的运作机制。隐喻的典型结构为"A 是 B"，而 A 和 B 分属于两个完全不同的范畴类别，是从一个概念域向另一个概念域的映射。因此，隐喻的一个显著特征是使两种本无联系的事物产生联系。这两个概念域在翻译学中一般被称为原文空间和译者空间。在翻译过程中，译者首先确定原文空间里所反映的客观世界，即触发物和目的物及其可能的认知联系，然后需要把原文空间的事物及其之间的认知联系转移到译者空间，也就是说，翻译的对等还是建立在客观事物之间的认知联系基础之上的[1]。在进行隐喻翻译时，实现认知上的对等是翻译映射成功的关键，因为读者对隐喻的理解是通过原语隐喻中包含的概念域在目标语概念中的映射来实现的，因此译者对翻译策略和翻译方法的选择就显得非常重要。

奈达把信息论与符号学引入翻译理论，提出"动态对等"的翻译标准。他指出："所谓翻译，是指从语义到语体在译语中用最切近而又最自然的对等语再现原语信息。"[2] 因此，基于隐喻的可认知性，在翻译时译者为了在译语中找到对应语，顺利实现从源语到译语的映射，通常会采用对等策略、转化策略和异化策略等。

一、对等策略

对等策略是指隐喻中从源域向目标域对等映射的策略。隐喻翻译中的语言转化实际上是进行又一次喻化认知的过程。这个过程包括译者在源域语言范畴的诸多特征中做出选择，然后用目标域范畴中选择的特征与之进行对应映射，即译语篇章是源语篇章在译语文化的再现。总的来说，翻译是两个认

---

[1]　孙亚. 语用和认知概论 [M]. 北京：北京大学出版社，2008：73.

[2]　Nida, E. A. *Language, Culture and Translation*[M]. 上海：上海外语教育出版社，1993：2.

知域之间的活动或关系，是源语篇章向译语篇章的映射。

人类在面对相同的客观世界时所获得的经验是相似的，由此产生的认知理解也同样存在较大的相似性，所以，不同民族的语言中也就会出现许多源域向目标域映射方式相同的隐喻。基于相同意象而建构的隐喻具有民族共通性，即隐喻的概念域可能具有对等映射的目标域。对于此类隐喻的翻译，为保持对等的风格，可以通过隐喻概念的对等映射方式，使用相同的概念域进行映射，也就是采用对等策略。所以在翻译时，可以通过寻找目标语中相同的认知意象进行直接翻译。

例如，"Misfortune never comes singly"可以译为"祸不单行"，"Time is money"可以译为"时间就是金钱"。采用对等策略进行翻译，一方面可以忠实地反映原文内容，实现对等映射，另一方面可以保留并传递原文隐喻所蕴含的文化色彩。

二、转化策略

语言作为文化的载体，受不同文化背景、历史渊源等因素的影响，因此不同的语言既会有相似之处，又会呈现出一定的差异。在翻译过程中，对于一些不能采用对等策略的隐喻，可以采用转化策略，使用译语中相应的隐喻表达进行转换翻译。

转化策略的运用首先要考虑民族文化的因素，特别是对一些文化负载词的翻译，如成语或俗语。文化是语言的环境，思维方式是沟通文化与语言的桥梁，同时对文化心理要素产生相应的制约作用；而隐喻则是其中富有独特的民族文化色彩的代表，不同的文化社会使其语言中的隐喻有很大的差异性[1]。

（一）替换隐喻形象

语言是人们对客观世界的认知经验进行组织的结果，而人类的经验源于人与自然、人与人之间的相互作用。不同民族在历史传统、社会环境、宗教信仰、心理与思维方式等方面存在巨大的差异。如果读者无法有效接受源语概念域的映射，就会导致认知处于不对等的状态，容易引发认知偏差。在这

---

[1] 孙继红. 认知隐喻与翻译策略 [J]. 大连海事大学学报（社会科学版），2011，10（3）：103.

种情况下，可以借助原文隐喻的含义，获取概念域中的译语隐喻，以译语中相似或相近的隐喻形象有效体现源语的隐喻表达，从而获得与原文读者同样或相似的反应。这样，使用目标域中的相关隐喻形象来替换源语域中的隐喻表达，从而达到意义对等。

例如，形容"事物迅速大量的出现"，汉语用"雨后春笋"，而英语则用"spring up like mushrooms"。由于英国不出产竹子，而且 bamboo 也是外来词，所以，在翻译"雨后春笋"时，要把"春笋"转换成英语读者熟悉的喻体 mushrooms，才能有效传递信息。

（二）省略隐喻形象

语言受到不同历史渊源、文化背景的影响，本身体现出巨大的差异性。文化以语言作为基本载体，在翻译时译者可能会遇到很多不可调和的矛盾。很多隐喻反映源语中的独特文化内涵，与目标语言文化相差甚远，如果进行对等翻译，对于缺乏相应文化背景的目标语读者而言，译文就会显得晦涩难懂，甚至会引起不同的联想。为了达到有效交际的目的，译者需要放弃源语的隐喻形式，结合译语文化推导出其中的映射意义并呈现出来，从而达到语用等效。

英语中的隐喻 to carry coals to Newcastle，字面意思为"背着煤去纽卡斯尔"。"纽卡斯尔"是英国著名的煤都，因此该短语一般用来指"多此一举"或"徒劳无功"。由于汉语中没有对应的映射，对于缺乏相关背景知识的读者而言，直译会造成理解上的障碍。为了便于读者理解，可以舍弃源语隐喻形式"纽卡斯尔"，直接取喻义。

三、异化策略

由于地域等差异，人们认知方式不同，在思维和语言表达中也有不同的表现，因而不同的语言之间存在不同程度的差异。在翻译时，有的差异可以通过灵活运用不同的翻译方法得以映射表达，但也有许多源语的隐喻在译语中出现空缺的情况。这种空缺大多与源语的隐喻中包含独特的历史文化信息和背景知识有关，遇到这种情况，就需要采用异化策略。

异化策略是移植原文中隐喻源域对目标域的映射，是以源语文化为归宿而进行的语际篇章意义的互相转换[1]。翻译是一种跨文化的交流活动，涉及信息与文化的交流。异化策略在一定程度上可以消除语言文化障碍，使译语读者能够有效获取源语信息。通过异化策略，源语文化得到较大程度的保留，译语读者也就能够了解到异域文化。不同语言背景的人具有不同的思维和认知方式，从而产生具有独特文化内涵的隐喻。因此，在翻译时若译语文化中不存在相同或相似的隐喻，可以采用异化策略。这样可以把具有独特文化内涵的隐喻移植到译语中，有利于源语文化的对外传播。

东西方文化对于动物有着不同的认知。西方文化认为，兔子是怯弱的象征，所以有隐喻表达 as timid as a rabbit，而在中国文化中，"老鼠"才是胆小的代名词，因此，译为汉语则为"胆小如鼠"。同样，在西方人眼中"马"是强壮的象征，而在中国人眼中"牛"更强壮。因此，英语表达 as strong as a horse 翻译成汉语则是"力大如牛"。

第三节　隐喻的翻译方法

翻译是两种语言之间的交际，不仅是语言转换的过程，而且也是文化交流的过程。其实质是能够突破不同语言之间的差异，从而实现两种文化之间的交流。隐喻是人们在类比和创造相似性联想的基础上，在不同认知域之间进行映射的过程。由于中西方文化存在巨大的差异，译者在翻译隐喻时会遇到诸多问题。译者只有具备深厚的文化底蕴，合理利用各种翻译策略和方法，处理好两种语言文化之间的差异，才能最大限度地译出隐喻所包含的文化内涵。隐喻翻译的常用方法主要有直译法、意译法、直译与意译结合法及音译法等。

一、直译法

认知是语言的前提，语言是人的认知与客观世界相互作用的结果。由于

---

[1] 孙继红.认知隐喻与翻译策略 [J].大连海事大学学报（社会科学版），2011，10（3）：102.

人类所处的自然环境具有相似性，不同民族对客观世界的认知体验具有一定的相似性。对于同一抽象事物的认知和理解，人们常常会选择相同或相似的喻体视角。因此，不同语言中存在着很多相似的隐喻。

直译以相同的认知心理为基础，通过隐喻概念域的对等映射，使译语读者获得相同或相似的认知反应和认知体验。如果两种语言中的隐喻所激活的目标一致，译者可以进行直译，实现隐喻认知在不同语言之间的迁移。直译法能够最大限度保留源语文化特征，开阔译语读者的文化视野，丰富译语的表达，促进两种文化间的交流。

例如，英语中的 to add oil to the flames 和 castle in the air 这两个表达，可以通过隐喻概念域的对等映射，在汉语中找到"火上浇油"和"空中楼阁"两个短语，故可以采用直译法。

二、意译法

由于不同语言与文化之间存在着巨大差异，有时源语中的文化负载词无法在译语中找到完全对应的词语，无论直译还是直译加注都可能导致隐喻所蕴含的文化信息丢失，这种情况下可以考虑采用意译法。

意译法是在理解词语表层意义的基础上，用译语的习惯表达把隐喻的深层含义表现出来，以达到交流的目的。这种译法基于原文隐喻的含义，通过译语读者较为熟悉的信息，使其可以从译文中得到相应的认知体验。在译语文化中，这种译法并不能实现源语隐喻的对等映射，必须通过译语中的对应隐喻进行翻译[1]。

例如，"Every man has a fool in his sleeve"若直译为"人人袖子里都装着傻瓜"，会让译语读者不知所云。因此，需要舍弃源语的语言形式和字面意义，以译语中的词语表达源语的文化信息，译为"人人都有糊涂的时候"，使译文与原文在内容上达成一致。

三、直译与意译结合法

由于各民族在社会环境、历史传统、宗教信仰等方面存在差异，与客观

---

[1] 文旭，肖开容.认知翻译学 [M].北京：北京大学出版社，2019：53.

世界的互相作用中获得的经验必然也会存在差异。这些差异同样体现在包括隐喻在内的语言表达中。在这种情况下，虽然源语中的隐喻跟译语中的隐喻不尽一致，但都体现了同样的认知，因此通常不是把原文中的喻体直接移植到译语中，而是采用译语的喻体翻译原文的隐喻，以方便译语读者接受隐喻信息，从而在新的认知语境中实现翻译等值[1]。在直译可能导致意思不清或误解时，应尽可能采取直译与意译相结合的方法进行翻译。

例如，"The conversation was on wings"句中出现的 on wings 让人联想到鸟儿在空中自由自在地飞翔。句子的隐含意思是：The conversation was unbounded, as free as a bird in the sky. 句中将"谈话"隐喻成"小鸟"，喻指谈话轻松愉快。若直译成"谈话像是长了翅膀一样"显然词不达意，因此可以考虑采用直译与意译结合法，译为：谈话变得轻松自如，无拘无束。

四、音译（加注）法

在跨文化交流中，音译（加注）法也较为常见。音译（加注）法是将源语的发音直接转换成译语相同或相近的语音，采用的译语词汇失去其自身的原意，只保留语音和书写形式。有时为了便于读者理解，会采用加注的形式予以补充。

隐喻通常蕴含着丰富的文化内涵，包括特有的民俗风情、典故、传说、历史事件等。在另一种语言中寻找对应的喻体进行翻译时，由于文化空缺，往往无法完全再现源语的文化信息。为了准确表达隐喻的意义，让译语读者获得相同或相似的认知反应，可采用音译（加注）法，补充说明隐喻蕴含的文化内涵。这样不仅可以保留源语的文化色彩，也可以帮助读者了解背景知识，方便对原文的理解。

例如，英语中的 Pandora's Box 译为"潘多拉的盒子"（比喻祸害的根源），Judas kiss 译为"犹大之吻"（比喻背叛行为、口蜜腹剑）。由于这些表达在汉语中出现空缺，译成汉语时常常需要采用加注法来补充相关背景知识或词语起源等相关信息，以便于读者理解。

[1]　张光明. 认知隐喻翻译研究 [M]. 北京：国防工业出版社，2010：116.

小　结

　　文化移植和语言沟通是实现翻译过程的表现，源语文化通过翻译得以重构，使一种语言中蕴含的意义及文化能够更好地传递至另一种文化中。因此，隐喻的翻译需要结合文本传递的信息，通过隐喻的映射，使译语读者获得相同或相似的认知反应和认知体验，从而实现传递信息的目标[1]。

　　本章从认知角度探讨影响隐喻翻译的因素，主要包括文化差异与心理差异。这些差异是翻译的障碍，需要在全面理解原文喻义的基础上进行适当处理，才能进行准确的翻译。本章还探讨了隐喻的翻译策略和方法。隐喻翻译不是语言形式的简单对应，也不是单纯的喻体转换过程，而是从思维到语言的互动过程，涉及文化、心理等多方面因素。因此，翻译隐喻时，译者需要在翻译策略的指导下，综合运用多种翻译方法，把源语的隐喻在译语中表现出来，从而最终达到信息传递和文化交流的目的。

---

[1]　黄金德. 认知语言学视域下的英汉翻译策略研究 [M]. 沈阳：东北大学出版社，2019：133.

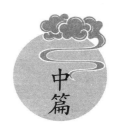

中篇

《素问》隐喻及英译

第三章 《素问》隐喻研究与英译本选择

《黄帝内经》是我国现存最早的医学典籍之一，是劳动人民长期与疾病做斗争的经验总结。书中提出许多重要的防病和治病原则，是中国传统医学的理论思想基础及精髓。但是由于《黄帝内经》成书年代较为久远，其中充满了各种隐喻，文辞深奥难懂，影响了对经文的理解。因此，对《黄帝内经》隐喻的研究将有助于准确理解把握中医独特的文化现象与思维方式，进而推动中医药典籍翻译和对外交流活动的开展。本章将介绍《素问》隐喻产生的原因与形成机制，以及隐喻的功能与类型。在此基础上说明选取《素问》四个英译本的依据，以便进行后续的译本对比研究。

第一节 《素问》隐喻的产生原因与形成机制

隐喻作为言语表达的修饰手段和认识理解客观世界的认知手段，是人类存在的重要基础之一。《素问》中出现的大量隐喻，充分体现了我国古代先哲和医家对生命科学的认知方式、思维方式和表达方式。因此，《素问》中隐喻的使用有其认知原因、心理原因和语言原因[1]。取象比类是中医学的一种基本思维方法，是中医理论建构的基本方法，甚至可以称为"中国式隐喻"的认知模式[2]。《易传》认为其整个过程包括观物、取象、比类、体道四个环节，

---

[1] 陈战，刘桂荣，刘晓杰.《黄帝内经》隐喻产生原因探析[J].中国中医基础医学杂志，2020，26（1）：5-7.

[2] 马子密，贾春华.取象比类——中国式隐喻认知模式[J].世界科学技术（中医药现代化），2012，14（5）：2085.

这正是《素问》隐喻的形成机制。

一、产生原因

《素问》隐喻的出现有着认知、心理和语言等诸多方面的原因。

1. 认知原因　在《黄帝内经》时代，限于当时的科学水平及认知方法，先民们需要利用隐喻的方式表达抽象的医理，借助更为熟悉的自然界事物和现象认识人类自身和人体内部的规律，即所谓的"以物度己""远取诸物"。先民们就是通过"取象天地，效法万物"的隐喻方式认识世界。

世界上许多传统医学，在很大程度上都是借助隐喻的思维方法进行建构的。尽管中医学在理论上与这些医学不尽相同，但是同样能够起到治病救人的作用。令人遗憾的是，很多传统医学已经消失，但是中医学依然屹立在世界东方，这与"天人合一"思想指导下的中医学隐喻思维密不可分。良好的临床疗效是中医学生存和发展的根本保证，如果缺乏这一点，中医学只能视为一种文化，而不能成为一门医学。

2. 心理原因　认知因素反映的是人类共同的认知过程和方式，而心理原因反映人脑内部与外部世界的相互作用。中医学基础理论在很大程度上是通过隐喻的方式构建而成的。一方面，在《黄帝内经》产生的时代，思维和语言相对"贫困"，所以古代医家"无奈"地选择了隐喻这种思维方式，表达对人体生命科学和疾病规律的认知。另一方面，隐喻思维可以帮助人们产生轻松自在的心理和"似曾相识"的感觉[1]，从而产生强烈的共鸣和认同感，因此对于古代医家们来说，选择隐喻的思维方式建构中医学经典理论，在当时的历史条件下是唯一且较为理想的选择。

3. 语言原因　隐喻首先表现为一种语言现象，是语言自身发展的结果。《黄帝内经》时代的先民们遵循"以己度物"的隐喻思维和认知方式，通过具体的、熟悉的意象命名万事万物[2]。在认识和阐释人体的构造、生理功能、疾病现象时，由于缺乏相关的词语与表达，先民们不得不采用"以物度己"，即"远取诸物"的隐喻方式，用以满足当时语言贫乏条件下的表达需要，于是《黄帝内经》中出现了大量的隐喻。"远取诸物"的隐喻思维被广泛应用于中

---

[1]　张沛. 隐喻的生命 [M]. 北京：北京大学出版社，2004：1.

[2]　维柯. 新科学 [M]. 朱光潜，译. 北京：商务印书馆，1989：222.

医学核心概念的命名上。例如，原本用于表示仓库、宫、府的"藏府"被用来表达人体器官，原本用于表示自然现象的"经络"被用来指代人体生命通道，原本用于表示生活用具的"权衡规矩"被用来形容四季脉象，原本用于表示古代官制的"君臣佐使"被用于说明制方原则等。

二、形成机制

《素问》隐喻的形成过程主要包括观物、取象、比类、体道四个环节。

1. 观物 "观"是对外界物象的直接观察和感受，"物"指的是外界的物象，"观物"即直接观察和感受客观世界中存在的事物或现象。观物是取类比象的前提条件。作为人类思维的"象"并非一直存在，而是需要人脑在观察客观事物的基础上不断进行类比和提炼。因此，首先要"观物"，然后才能"取象"。通过观物，人们获得对事物或现象的初步印象或感觉，并在头脑中保存记忆，在某些条件的刺激下可以利用这些印象或感觉取象比类。

2. 取象 "取"是对外界的物象在"观"的基础上进行概括、提炼及创造，"象"则是对所观物象的再现，它不仅指自然万物的外在形态，更注重于表现其内在特征。"取象"就是通过不断地观察和感知自然界中客观存在的事物或现象，在此基础上不断总结和提炼事物或现象的内在"意象"。"象"既可以是抽象的，也可以是具体的。例如，卦象就是一种相对抽象的"象"，是从诸多具体事物中抽象出来的普遍共性，用于阐释和指导世间万物。相比之下，脉象就相对具体。由于脉比较难以捉摸，古人便将脉隐喻为熟悉的具体事物或者生活场景。

3. 比类 指对需要认知的事物与已经提取的"象"进行比较和类比，尽可能发现二者之间的某些相似性，继而将对已知"象"的相关认知转移到有待认知的事物上，从而获得对该事物的功能或属性的认知[1]。比类能够帮助贯通融会医学道理，在冥冥莫测中掌握疾病的变化。中国古代强调天人合一，《素问》也反复强调习医者不仅需要"中知人事"，更需要"上知天文，下知地理"。从中医学的角度来说，取象比类是对人体和宇宙万物进行认知的重要方式之一，通过比较和归类人体的生理和病理现象与宇宙万物的属性和特点，

---

[1] 兰凤利. 取象比类——中医学隐喻形成的过程与方法 [J]. 自然辩证法通讯，2014，36（2）：101.

帮助人们不断加深对人体生理和病理规律的认识。

4. 体道　是取象比类的最后环节，也是最重要的环节。所谓"体道"，就是通过"喻"的方式开展比较和类比，从而发现事物的规律。体道主要体现在取象命名、指导医疗实践和获取新知三个方面。取象命名是指利用取象比类的隐喻思维方式命名中医学的核心概念，从而建构中医学理论体系。指导医疗实践是指古代医家借助"有诸内者，必形诸外"的认知方式，"司外揣内""司内揣外"，以象测藏，为辨证施治做好准备。获得新知是指根据已获取的"象"推测未知的领域，从而推动中医学不断取得新的发展和进步。"科学隐喻能够产生重要的科学发现，甚至可能引发科学革命。隐喻化的本质是发散性和创造性，科学家使用隐喻主要为了理论创新"[1]。

在运用取象比类的隐喻思维解决问题时，通常并不能一次性地完成"先取象""后比类"两个思维阶段。医家在认识疾病的过程中，首先通过望闻问切了解患者的症状，开始取象，然后进一步深化取象思维，进行比类认识；继而将比类的结果与再次获取的新的"象"进行比类。上述过程可能需要进行多次反复循环——每次运用"取象比类"的定性思维都是进行了一次维度调整，都在一定程度上消除不同事物之间的差异性，也是在一步步地向着"治病救人"的目标接近——这样就大大提高了取象比类结果的准确性。

取象比类是中医学的核心方法论。在中医学基本概念的形成、医理阐述和临床发展过程中，"观物－取象－比类－体道"四大环节贯穿始终，"象－比－喻"的思维方式也得到充分体现，最终形成了包含着复杂隐喻体系的中医学语言。因此可以说，中医学本身就是在语言化和隐喻化的过程中逐渐形成的，可以称得上是一种语言医学体系。

第二节　《素问》隐喻的功能与类型

在医学实践中，先民们不断发现新的事物、新的联系和规律，不断提出

[1]　郭贵春. 隐喻、修辞与科学解释 [M]. 北京：科学出版社，2007：36.

新的概念和理论，如何将这些内容清楚表达出来便成为一大难题。在这一过程中，隐喻发挥了重要的作用。它不仅为中医概念的表达提供了恰当的语言形式，更重要的是通过隐喻达到了认知的目的。根据源域的不同，《素问》隐喻可以分为四种类型：空间隐喻、本体隐喻、结构隐喻和社会关系隐喻。

一、功能

《素问》隐喻主要具有语言表达、修辞和认知等方面的功能[1]。

1. 语言表达　隐喻是人类表达新意义的重要手段之一，借助传统语言系统中已经存在的词汇表述新理论或概念成为一种经济而有效的选择[2]。《黄帝内经》成书时期，中医语言尚处于原始阶段，亟需创造出大量的全新词汇来表达中医学的概念和范畴。为了解决词汇匮乏与大量需求之间的矛盾，人们不得不发挥想象力，通过相似性的心理联想，寻找概念之间存在的内在联系，借用已经存在的词汇以跨域映射的方式呈现新的含义，从而形成词汇的隐喻用法。例如，中医病因的"六淫"概念就是以自然隐喻的方式形成的。究其实质，就是将原本用于表述自然界中气候因素的词汇的意义进行扩大和延伸，使之成为中医学的概念。《素问》探讨的是人体复杂的生理、病理活动，很多时候难以直接用言语表达。借助隐喻进行表达不失为一种简洁而有效的方法。由此，一方面体现人类思维的经济性原则，另一方面也使中医概念呈现出一词多义、范畴界定模糊的特点。

2. 修辞　隐喻作为一种修辞手法，必然会表现出一定的美学价值。隐喻具有修辞功能，可以增加间接性和生动性，可以创新，可以使语言温和、精练、优雅[3]。《素问》中使用了大量的隐喻，使这部中医经典著作表现出强烈的形象性、诗意性和艺术性。例如，在论述面部色泽的变化与五脏之气盛衰的关系时，《素问·五脏生成》云："五脏之气，故色见青如草兹者死，黄如枳实者死，黑如炲者死，赤如衃血者死，白如枯骨者死，此五色之见死也。青如翠羽者生，赤如鸡冠者生，黄如蟹腹者生，白如豕膏者生，黑如乌羽者生，此五色之见生也。"此处运用一系列与色泽相关的隐喻介绍色诊，医家可

[1]　陈战.《黄帝内经素问》隐喻研究[M].北京：人民卫生出版社，2021：46-49.
[2]　郭贵春，安军.隐喻与科学理论的陈述[J].社会科学研究，2003，25（4）：3.
[3]　束定芳.隐喻学研究[M].上海：上海外语教育出版社，2000：113-117.

以根据五种色泽判断五脏的死证或者有生气的情况。由此可见，隐喻帮助人们展开丰富的想象和联想，增强中医语言表达的趣味性、生动性和形象性，并使隐喻具备了一定的审美价值，让人产生耳目一新的感觉，引起读者的共鸣，达到很好的修辞效果。

3. 认知 隐喻是人类的一种基本认知方式。在隐喻的认知作用下，人们可以通过已获取的对某一领域的经验来认知另一领域，利用对较为熟悉的领域形成的经验认识不熟悉或较难把握的领域，从而形成某种态度，并采取相应的行动[1]。《素问》借助隐喻的认知方式建构了中医学的基础范畴和核心概念，为中医理论的表达提供了合适的语言形式，例如脏腑、心火、肝风、气海、四气（寒、热、温、凉）、五味（辛、甘、酸、苦、咸）等。隐喻可以帮助解释人体的各种生理表现，阐述疾病发生、发展和变化的规律，从而指导临床诊断和治疗。另外，《素问》运用人类社会中表达情志活动的"喜怒忧思悲恐惊"来隐喻引起疾病的因素。《素问·阴阳应象大论》指出"怒伤肝""喜伤心""思伤脾""忧伤肺""恐伤肾"等，说明情志活动过度剧烈，超越人体的承受限度，必然会影响脏腑的气血功能，导致全身气血紊乱。

二、类型

《素问》隐喻主要包括空间隐喻、本体隐喻、结构隐喻和社会关系隐喻等四种类型。

1. 空间隐喻 也叫方位隐喻，是指同一系统内部参照上－下、内－外、前－后、深－浅、中心－边缘等空间方位组织起来的隐喻概念，是以空间概念为源域向目标域进行映射，进而获得引申和抽象意义的认知过程。在《素问》中具体表现为"上－下"空间隐喻、"内－外"空间隐喻。根据其隐喻含义，"上－下"空间隐喻可以分为表示时间、数量、地位、状态或趋势、范围等，"内－外"空间隐喻可以分为表示运行状态、范围、色诊和脉诊、房事等。

2. 本体隐喻 也叫实体隐喻，是人类在体验物质实体的基础上，将抽象而模糊的思想、感情、心理活动、事件、状态等无形的概念，看作熟知的、

---

[1] 束定芳 . 隐喻学研究 [M]. 上海：上海外语教育出版社，2000：134.

具体的、有形的实体，从而可对其进行指称、量化、识别其特征及原因等。《素问》中存在大量的本体隐喻，类型非常丰富，具体表现为自然隐喻（如天、地、日、月、海、土、风、水、火、溪、谷）、容器隐喻（如身体、脏腑、口、户）、动物隐喻（如鱼、虫、鸡、鸟、虎、驹）、植物隐喻（如榆荚、薏苡子、散叶、草木、黍米、大豆）等。

3. 结构隐喻　指以一种结构清晰的概念来建构另一种结构模糊的概念，使两种概念相叠加，从而能够将谈论某一概念各方面特征的词语用于谈论另一个概念。一般而言，使用源域中具体的、已知的或比较熟悉的概念去类比目标域中抽象的、未知的或比较生疏的概念。在《素问》中具体表现为隐喻构建了阴阳学说、五行学说、精气学说、藏象学说等。另外，其中大量的战争隐喻也属于结构隐喻，用以说明致病因素的性质和侵袭方式、预后不良或疾病恶化等。

4. 社会关系隐喻　是指参照社会生活中用来表达人际关系的各种具体或抽象概念所形成的中医隐喻概念，如君臣、父母、母子、夫妻、主客等。在《素问》中，社会关系隐喻具体表现为官职隐喻、父母隐喻、母子隐喻等，用以隐喻人体不同的构成部分之间的关系、"胜复之气"在一年中的不同变化和不同器官的功能等。

第三节　《素问》英译本的选择

自 1925 年以来，《黄帝内经》的英译工作和相关研究已有近百年时间，国内外已出现 20 多个不同版本的英译本。根据译者的不同身份和学术背景，本书选择其中的四个典型英译本进行对比研究。

一、李本：*Yellow Emperor's Cannon of Medicine · Plain Conversation*

作者李照国是著名的中医药翻译家，一直致力于中医名词术语标准化、中医药翻译与国际传播工作，出版专著二十余部，译著三十余部，发表各类论文数百篇。

李本由李照国历经二十余年的不懈努力最终完成，于 2005 年由世界图书出版西安有限公司出版，2007 年入选国家新闻出版署《大中华文库》工程。李本为《素问》全译本，共三册，采用中英文对照的形式，包含中文原文、现代汉语译文和英文译文。李本的目标读者为对中医有浓厚兴趣但是缺乏系统知识的西方读者，以向西方国家传播中医药文化为目的，遵循"译古如古，文不加释"的翻译思想，避免以今释古及过度解读与阐释，更侧重异化策略，最大限度地保持原作的写作风格和思想内容，保留和传递原文的文化内涵。

李照国兼具英语语言文学和中医学双重学术背景，对中医概念、医理及思维方式的理解较为准确和深入，译本在传达医学知识的同时具有文化厚度与深度，语言更多地呈现学术性。在对隐喻内容的处理上，李本力求文字简练、语法准确、表述清晰明了，以实现阐释中医知识和传递中医文化的双重目标，在众多译本中极具代表性。

二、威本：*The Yellow Emperor's Classic of Internal Medicine*

作者威斯（Ilza Veith），是美国医史学家、加利福尼亚大学生命科学和精神病史系终身荣誉教授，精通五国语言，包括中文和日语。

威本是威斯在美国约翰·霍普金斯大学医学史研究所（Institute of the History of Medicine of the Johns Hopkins University）攻读博士学位期间对有机化学家林达沃（J. W. Lindau）的《黄帝内经》翻译遗稿进行研究和重译的学术成果，所选版本为京口文成堂摹刻宋本《黄帝内经》，以博士学位论文的形式完成。1949 年，由威廉姆斯和威尔金斯出版社（Baltimore: Williams &Wikins）首次出版，后经修订，多次再版。本书选用的版本为台湾南天书局有限公司出版（1982 年版）。

威本为节译本，包括《素问》前 34 章内容，主要从医史学的角度对这部中医经典巨著进行初步介绍，尝试展现《黄帝内经》在医学史上的重要地位和价值，帮助西方读者了解《素问》的主要内容，几乎不涉及文学、语言学等方面的内容。威本由引言、前言、目录、正文、致谢等五部分组成，其中正文部分主要包括简介、附录、参考文献、译文和索引，内容较为详尽和丰富。

威本算得上《素问》翻译史上第一个真正意义上的英译本。译本主要运用异化的翻译方法，同时采用夹注和脚注补充翻译。该译本虽非全译本，但由于译者是以英语为母语的美国学者，译文符合英语国家读者的心理习惯和语言习惯。尤其在对隐喻的处理上，具有文字优美、用词丰富、行文流畅的特点，译文可读性较强，在众多国外译者的《素问》英译本中颇具特色。

三、文本：*Huang Di Nei Jing Su Wen: An Annotated Translation of Huang Di's Inner Classic — Basic Questions*

作者文树德（Paul Ulrich Unschuld），是德国著名的医史学家和汉学家。1969 年开始研习中医药学，1986 年任慕尼黑大学医史研究所所长，主要著作有《中国医学：药学史》《中华帝国的医学伦理》《中国医学思想史》，主要译著有《难经》《黄帝内经素问译注》等。2017 年获得中国出版业颁发的第十一届"中华图书特殊贡献奖"。

文本由文树德与美国学者田和曼、中国学者郑金生合作完成，2011 年由加州大学出版社（University of California Press）出版。该译本分上、下册，将《素问》的 79 章进行全译。文树德致力于"产生出第一部语义正确的《素问》英文全译本以及一个有助于将来对原文研究工作的研究工具"[1][2]。秉承这种理念，该译本结合文献学、医史学及人类学的方法，参考三千余篇论文，极度注重语言和内容的考据。译本集翻译和评注于一体，大量运用注释提供相关历史文献资料，从词源或不同中医流派的理解等方面对翻译内容进行补充，篇幅宏大，内容详尽，在语言形式、内容、风格方面最大限度地保留《素问》之原貌，再现其文化、历史、医学价值，是典型的学术研究型译本，在欧美和国内颇受肯定和欢迎。

文树德主张要忠实原著，原汁原味地翻译中医经典古籍。翻译术语时要一丝不苟地探究语源，重视隐喻和比象手法在具体语境中的应用。在文本中，术语多用直译的方法，尽可能保证形式和内容都与原文一致，尤其是保护中文术语中原本存在的比象和隐喻。

[1] Paul U. Unschuld. *Huang Di Nei Jing Su Wen. An Annotated Translation of Huang Di's Inner Classic–Basic Questions*[M]. University of California Press. Berkeley and Los Angeles, 2011: 10.

[2] Paul U. Unschuld. *Huang Di Nei Jing Su Wen. Nature, Knowledge, Imagery in an Ancient Chinese Medical Text*[M]. University of California Press. Berkeley and Los Angeles, 2003: Ⅹ – Ⅻ.

四、吴本：*Yellow Emperor's Canon of Internal Medicine*

作者吴连胜、吴奇父子，是在美国行医的中医师。吴奇早年就读于天津中医学院，毕业后在天津中医药大学第一附属医院工作。1988 年受聘于美国旧金山中医针灸大学，并于 1989 年考取美国加州针灸执照。吴连胜 1995 年移居美国。吴氏父子长期从事中医临床工作，具有丰富的实践经验和深厚的理论水平。

吴本最早在美国出版，1996 年荣获第三届世界传统医学大会最高荣誉金奖。1997 年由中国科学技术出版社在中国出版，为中国大陆第一个《黄帝内经》英译本，源语文本为唐代医学家王冰的《补注黄帝内经素问》。该译本采用英汉对照的形式，适应了中国的时代发展和市场需求，便于读者学习和研究。本书选用译文来自 1997 年版本。

吴本译文风格独特，前无序言，后无附录，不标注文献来源，衍文略去不译，翻译更侧重采用以目的语文化为导向的归化策略，并不属于传统意义上的学术研究型译本。吴本侧重临床实用，在语言运用上没有过多考究，因此译本的行文朴实易懂，更贴近临床的阅读需求，减少行医阻碍，扩大了传播的广度，应该是指导学生学习的应用型版本 [1]。该译本注重展现中医的临床实践价值，操作性和指导性较强，受到非学术研究领域读者的欢迎。

小　结

《素问》隐喻的产生具有一定的历史原因。在认知方面，先民们利用"取象天地，效法万物"的隐喻方式表达抽象的医理，借助熟悉的自然界事物和现象认识人类自身和人体内部的规律。在心理方面，隐喻在本质上倾向于寻找不同感觉、经验和认识领域之间存在的相似之处，使人们产生强烈的共鸣和认同感。在语言方面，先民们采用"远取诸物"的隐喻方式，借用现成

---

[1]　杨渝，陈晓 .《黄帝内经》英译文本分类述评（1925—2019）[J]. 中医药文化，2020，15（3）：41–43.

的词语或方式表达特定概念或者新概念，满足当时语言贫乏条件下的表达需要。取象比类是中医学的核心方法论，观物、取象、比类、体道四个环节是《素问》隐喻的形成机制。

《素问》隐喻表现出较强的功能。《素问》隐喻为中医概念的表达提供了语言表达手段，利用已有的词语表达中医学的概念和范畴，增强中医语言表达的趣味性、生动性和形象性。同时，《素问》大量运用隐喻的认知方式，建构了中医学的核心概念，启发人们探索人体和世间万物之间的联系，为观察和认识人体提供独特的思维方式。根据源域的不同，《素问》中的隐喻可以分为四种类型：空间隐喻、本体隐喻、结构隐喻和社会关系隐喻。

《素问》在国内外的英译本有 20 多个版本。李照国、威斯、文树德、吴连胜和吴奇等译者的生活环境和学术背景不同，各自的译本也各具特色，对隐喻的处理方式也各有千秋，自然也就成为进行隐喻英译对比研究的对象。

第四章　空间隐喻及英译

空间隐喻，也叫方位隐喻，是指同一系统内部参照上－下、内－外、前－后、深－浅、中心－边缘等空间方位组织起来的隐喻概念[1]，是以空间概念为源域向目标域进行跨域映射，进而获得抽象意义和引申意义的认知过程。空间对于人们生存来说必不可少，因此成为较早产生的、可以直接理解的最基本概念之一。

运用空间隐喻可以将空间中存在的各种关系和性状跨域投射到非空间的关系和性状上。这样不仅可以使原本未知的、抽象的概念变得更为熟悉、更为具体，而且能够不断地丰富读者的想象力，使本来没有关系的事物建立某种关联。莱考夫和约翰逊认为，方位隐喻的来源是直接的身体体验，体验的基础可以从社会物质化的环境中寻找[2]。人们通过身体由近及远地感知周围的空间；在此过程中，人们不断地观察周围世界，并和周围的人和事物相互交流，从而获得大量体验，清楚地了解人体的各个部分，以及与外部世界的相互关系。人们可以运用各种感官去直接感知空间，但却无法直接感知时间等抽象概念，于是人们便通过空间隐喻借助空间概念来描述时间、范围、数量、情绪、身体状况、社会地位等抽象概念。因此，空间隐喻是人类认知世界的最基本方式之一，在人类的认知活动中发挥着重要的作用。

按空间方位的不同，《素问》中的空间隐喻可以分为两大类："上－下"空间隐喻和"内－外"空间隐喻。

---

[1]　孙毅. 认知隐喻学多维跨域研究 [M]. 北京：北京大学出版社，2013：66.

[2]　Lakoff, G. & Johnson, M. *Metaphors We Live By*[M]. Chicago: University of Chicago Press, 1980:15–16.

第一节 "上 – 下"空间隐喻及英译

"上 – 下"原本表示空间位置的高低，后来逐渐用来隐喻其他概念。"上"常用来隐喻高兴、健康、有力量、数量多、社会地位高、美德以及理性等；而"下"则恰恰相反，常用来隐喻悲伤、疾病、死亡、缺乏力量、数量少、地位低下、邪恶以及情绪化等[1]。

《素问》中出现大量表达"上 – 下"空间概念的词语，根据其隐喻含义，可以分为时间、数量、地位、状态或趋势、范围等五类。下面将对比和分析四个译本关于"上 – 下"空间隐喻的英译方法和译文特点。

一、时间

在《素问》中，"上 – 下"这对空间范畴通过跨域映射用于表示时间概念，较早为"上"，较迟则为"下"。

1. 余闻上古之人，春秋皆度百岁……（《素问·上古天真论》）

释义：我听说上古时代的人，他们年龄都能超过百岁……

李本：I am told that people in ancient times all could live for one hundred years...

威本：I have heard that in ancient times the people lived (through the years) to be over a hundred years...

文本：I have heard that the people of high antiquity, in [the sequence of] spring and autumn, all exceeded one hundred years...

吴本：I am told the people in ancient times could all survive to more than one hundred years old...

句中的"上"不是指空间位置的高低，而是指时间概念。"上古"指远古，即人类生活的早期时代。"上古之人"指在远古时代生活的人。

文本采用直译法，将"上古"译为 of high antiquity。antiquity 意为"古

---

[1] Lakoff, G. & Johnson, M. *Metaphors We Live By*[M]. Chicago: University of Chicago Press, 1980:15–16.

代"，在英语文化中尤指古希腊和古罗马时期，措辞古朴、正式；high 凸显时间的久远，准确形象地传达出"上"的隐喻含义。因此文本成功完成两种语言和文化的转换，实现有效交际。

李本、威本和吴本均采用意译法，将"上古"译为 in ancient times（古代）。句中"上"强调时间的久远，而 in ancient times 所指过于宽泛，因此三个译本在内容上均接近原文，但都没有译出"上"的隐喻内涵，未能保留原文的隐喻特色。

2. 肝病者，平旦慧，下晡甚……（《素问·脏气法时论》）

释义：患有肝病的人，在天刚亮（属寅卯）的时候，会感到好些，到了傍晚（属申酉）的时候，病情就会重些……

李本：Liver disease gets improved in the morning, worsened in the evening...

威本：Those who have a disease of the liver are animated and quick-witted in the early morning. Their spirits are heightened in the evening...

文本：In the case of liver diseases, [the patient] feels better at dawn. [The disease] becomes serious in late afternoon...

吴本：The patient with liver disease will turn to the better at dawn, turn to the worse at dusk...

句中的"晡"，即晡时，下午三点至五点。下晡，即五点以后。"下"亦用来指代时间概念。

四个译本均对"下晡"进行了意译。李本和威本译为 in the evening，文本译为 in late afternoon，而吴本译为 at dusk。这三个短语的意思相近，都较为准确地传达出"下晡"的基本含义，但却未能表达出"下晡"的文化内涵。威本对"下晡甚"的理解出现了错误，将其译为 their spirits are heightened in the evening（晚上精神振奋起来），属于误译。

句式结构上，李本和吴本采用和原文相似的结构，句式工整流畅，行文简洁清晰，易于读者理解。文本则把原句分解成并列句，稍显松散；陈述对象（the patient 和 the disease）的变化使译文在连贯性上逊于原句。

二、量级

《素问》中，"上－下"这对空间范畴也被用于表示数量的多少。数量多于某个数字为"上"，少于某个数字则为"下"。

1. 故人迎一盛……四盛已上为格阳。（《素问·六节藏象论》）

释义：人迎脉搏大一倍……大四倍以上称为格阳于外。

李本：If [the pulse of] Renying is one time greater [than usual]... [if it is] more than four times greater [than usual], [it] causes Geyang (blockage of Yang).

威本：When people have one pulse full and abundant... When four pulses are full and abundant, the disease has come to an end and the powers above act as regulators of Yang.

文本：Hence, when [the movement in the vessels] at man's facing is once over [normal] fullness... When it is four times over [normal] fullness or more, [the disease] is "obstructed yang".

吴本：When the Renying pulse (the pulse of the cervical arteries lateral to the thyroid cartilage... when the Renying pulse becomes acute more than four fold greater than the Cunkou pulse, it indicates that Yang is abundant to the utmost which can no more communicate with Yin, and in this case, it is called "Yang being rejected".

"上"隐喻为量级，表示数量上多于、大于某个数字。

李本和吴本采用意译法，将"以上"译为 more than... greater than，正确解读原文，实现了"上"由空间范畴向量级范畴的映射。李本在句式的处理上也较为成功，使用和原文一致的排比句，句式工整，层次清晰，简洁明了。吴本亦使用排比句，并对"格阳"做了较为详尽的解释，便于读者理解。但和李本相比，语言稍显繁琐。

文本采用直译和意译相结合的方法，将"以上"译为 over... or more，较准确地实现了语言转换，达到有效交际目的。

威本将"以上"直译为 above，单就这一词来说，威本成功实现了语言转换，但对"人迎""盛"等关键词的错误理解导致对整句话的理解出现偏差，出现误译。

2. 人一呼脉四动以上曰死。（《素问·平人气象论》）

释义：若人一呼，脉的跳动在四次以上的必死。

李本：[If] a person's pulse beats over four times within one exhalation, it is fatal.

威本：When a person has one exhalation to four movements of the pulse above, it means that death will follow.

文本：When man exhales once and his vessels exhibit four movements or more, that is called "fatal".

吴本：If the pulse beats four times in an exhalation... the patient will die.

"四动以上"指脉的跳动次数在四次以上。

李本采用直译法，译为 over four times；而文本采用意译法，译为 four movements or more。两种译法都正确地解读了原文，准确地实现语言转换，完成有效交际。李本将"上"译为 over，保留了"上"的文化内涵，同时还成功实现了两种文化之间的转换。在句式结构上，李本和文本都使用"从句＋主句"的复合结构。李本借助介词 within，使行文更为简洁，语义关系更加清楚。文本的从句由两个独立句组合而成，句式略显松散。

威本中，"脉四动以上"被译为 four movements of the pulse above（上面脉的四次跳动），above 用来修饰 the pulse，而不是 four movements，显然是对原文的误读，属于误译。

吴本中，"四动以上"被简单地译为 four times，没有译出"以上"，出现了漏译。

三、地位

在《素问》中，原本表示空间概念的"上－下"还被隐喻为社会地位的高低。社会地位高为"上"，相反，社会地位低则为"下"。

1. 夫上古圣人之教下也，皆谓之虚邪贼风，避之有时。（《素问·上古天真论》）

释义：上古时代的圣人，教导他的下属们说，对于能损伤人体的虚邪贼风，要适时地加以回避。

李本：When the sages in ancient times taught the people, they emphasized [the importance of] avoiding Xuxie (Deficiency–Evil) and Zeifeng (Thief–Wind) in good time.

威本：In the most ancient times the teachings of the sages（圣人）were followed by those beneath them; they said that weakness and noxious influences and injurious winds should be avoided at specific times.

文本：Now, when the sages of high antiquity taught those below, they always spoke to them [about the following]. The depletion evil and the robber wind, there are [specific] times when to avoid them.

吴本：In ancient times people behaved according to the teaching of preserving health of the sages: All evil energies of various seasons are harmful to people, they attack the body when it is in general debility, and they should be defended anytime and everywhere.

句中的"下"与社会地位高的"圣人"相对，用于指社会地位较低的人，即百姓。

英语中的 beneath 和 below 也具有"社会地位低"的隐喻含义。威本和文本对"下"进行直译，分别译为 those beneath them 和 those below。语言简洁准确，不仅成功地实现有效交际，还最大限度保留了原文的文化内涵。

李本和吴本采用意译法，将"下"译为 people。但是，people 在英语中是"人"的总称，和 thing 相对应，既包括地位高的人，又包括地位低的人。因此，将"下"译为 people，从语言转换上来说并不准确，同时也丢失了"下"在原文里特有的文化内涵。

2. 故主明则下安。（《素问·灵兰秘典论》）

释义：君是最主要的。它如果得力，下边就能相安，这是根本的道理。

李本：If the monarch (the heart) is wise (normal in functions), the subordinates (the other organs) will be peaceful (normal in function).

威本：When the monarch is intelligent and enlightened, there is peace and contentment among his subjects.

文本：Hence, if the ruler is enlightened, his subjects are in peace.

吴本：As the heart is the monarch in the organs, it dominates the functions of the various viscera, so when the function of heart is strong and healthy, under its unified leadership, all the functions of the various viscera will be normal.

句中"主"指君主，"下"与之相对，指君主的各级臣子、臣民。

李本采用意译法，将"主"和"下"分别译为 monarch 和 subordinates，但在这个具体的语境中，"君"同时还表示心脏，"下"表示除心脏之外的其他器官，因此李本又在 monarch 和 subordinates 的后面补译出 the heart 和 the other organs，表意准确。

威本和文本皆将"下"意译为 his subjects，准确译出"臣民"的隐喻内涵。

吴本对"主"和"下"进行意译，译为 the heart 和 the various viscera，语义表达清楚，便于读者理解。

总的来说，李本语言简练，表意准确，句式结构基本和原文保持一致，与其他三个译本相比，更胜一筹。

四、状态或趋势

在《素问》中，"上 – 下"空间范畴还被隐喻为气血在人体中的运行状态或趋势，说明致病邪气的性质，描述病位，解释病机等。一般来说，疾病侵袭人体为上，而疾病渐愈为下，具有明显的中医学特点。

1. 是故冬至四十五日，阳气微上，阴气微下。（《素问·脉要精微论》）

释义：四时阴阳的情况，冬至一阳生，到四十五天，阳气微升，阴气微降。

李本：During the forty-five days from the Winter Solstice [to the Beginning of Spring], Yangqi is gradually ascending while Yinqi is gradually descending.

威本：Winter lasts for forty-five days, and during that time the influence of Yang, the element of light and life, is weak in the upper pulse and the influence of Yin is weak in the lower pulse.

文本：Hence, during the 45 days [following the term]"winter solstice"，the yang qi is feeble and ascends and the yin qi is feeble and descends.

吴本：The conditions of Yin and Yang in the four seasons are: the first Yang generates on the winter solstice, and on the forty-fifth day after it, the Yang-energy ascends slightly and the Yin-energy descends slightly.

句中的"上"和"下"已经不再单纯表示方位，而是表示阳气和阴气向上或向下的运行状态。

李本、文本和吴本均采用直译法，将"上"和"下"译为 descend 和 ascend，较好地实现了由空间范畴向趋势范畴的映射，准确再现原文信息，完成有效交际，同时成功实现两种文化之间的转换。

威本译为 in the upper pulse 和 in the lower pulse，仍将"上"和"下"视为空间范畴概念，对原文理解出现错误，属于误译。

在句式上，威本、文本和吴本使用 and 连接前后两个句子，李本则使用 while。while 更能形象地表现出阳气和阴气两种截然相反的运动趋势的对比关系。因此，与其他三个译本相比，李本的句意逻辑关系更清晰，译文更出色。

2. 色见上下左右，各在其要，上为逆，下为从。（《素问·玉版论要》）

释义：客色的变色，呈现在鼻部上下左右，必须注意分别察看它的不同特点。病色向上移的为逆，向下移的为顺。

李本：[The changes of countenance] on the upper, lower, left and right [parts of the face] indicate the main changes of diseases respectively. The upper is Ni (unfavorable) and the lower is Cong (favorable).

威本：The appearance and complexion must be watched high and low, to the left and to the right, for each has its significance. When the color rises it indicates rebellion; when it recedes it indicates submission.

文本：The complexion, how it appears above and below, on the left and on the right, all this [can be found] in these essentials. Above is opposition; below is compliance.

吴本：One should observe carefully the guest colour appears on the upper, lower, left or right side of the nose to discover its movement. When it moves upwards, it is in the reverse direction; when it moves downwards, it is in the agreeable direction.

句中的"上"和"下"隐喻为运动趋势，分别指病色向上或向下移行。吴本将"上"和"下"分别直译为 moves upwards 和 moves downwards，既实现语言和文化的转换，又实现有效的交际。在句式结构上，吴本使用 when 引导的表示条件关系的从句＋主句这一复合句式，虽然与中文句相比，结构稍显复杂，但逻辑关系和句意更为清晰。

李本和文本均采用直译法，将"上"和"下"分别译为 the upper/the lower 和 above/below。二者均未译出"上"和"下"的隐喻含义，因此语言转换不够准确，影响交际目标的完全实现。

威本采用直译和意译相结合的方法，将"上"直译为 rises，将"下"意译为 recedes。rise 可以准确形象地表达病色向上的运动趋势，但 recede 的含义是"渐渐远离，渐渐远去"，和"下"的意思并不完全相符，因此译不达意。

3. 十二日厥阴病衰，囊纵少腹微下。（《素问·热论》）

释义：到第十二天，厥阴病减轻了，阴囊也松缓下来，少腹部也觉得舒服。

李本：In twelfth day, Jueyin disease alleviates, the scrota become relaxed and hang slightly from the lower abdomen.

威本：On the twelfth day the absolute Yin becomes less sick, the scrotum slackens, the [swelling of the] stomach is reduced.

文本：On the twelfth day, the disease in the ceasing yin [conduits] weakens. The scrotum slackens, and the lower abdomen moves down slightly.

吴本：On the twelfth day, the disease of Jueyin will be recovered, the scrotum becomes relaxed, the lower abdomen becomes comfortable.

句中的"微下"，指少腹微微下垂的状态。

威本和吴本采用意译法，将"少腹微下"分别译为 the swelling of the stomach is reduced（胃肿胀减轻）和 the lower abdomen becomes comfortable（少腹变得舒服）。与威本相比，吴本语言更为准确，但因为中西方文化差异，吴本放弃了"下"隐含的中医文化内涵。

文本采用直译法，将"少腹微下"译为 the lower abdomen moves down slightly（少腹轻微下移）。不过，读者可能无法理解这句话的隐含意义：the lower abdomen becomes comfortable（少腹变得舒服）。因此，语言的转换并不十分准确，影响交际目标的完全实现。

李本中，"囊纵少腹微下"译为 the scrota become relaxed and hang slightly from the lower abdomen，将"少腹下垂"译为"阴囊下垂"，出现误译。

4. 尽气闭环，痛病必下。（《素问·诊要经终论》）

释义：邪气一去，穴孔合闭起来，痛病也就消除了。

李本：[The Acupoints needled] should be closed after the dispersion of pathogenic factors and the disease heals [soon afterwards].

威本：And since the circulation of the air is also obstructed, there is extreme pain, and diseases are brought about which must be expelled.

文本：Pain and disease must subside.

吴本：When the evil-energy is removed, the hole of the acupoint is closed, the pain will be eliminated.

"痛病必下"指的是"病痛之气便下行而愈"[1]。"下"的意思为"治愈，消除"。李本、文本和吴本均对"下"进行意译，分别译为 heals、subside 和 be eliminated。三位译者都正确解读"下"的隐喻含义，语言转换较为准确，能够实现有效交际，美中不足是放弃了"下"的中医文化内涵。

威本译文的意思为：由于空气的流通也受到阻碍，因此存在极度的疼痛，并且导致必须将其排出的疾病。这是对原文的错误理解，属于误译。

在句子结构上，文本漏译"尽气闭环"。李本将前后两句译成 and 连接的两个并列句，后半句使用主动语态，更符合中国人的思维方式。吴本采用"when 引导的从句＋主句"复合结构，三处使用被动语态，句意逻辑关系更为清晰，易于读者理解，更符合西方人的行文风格 [2]。

5. ……名曰肺痹，发咳上气。（《素问·玉机真脏论》）

释义：……这就是肺痹，发为咳嗽上气。

李本：...cause Feibi (Lung-Bi Syndrome) [with the symptoms of] cough and adverse flow of Qi.

威本：...and then its name is numbness of the lungs, which emit a cough of the upper respiratory tract.

文本：It is [now] called "lung block". It developed cough and rising qi.

吴本：...to cause lung-bi-syndrome, and cough and adverseness of lung energy will occur.

"上气"是由肺气不利所致，此处的"上"隐喻为运动趋势，指病气上行。

[1] 山东中医学院，河北医学院 . 黄帝内经校释 [M]. 北京：人民卫生出版社，1982：202.
[2] 罗茜，周媛，李涛安 . 概念整合视角下《黄帝内经》空间隐喻英译研究 [J]. 中医药导报，2019，25（18）：140.

李本和文本均采用意译加音译的方法，将"上气"分别译为 adverse flow of qi 和 rising qi。两个译本都译出"上"的隐喻含义，但李本更为准确，因为 adverse flow 强调"病气上行"实际上是气的一种不正常的运动趋势。

威本将"上气"译为 the upper respiratory tract（上呼吸道），属于误译。

吴本译为 adverseness of lung energy（肺气不利），但这是导致"上气"的原因。"上气"一词并没有译出，因而译不达意。

6. 四变之动，脉与之<u>上下</u>。（《素问·脉要精微论》）

释义：脉搏的往来上下与这四时的变迁是相应的。

李本：The changes of pulse conditions also correspond to such variations in the four seasons.

威本：This change of the four seasons influences the upper and lower pulses.

文本：The movement [of the qi] during the four [seasonal] changes: the [movement in the] vessels rises and descends with them.

吴本：The coming and going and the ups and downs of the pulse are corresponding with the variations of the four seasons.

句中"上下"隐喻为运行状态，指人体脉象的升降沉浮。

李本采用意译法，将"上下"译为 the changes。吴本采用直译和意译相结合的译法，译为 the coming and going and the ups and downs。两个译本都能够较准确地传达出"上下"的隐喻含义，既成功完成语言的转换，又可以实现有效交际。

文本采用直译法，将其译为 rises and descends。然而句中的"上下"指脉象的所有变化，不仅仅包括脉象的升和降（rises and descends），因此不免有以偏概全之嫌，语言转换不够准确。

威本将"上下"译为 the upper and lower pulses（上面的和下面的脉搏），对原文理解有误，属于误译。

五、范围

《素问》中，"上""下"既可以指人体的头部和脚，也可以指人体的上下身，还可以指天地。

1. 故<u>上下</u>至头足，不得主时也。(《素问·太阴阳明论》)

释义：从头至足，无处不到，所以不单主一个时季。

李本：That is why [it transports nutrients] from the upper to the lower and from the head to the feet. [So it] does not dominate just in one season.

威本：Thus above and below, the head and the foot, cannot be directly influenced by the (temperature of) the four seasons.

文本：Hence, in the upper and lower [parts of the body] it reaches head and feet; it cannot rule [only one specific] season.

吴本：It takes effect on the head, foot and everywhere of the body, ...it does not dominate an individual season specifically.

句中"上下"表示范围的大小，指人体从头至足，无处不到。

李本采用直译法，将"上下"译为 from the upper to the lower，准确再现"从上到下"之义，实现有效交际，同时成功完成文化转换。

吴本采用意译法，将"上下"隐喻转化为其本义，译为 everywhere of the body，语言转换较为准确，能够实现有效交际，但却放弃了"上下"的文化内涵。

威本和文本对"上下"进行直译，分别译为 above and below 和 in the upper and lower。威本中 above and below 和 the head and the foot 并列作句子主语，但 above and below 不是名词性短语，无法充当主语，应该属于语法错误。文本的 in the upper and lower 虽然完成语言的转换，但是语言不及李本准确，没有凸显"无处不到"的含义，因此无法完全达到交际目的。

2. <u>上下</u>不并，良医弗为。(《素问·生气通天论》)

释义：如果病到上下之气不能相通，到那时，即使高明的医生也是治不好的。

李本：[If] the upper [part of the body] cannot communicate with the lower [part of the body], even excellent doctors are helpless.

威本：...then the upper and the lower (parts of the body) cannot communicate; and even skillful physicians are then not able to help.

文本：When [a stage is reached where] above and below have lost their union, then [even] a good physician cannot do anything about it.

吴本：When the condition is serious, the Yin and Yang energies will be unable to communicate with each other, which will make even a good doctor can do nothing with it.

句中的"上下不并"指上下不通，阴阳之气阻隔[1]。"上下"表示范围，指人体的上部和下部，泛指整个人体。

李本和威本采用直译法，将"上下"译为 the upper part of the body 和 the lower part of the body。从语言上来说，译本较为准确，但是未能译出"阴阳之气阻隔"这一隐含意义，导致读者可能并不能真正理解"上下不并，良医弗为"的意思。因此，李本和威本虽然完成语言转换，但并没有完全达到交际目的。

文本同样采用直译法，将"上下"译为 above and below，但这个短语无法充当主语，属于语法错误。

吴本对"上下"进行意译，译为 the Yin and Yang energies，未能准确译出"上下"表示人体上部和下部的隐喻内涵，故译不达意。

3. 九候之相应也，上下若一，不得相失。（《素问·三部九候论》）

释义：九候之间，应该相互协调，上下如一，不得互相参差。

李本：[The pulse states] in the Nine Divisions should be in harmony and unity and should not be in disharmony.

威本：The nine subdivisions must respond to each other. The upper ones and lower ones must work as though they were one; they must not fail each other.

文本：As for the mutual correspondence of the nine indicators, above and below [should be] like one. It must not be that they do not conform with each other.

吴本：The nine sub-parts should be harmonious and be in accordance with each other and must not be uneven.

句中的"上下"指九候的上部和下部，泛指九候的整体。

李本和吴本采用意译法，分别译为 the Nine Divisions 和 the nine sub-parts，基本译出"上下"的隐喻含义，实现有效交际。李本在 the Nine Divisions 前面补译出 the pulse states，在内容表达上比吴本更加详细准确，更易于

---

[1] 山东中医学院，河北医学院 . 黄帝内经校释 [M]. 北京：人民卫生出版社，1982：41.

读者理解。

威本采用直译法，将"上下"译为 the upper ones and lower ones，既实现语言和文化的转换，又达到交际目的。

文本同样采用直译法，将"上下"译为 above and below，虽然完成了语言的转换，但从语法上来说，above and below 不是名词性短语，无法在句中充当主语，属于语法错误。

4. 上下相召奈何？（《素问·天元纪大论》）

释义：天地阴阳相互感召是怎么一回事呢？

李本：How do the Upper (Heaven–Qi) and the Lower (Earth–Qi) interact with each other?

文本："Above and below call on each other",what does that mean?

吴本：What is the condition when the heaven and earth inspiring each other?

"上"指天气，"下"指地气。召，犹招也，此指感召。"上下相召"即天气和地气相互感召。

李本采用直译加注法，将"上下"译为 the upper (Heaven–Qi) 和 the lower (Earth–Qi)。通过注释 Heaven–Qi 与 Earth–Qi 对 the upper 和 the lower 的内涵意义进行解释，帮助读者更好地理解原文。

文本将"上下"直译为 above and below，而吴本则意译为 the heaven and earth。由前面的分析可知，句中"上"和"下"并非指"天"和"地"，而是指"天气"和"地气"。因此，两个译本的语言转换都不够准确，导致译不达意。此外，文本中，above and below 并非名词性短语，无法在句中充当主语，出现语法错误。

第二节　"内 – 外"空间隐喻及英译

"内 – 外"原本用于表示空间位置，但是在《素问》中多处用于隐喻其他概念。"内"常被用来隐喻病邪侵犯人体的运行状态，还用来表示范围、脉诊和房事等；而"外"则常用来隐喻病邪侵犯人体的运行状态和范围。下面将从翻译方法、语言和文化转换、句式结构等方面对"内－外"空间隐喻的英译进行对比和分析。

一、运行状态

《素问》中，"内－外"空间范畴用于隐喻病邪在体内的运行状态、说明致病邪气侵犯人体的路径、描述疾病发生的位置、阐释疾病发生的机理等。

1. 贼风数至，虚邪朝夕，内至五脏骨髓，外伤空窍肌肤。（《素问·移精变气论》）

释义：贼风虚邪不断侵袭，就会内里侵犯到五脏骨髓，外面伤害孔窍肌肤。

李本：Besides, Zeifeng (Thief-Wind) frequently attacks and Xuxie (Deficiency-Evil) repeatedly invades, internally into the Five Zang-Organs and bone marrow, and externally into the orifices, skin and muscles.

威本：Evil influences strike from early morning until late at night; they injure the five viscera, the bones and the marrow within the body, and externally they injure the mind and reduce its intelligence and they also injure the muscles and the flesh.

文本：The robber wind frequently reaches [them]. The depletion evil [is present] in the morning and in the evening; internally it reaches to the five depots, to the bones and to the marrow; externally it harms the orifices, the muscles, and the skin.

吴本：When the thief-evil invades unceasingly, the patient's viscera and bone marrow will be hurt inside, and the orifices and muscle will be hurt outside.

句中"内"和"外"具有"向内"和"向外"之义，说明病邪在体内的运行路径，描述病邪侵袭人体的部位，包括五脏六腑、骨髓、经脉等。

四个译本对"内"和"外"均采用直译法。李本和文本分别译为 internally 和 externally，威本译为 within the body 和 externally，而吴本译为 inside 和 outside。四位译者都正确解读原文，译出"内""外"的隐喻含义，实现有效交际和文化转换。但是，威本将"内"译为介词词组 within the body，"外"译为副词 externally，形式上不如其他三个译本工整。

在句式结构上，李本基本与原文保持一致，使用主动语态，句式简洁，

《黄帝内经素问》隐喻英译对比研究

48

句意清晰。吴本则将原文的主动句式转换成被动句式，更符合英语的行文风格。威本和文本的句式稍显繁琐，给读者的理解带来不便。

2. 风气藏于皮肤之间，内不得通，外不得泄。（《素问·风论》）

释义：风气侵入人体的皮肤里面，既不能在内部流通，又不能向外部疏泄。

李本：[When attacking the body,] wind tends to stay [in the region] between the skin [and the muscles] and is difficult to penetrate inside or escape to the outside.

文本：When wind qi is stored in the skin, it cannot penetrate into the interior and it cannot flow away to the outside.

吴本：When the wind-evil invades into the skin, it can not be dispersed to the interior, nor can it be diffused to the exterior.

句中"内"和"外"表示"向内"和"向外"之义，描述风气在体内的运行路径。

三个译本均采用直译法，李本译为 penetrate inside 和 escape to the outside，文本译为 penetrate into the interior 和 flow away to the outside，吴本译为 dispersed to the interior 和 diffused to the exterior。三个译本都使用"动词＋副词（如 inside）或介词短语（如 to the outside）"的类似结构，将原文中的"内－外"空间隐喻转化为运动趋势，语言转换较为准确，同时成功实现交际目标和文化的转换。

李本补译出 When attacking the body 和 in the region，句意更为清晰，便于读者理解。

吴本将"内"和"外"译为 to the interior 和 to the exterior，二者前后呼应，形式上工整悦目，读起来朗朗上口，为最佳译本。

3. 肾汗出逢于风，内不得入于脏腑，外不得越于皮肤。（《素问·水热穴论》）

释义：当汗出的时候，遇到风邪，汗孔骤闭，余汗未尽，向内不得回到其脏，向外不能泄于皮肤。

李本：Invasion of wind during sweating cannot deepen into the Zangfu-Organs or get out of the skin.

文本：When sweat leaves the kidneys and encounters wind, internally it cannot enter the depots and palaces and externally it cannot transgress beyond the skin.

吴本：When the wind-evil invades the body during the sweating, his sweat pores will close all of a sudden, as the perspiration has not completed, the sweat can not return to its viscus inside, neither can it be discharged to the skin outside.

句中"内"和"外"表示汗在体内的运行路径，具有"向内"或"向外"之义。

三个译本均采用直译法，李本译为into和out of，文本译为internally和externally，吴本译为inside和outside。这些表示方位的介词或副词与相关动词搭配（如deepen into，internally...enter，discharge...outside等），形象地描绘出汗的运行路径，因此三个译本对"内"和"外"隐喻含义的翻译都较为准确。

句中"内"和"外"的施动者应是"汗"（sweat），李本误解为invasion of wind，出现了误译。

吴本采用增译的方法，增加原文中隐而未明的内容his sweat pores will close all of a sudden, as the perspiration has not completed（汗孔骤闭，余汗未尽），句意更加清晰，易于读者理解。

文本采用和原文基本相同的句式，与吴本相比，行文更简洁。

总的来说，文本和吴本都较好地达到有效交际的目的，但译文中多处使用西医术语解释中医内容，放弃了原文的文化内涵。

4. 以息方吸而内针。（《素问·八正神明论》）

释义：要在病人吸气的时候进针。

李本：The insertion of the needle [when the patient] just breathes in.

威本：One must apply it when the breath is being inhaled. Then the needle must be inserted, and it must be repeated when the breath is being inhaled again.

文本：When the breathing is just (fang) [in a state of] inhaling, then one inserts the needle.

吴本：The inserting of the needle at the time when the patient just inhales.

本句说明如何把握进针的时机，其中"内"用作动词，意为"向里进"，"内针"即为"进针"。

四个译本均将"内"意译为insert。李本和吴本分别使用insert的名词形式 insertion 和动名词形式 inserting 表示"内"。与 insertion 相比，inserting 强调动作，更准确地表达出"内"用作动词的隐喻含义，因此吴本的语言转换更为准确。

威本的句式稍显拖沓，句中的逻辑关系也不甚清晰。根据原文内容，可将 one must apply it 删去，将 when the breath is being inhaled 和 the needle must be inserted 组合在一起，形成一个主从复合句，这样句式更紧凑，句意也更清晰。

文本将"内"译为动词 insert，将"方"译为汉语拼音 fang，并在后面进行解释，译文语言准确，能够实现有效交际，同时还保留了一定的文化特色。

二、范围

《素问》中，"内 – 外"空间范畴用于表示范围。

1. 游行天地之间，视听八达之外。（《素问·上古天真论》）

释义：悠游于天地之间，所见所闻，能够广及八方荒远之外。

李本：...and roaming around on the earth and in the heavens. So they could see and hear [things and voices] beyond the eight directions.

威本：They roamed and travelled all over the universe and could see and hear beyond the eight distant places.

文本：They roamed between heaven and earth and their vision as well as their hearing went beyond the eight reaches.

吴本：They travelled extensively and to hear and see things in distant places.

句中"外"是一个范围概念，"八达之外"说明中古至人游历丰富，见闻广博。

李本、威本和文本均采用直译法，将"外"译为 beyond，较为准确地译出"外"的隐喻含义。然而，由于中西方文化的巨大差异，三个译本将"八达之外"分别译为 beyond the eight directions、beyond the eight distant places 和 beyond the eight reaches，这并不符合英文中"遥远的地方"的表达习惯。因此，这三个译文均译不达意，无法达到有效交际的目的。

吴本对"八达之外"进行意译，译为 in distant places，用词地道准确，通俗易懂，但却放弃了"八达之外"的文化内涵。

2. 热气盛，藏于皮肤之<u>内</u>，肠胃之<u>外</u>，此荣气之所舍也。（《素问·疟论》）

释义：热气过盛，藏在皮肤之内，肠胃之外，也就是邪气居于营气之内。

李本：This [disease]...lingers inside the skin and outside the intestines and stomach where Rongqi (Nutrient-Qi) is housed.

文本：The heat qi abounds; it is stored inside the skin and outside of the intestines and the stomach. {This is where the camp qi lodges.}

吴本：When the heat is overabundant, it will hide in the skin and beyond the stomach and intestine, ie., the evil-energy will reside in the Ying-energy.

句中"内"和"外"都表示范围，说明病邪侵袭人体的路径和留藏的部位。

李本和文本均采用直译法。李本译为 inside 和 outside，文本译为 inside 和 outside of。两个译本都准确再现原文的隐喻含义，但如将文本中 outside 后面的 of 去掉，行文会更简洁，形式也更工整。

吴本同样对"内"和"外"进行直译，分别译为 in 和 beyond。在英文中，beyond 侧重表达"超出""超越"之意，表示地理范围指"在……较远的一边"，因此使用 beyond the stomach and intestine 表达"肠胃之外"，在语言转换上不够准确。

三、色诊和脉诊

《素问》中，"内""外"还可以用来表示诊断方法，"内"表示脉诊，"外"表示色诊。

1. 外内相得，无以形先……（《素问·宝命全形论》）

释义：同时还要色脉相参，不能仅看外形，必须将症状吃透，达到纯熟的地步才能给人治病。

李本：Both the external [manifestations] and the internal [changes] must be taken into consideration, avoiding giving first priority to the external [manifestations].

威本：But one should rely upon one's combined examinations of the external and the internal circumstances, and one should not rely upon past experience.

文本：Outer and inner [should] agree with each other, and no priority should be given to [the patient's] physical appearance.

吴本：Examine the pulse condition of the patient, be sure the pulse of the exhausted visceral-energy is existing and must not examine the outer appearance of the patient only.

句中"外内"表示中医学的两种诊断方法，"外"指察色，"内"指诊脉。

李本和威本都采用意译法。李本将其译为 the external manifestations and the internal changes，威本译为 examinations of the external and the internal circumstances。两个译本中所使用的 manifestations、changes 和 circumstances 意义过于宽泛，语言转换不够准确，未能传达出"外"和"内"的隐喻含义，影响有效交际。

吴本同样采用意译法，将其译为 examine the pulse condition of the patient 和 examine the outer appearance of the patient，不仅准确再现原文信息，还传递了中医的文化内涵。但吴本在句式处理上比较随意，使用两个祈使句，而且 must 的前面缺少主语，不符合书面语的行文特点。

文本采用直译法，将"外内相得"译为 outer and inner should agree with each other，虽然在语言上最大限度地和原文保持一致，但由于没有表达出"外内"的具体所指，影响译文的可读性。

2. 所以不十全者，精神不专，志意不理，外内相失，故时疑殆。(《素问·征四失论》)

释义：之所以不能得到十全的疗效，是由于精神不能集中，思想上不加分析，又不能参合色脉，因此时常产生疑问和困难。

李本：The reason that doctors cannot achieve perfect [result in treating diseases lies in the fact that they] cannot concentrate [their] mind, make logical analysis and take both the external [manifestations] and the internal [disorders] into consideration. That is why [they are] frequently confused and fail [in treating diseases].

文本：The reasons why there is no success in all [cases treated are the following:] when the essence spirit is not concentrated and when the mind lacks understanding, outside and inside lose mutual correspondence. Hence, [practitioners] often encounter uncertainties and dangers.

吴本：The failure of achieving a perfect curative effect is due to the inability of concentrating one's mind, fail to do any mental analysis and unable to know the channels' conditions by inspecting the complexion. Thus, perplexity and trouble often occur.

句中"外内"亦指色诊和脉诊。李本采用意译法，译为 take both the external manifestations and the internal disorders into consideration。译文中的 manifestations 和 disorders 意思过于宽泛，无法准确表达出"外内"色诊和脉诊的隐喻含义，可能会使读者产生疑惑，无法达到有效交际的目的。

吴本同样采用意译法，译为 know the channels' conditions by inspecting the complexion（通过察看肤色了解经脉的状况），这与原文的意思并不十分相符。"外内"是两种并行的诊断方法，应是并列关系，因此应译为 examine the channels' conditions and inspect the complexion。此外，分析句子结构可知，吴本中 due to 的宾语为 the inability，fail 和 unable，但是 fail 和 unable 分别是动词和形容词，不能作介词 to 的宾语，因此属于语法错误。

文本为保留原文的语言风格，将"外内"直译为 outside and inside，致使"外内"的隐喻含义无法在译文中直接体现，影响读者理解。

四、房事

《素问》还经常使用"内"来表示房事。

1.……**名曰肺痹，寒热，得之醉而使内也**。（《素问·五脏生成》）

释义：……这种病叫作肺痹；它的致病原因是寒热，并在醉后入房。

李本：...known as Feibi (Lung-Bi Syndrome). It is caused by cold-heat and sexual intercourse after drinking of alcohol.

威本：The name of the disease is "numbness（痹）of the lungs" and the external evidences are chills and fevers. This disease is caused through toxicity which influences the inner body.

文本：This is called lung block, as well as cold and heat. One gets it when one is drunk and then sends inwards.

《黄帝内经素问》隐喻英译对比研究

吴本：The disease is called lung bi-syndrome, which is caused by cold and heat and the conducting sex intercourse after being drunken.

句中"内"指房事。

李本和吴本对"内"进行意译，分别译为 sexual intercourse 和 the conducting sex intercourse。两个译本均正确解读原文，译出"内"的隐喻含义。在语言运用上，李本比吴本更为规范。吴本过于口语化，intercourse 的前面应该使用形容词 sexual 作定语，而非 sex，将 the conducting sex intercourse 改为 the conducting of sexual intercourse 更符合书面语的行文特点。

威本将"内"意译为 inner body。译者对全句的理解出现错误，导致误译，未能准确译出"内"的隐喻内涵。

文本将"内"直译为 inwards，又在注释中对 send inwards 做了进一步的解释，即 have sexual intercourse，既保留原文的语言特色，又准确地译出"内"的隐喻含义。

2. 故《下经》曰：筋痿者，生于肝，使内也。（《素问·痿论》）

释义：所以《下经》说：筋痿的病生于肝，是由于入房过度引起的。

李本：So [the canon in ancient times entitled] *Xiajing* said, "Jinwei (Sinew-Flaccidity) originates from the liver and is induced by excessive sexual intercourse."

文本：Hence, the *Lower Classic* states: "Sinew limpness is generated by sending inwards."

吴本：So, it is stated in the:《Lower Classics》, "the tendinous bi-disease is caused by excessive sexual activities".

句中"内"亦指房事[1]。李本对"内"进行意译，译为 excessive sexual intercourse，对"筋痿"采用音译加注法，既保留中医文化特色，又便于读者理解。整个译文语言准确，行文简洁，达到有效交际的目的。

吴本同样采用意译法，译为 excessive sexual activities，准确译出"内"的隐喻含义。但吴本在标点和语言使用上出现一些错误，*Lower Classics* 前面的冒号应该去掉，英文书名应该使用斜体，而不是中文的书名号，其后的逗号应该改为冒号。这些错误严重影响译文的质量和可读性。

---

[1] 山东中医学院，河北医学院.黄帝内经校释[M].北京：人民卫生出版社，1982：576.

文本将"内"直译为 inwards，又在注释中对 inwards 做了进一步解释，即 enter the women's chambers (i.e., sexual intercourse)，既在语言和句式上和原文保持一致，又便于读者理解。

小　结

本章介绍《素问》中的两类空间隐喻："上－下"空间隐喻和"内－外"空间隐喻。其中，"上－下"空间隐喻主要用来表示时间、量级、地位、状态或趋势、范围等，"内－外"空间隐喻主要用来表示运行状态、范围、色诊和脉诊、房事等。

翻译是译者的创造性劳动，译文是原文本和译者理解共同作用的结果[1]，因此译者这一主体在翻译过程中起着至关重要的作用。人类生活的外部环境的共性及其自身生理结构的共性决定了来自不同语言文化背景的人对同一事物可以有相同或相似的心理认知图式，从而为两种语言之间的直译提供可能。例如，"上－下"这对空间方位概念在英语和汉语中均可隐喻为范围、地位等概念，"内－外"均可表示运行状态，因而四位译者对此类空间隐喻多采用直译法。

然而，四位译者来自不同的社会文化背景，受自身知识结构、文化底蕴等因素的影响，对各类空间隐喻的认知解读不尽相同，进而导致翻译方法的差异和译文质量的良莠不齐。例如，汉语中"内"可以表示房事，这一隐喻含义是汉语特有的，带有明显的中医学特色，英文中找不到直接对应词，因此英译时只能进行意译。李照国精通古典文化，具有中医和英语的双重教育背景；吴连胜父子是美籍华人，长期在美国从事中医工作；文树德是著名的汉学家和医史学家。因此，他们基本能够正确解读此类隐喻，译文中成功实现两种语言之间的转换，达到交际目的。威斯虽是一位医史学家，但其长期生活在国外，接受国外的教育，对此类空间隐喻的认知解读出现偏差，翻译

[1]　孙亚.心理空间理论与翻译[J].上海科技翻译，2001（4）：14.

中未能译出此类隐喻的真正含义，出现多处误译。

　　总之，李本得益于译者深厚的中医文化功底和精湛的语言技能，译文中对空间隐喻的认知解读出错率最低，而且语言准确凝练，句式简洁紧凑。因而，与其他三个译本相比，李本译文质量最高。

第五章　本体隐喻及英译

　　本体隐喻是人类在体验物质实体的基础上，将思想、感情、心理活动、事件、状态等抽象的、模糊的、无形的概念看作具体的、熟知的、有形的实体，从而可以对其进行指称、量化，识别其特征及原因等。不同的概念之间由此形成一种相互关联的认知方式。借助于这种认知方式，人类可以对事物、体验和进程予以概念化并赋予其确定的物理属性，从而不断丰富、发展和升华对主客观世界的认知。本体隐喻是一种最为常见的隐喻，它将抽象的经验对象视为有形的实体，并进行范畴化、类别化和量化的改造；客观世界中存在着各种实体和物质经验结构，这些都为人们理解和认知另一经验对象提供了必要的物质基础 [1]。

　　《素问》中存在类型丰富的本体隐喻，主要包括自然隐喻、容器隐喻、动物隐喻、植物隐喻等。其中，自然隐喻是最常见的本体隐喻，使用天、地、日、月、风、水、火等自然现象的具体概念解释致病因素等抽象概念；容器隐喻是最典型和最具代表性的本体隐喻，运用府、仓、家、舍、室、器等直接或间接表达容器的词汇及门、内、外、中、开、闭等表达容器功能或属性的词汇解释中医理论体系中的脏腑、腠理、孔窍、腧穴等复杂的概念；动物隐喻以各种动物及其特征为喻体，用来指称或表征需要说明或陈述的人或物 [2]；植物隐喻则使用植物的整体、构成部分或生长状态表现脉象、病理变化、外候、大小、形状等内容。此外，"增水行舟""提壶揭盖"等治法和针灸经穴的隐喻性命名等基本上也属于本体隐喻。

　　本章选取《素问》中的部分自然隐喻、容器隐喻、植物隐喻和动物隐

---

[1]　谢之君 . 隐喻的认知功能探索 [M]. 上海：复旦大学出版社，2007：45.

[2]　孙毅 . 认知隐喻学多维跨域研究 [M]. 北京：北京大学出版社，2013：66.

喻，对四个译本的翻译方法、风格及语言特点进行较为详细的解析和对比，分析其在译法选取、目标侧重、语言使用、文体风格等方面的异同，探讨各自的优势和不足。

第一节　自然隐喻及英译

自然隐喻是《素问》中最常见的一种本体隐喻。它是指人们将用于表达自然现象的各种具体概念作为始源域，如天、地、日、月、海、土、风、水、火、寒、暑、湿、燥、云、雾、星、雨等，投射到各种抽象而复杂的目标域之中。从隐喻认知的角度来看，人们常常用肉眼能够观察到的、容易理解的、熟悉的东西来解释说明肉眼无法看到的、不容易理解的东西，也就是用最基本的具体概念或范畴来解释那些人们并不熟悉的抽象概念或范畴。古代医家借助各种自然现象来帮助认识人体，阐释人体器官的部位及功能，隐喻致病因素，为认识人体和治疗疾病提供了最经济、最有效的表述形式。

本节选取《素问》原文中所涉及的天地、日月、海、土、风、水、火和溪谷等八个类别自然隐喻的内容，对四个译本的翻译方法和特点进行分类对比研究。

一、天地

"天"本指人类生存范围（地球）以外的空间；"地"本指地球表面最下方，贴近地壳的表面部分。在《素问》中，涉及"天地"的隐喻非常多，意义也非常繁杂。"天"经常用来隐喻至高无上的地位、寿命长久、人体的上部等，而"地"则用于隐喻女性的月经、寿命长久、人体的下部等。

1. 昔在黄帝，生而神灵……成而登天。（《素问·上古天真论》）

释义：古代的轩辕黄帝，生来就很聪明……到了成年就登上了天子之位。

李本：Huangdi, or Yellow Emperor, was born intelligent... When growing up, he became the Emperor.

威本：In ancient times when the Yellow Emperor was born he was endowed with divine talents... when he became perfect he ascended to Heaven.

文本：In former times there was Huang Di. When he came to life, he had magic power like a spirit... After he had matured, he ascended to heaven.

吴本：Yellow Emperor of ancient time, was bright and clever when he was born... He became an emperor when he grew up.

句中"黄帝"指轩辕黄帝，被尊称为"天子"。人们利用对自然界中"天"的认知来隐喻现实生活中至高无上的"天子"，"成而登天"隐喻轩辕黄帝在成年之后登上天子之位。

李本和吴本采用意译法，将"登天"译为 became the/an emperor，准确理解原文的内涵意义。名词 emperor 意为"皇帝，君主"，"皇"为远古传说中英明盖世的部落酋长，"帝"为人们想象中主宰万物的天神。自秦王嬴政后，"皇帝"成为至尊的称号，变成中国历代封建君主的专用称谓[1]。因此在一定程度上 emperor 可以代替表达原文"天子"之义。

威本和文本采用直译法，将"登天"译为 ascend to heaven。由于中西文化差异，ascend to heaven 蕴含的内容与"登天"成为天子的文化对应关系稍弱，可能会给读者带来阅读障碍，造成理解偏差。

2. 二七而天癸至……故有子。（《素问·上古天真论》）

释义：到了十四岁时，天癸发育成熟……所以能够生育。

李本：At the age of fourteen, Tiangui begins to appear...Then she...is able to conceive a baby.

威本：When she reaches her fourteenth year she begins to menstruate... thus the girl is able to give birth to a child.

文本：With two times seven, the heaven *gui* arrives... hence, [a woman] may have children.

吴本：Her Taingui (the substance necessary for the promotion of growth, development and reproductive function of human body) appears at the age of fourteen (2×7)... As all her physiological conditions being mature, she can be pregnant and

[1] 楚欣. 司马迁笔下的秦始皇 [J]. 炎黄纵横，2016，24（6）：53-54.

bear a child.

句中用"天癸"隐喻能够促进生殖机能的物质，指女子的月经。

李本采用音译法将"天癸"译为 Tiangui，文本则使用直译加音译的方法译为 heaven *gui*。两者都保留了原文的语言特色，但是不利于读者对"天癸"的理解，会给读者带来一定的阅读障碍。

威本将"天癸"意译为 menstruate，意为"月经"，准确传递原文的内涵意义，但未能保留汉语言文化特色；吴本采用音译加注法将其译为 Taingui (the substance necessary for the promotion of growth, development and reproductive function of human body)，音译法保留了原文的语言特色，注解帮助读者理解原文，但美中不足的是注解过于冗长。

3. 天癸竭，地道不通，故形坏而无子也。（《素问·上古天真论》）

释义：天癸枯竭，月经断绝，所以形体衰老，不能再生育了。

李本：...and menstruation stops, she becomes physically feeble and is no longer able to conceive a baby.

威本：Her menstruation is exhausted, and the gates of menstruation are no longer open; her body deteriorates and she is no longer able to bear children.

文本：The heaven *gui* is exhausted. The way of the earth is impassable. Hence, the physical appearance is spoilt and [a woman can] no [longer] have children.

吴本：...her menstruation severs as her Taingui being exhausted. Her physique turns old and feeble, and by then, she can no more conceive.

句中女性的子宫被喻为自然界的"（土）地"，"地道"用来隐喻"月经"，女性月经绝止的生理现象则被喻为"地道不通"。

李本将"天癸竭，地道不通"合并意译为 menstruation stops，意为"月经停止"。遗憾的是，译文未能译出"地道"，舍弃了原文隐喻，不利于读者理解其文化内涵。

吴本将其意译为 menstruation severs，意为"月经断开"，未能实现译文与原文的文化对应，不利于读者对"地道"一词在意义上的构建。

文本将"地道"直译为 the way of the earth，仅表示出其字面意思，未能传递"地道"与月经的文化意义关系，给读者带来理解障碍。

威本将"地道"意译为 the gates of menstruation。gate 意为"门"，与原

文意思较为接近，虽然在一定程度上影响源语文化的独特色彩，但是相较而言，在保证目的语读者的阅读效果方面有一定优势。

4. 此其天寿过度，气脉常通，而肾气有余也……而天地之精气皆竭矣。（《素问·上古天真论》）

释义：这是由于他禀赋较强，自然的寿限超过一般规律，虽已年老，但他的气血筋脉照常畅通，肾气较常人有余……到了这个岁数，天地所赋予的精气，也都竭尽了。

李本：This [is due to the fact that their] Tianshou (Life-Span) exceeds [that of the others], their Qi and blood are always smooth in circulation and their Shenqi (Kidney-Qi) is in excess...

威本：Those are men whose natural limit of age is higher. The vigor of their pulse（气脉）remains active and there is a surplus of secretion of their testicles (kidneys)...because at that time the essence of Heaven and Earth will be exhausted.

文本：In this case the life span [allotted] by heaven exceeds the norm. The qi passes through the vessels as usual and the qi of the kidneys has a surplus... when the essence qi of heaven and earth are all exhausted.

吴本：This kind of people has a richer natural endowment of primordial kidney energy, and has a better postnatal recuperation to health...When the essence and vital energy of a man or woman being exhausted, it is also impossible for them to have any child.

句中"天寿"指先天禀赋，"天地"指男女，"天地之精气"隐喻"高寿男子"和"高寿女子"的先天精气，即肾气。

威本将"天寿"译为 natural limit of age（年龄的自然限度），较符合原文的意思，但不利于读者对"天"字的意义构建和对文化内涵的理解。

吴本将原文第一句进行合并解释，译为 a richer natural endowment of primordial kidney energy，将"先天禀赋强"作为"肾气足"的修饰语。然而，原文中"天寿过度，气脉常通"与"肾气有余"为因果关系，此处表达不够贴切。

李本采用音译加注法将"天寿"译为 Tianshou (Life-Span)。life-span 意为"寿命"，既在形式上和原文保持一致，又能帮助读者理解该词的内涵，贴切准确，较好地表达出原文的内容。

文本将"天寿"译为 the life span [allotted] by heaven。allot 意为"分配"，此译文可理解为上天分配的寿限，形象生动地描述寿限的特点，即客观自然。两者均能较好地表达原文精髓，便于读者理解。

李本未译"而天地之精气皆竭矣"。威本、文本分别将"天地"直译为 Heaven and Earth 和 heaven and earth，在形式上均与原文建立初步的对应关系，但未能表达出"男女"之内涵意义。吴本将"天地"译为 a man or woman，基本实现意义的传递，但未能保留原文特色，影响读者对"天地"形式和文化内涵的双重构建。

5. 若夫法天则地，随应而动，和之者若响，随之者若影。（《素问·宝命全形论》）

释义：如果能够按照天地阴阳的道理，随其变化而施针疗，就能取得如响应声，如影随形的疗效。

李本：[If the treatment is given] in accordance with the law of the heavens and the earth and is modified flexibly, [the curative effect will be like] sound following the explosion and shadow accompanying the body.

威本：Since these methods are those of Heaven, the Earth follows and adjusts its action. Those who are in harmony are like an echo; those who are in accord with these methods are like shadows.

文本：Now, when one takes heaven as law and the earth as rule and when [one's] activities follow what is corresponding [to them, then] harmony with [heaven and earth] will be like an echo and following [heaven and earth] will be like a shadow.

吴本：If one can apply the acupuncture therapy according to the principle of the variations of Yin and Yang of heaven and earth, the curative effects will be obtained as a matter of course.

句中"天"和"地"隐喻天地阴阳盈虚消长的道理，即自然规律。

李本、威本和文本均将"天""地"译为 heaven 和 earth，仅在用词形式上略有不同。李本使用 heaven 的复数形式 the heavens（天空），书面色彩浓厚。威本使用首字母大写的形式译为 Heaven 和 the Earth，起到一定的强调作用。文本使用小写形式 heaven and earth，优势不是很明显。三个译本虽做到形式上与原文对应，但均未能准确地诠释词语本身蕴含的隐喻，不利于读者对"天""地"在文化内涵和意义上进行构建。

吴本运用直译法并补译出 the variations of Yin and Yang of heaven and earth，体现"天""地"隐喻阴阳变化的自然规律，实现意义的传递，但是行文略显拖沓，不够简洁。

6.……地以候地，天以候天，人以候人。（《素问·离合真邪论》）

释义：……从下部脉来诊察下焦，从上部脉来诊察上焦，从中部脉来诊察中焦。

李本：The earth displays the earth, the heavens display the heavens and man displays man.

威本：The Earth has the climate of the Earth, and Heaven has the climate of Heaven. Man harmonizes these (climates) within his bowels...

文本：The earth serves to examine the earth; heaven serves to examine heaven; man serves to examine man.

吴本：...nor can he discern the upper and the lower part and prick rashly...

在"天人合一"观念的指导下，句中"天""地""人"分别用于隐喻人体的上、中、下三部以及这三部的上、中、下位置。

李本、威本和文本均使用 heaven 和 earth 表达"天"和"地"，只是用词形式上稍有不同。李本使用复数形式 the heavens，意思为"天空"，较为书面化。威本使用首字母大写形式 Heaven 和 the Earth，有突出强调作用。文本使用小写形式 heaven and the earth，没有特别之处。三个译本虽然在形式上与原文对应，但未能准确地诠释词语本身蕴含的文化内涵，表达不够明确，未能解释清楚"天地"指代的上部脉、下部脉和上焦、下焦。这会让读者不知所云，无法准确把握源语所要传递的信息。

吴本将"天"和"地"意译为 the upper and the lower part，虽便于目的语读者理解，但未能保留原文的语言特色，也不能帮助读者准确理解"天"和"地"的隐喻意义。

二、日月

"日"指太阳，银河系的恒星之一，是太阳系的中心天体，地球和其他

《黄帝内经素问》隐喻英译对比研究

行星都围绕它旋转，并从它获得光和热。"月"指月亮，是环绕地球运行的一颗卫星，也是离地球最近的天体。在《素问》中，"日"被用来隐喻阳光、光明、阳气、面色等，而"月"则被用于隐喻脉搏的阴阳变化、女性的月经（月事）等。

（一）面色和脉象

1. 色以应日，脉以应月。（《素问·移精变气论》）

释义：气色就像太阳一样有阴有晴；而脉息像月亮一样有盈有亏。

李本：[The changes of] the countenance are just like [the changes of] the sun and [the changes of] the pulse are just like [the changes of] the moon.

威本：The complexion corresponds with the sun; the pulse corresponds with the moon.

文本：The complexion is that by which [a physician establishes] correspondences to the sun. The [movement in the] vessels is that by which [a physician establishes] correspondences to the moon.

吴本：The complexion is like the sun, which has different conditions in the fine days and the cloudy days, and the pulse is like the moon, which has different conditions of wax and wane.

此句以"日"之明晦和"月"之盈亏分别隐喻"面色之明暗"和"脉搏之沉浮"。

威本和文本均将"日"和"月"直译为 the sun 和 the moon，未能对日、月的特点进行具体说明，读者理解起来存在困难。

李本补译出 the changes of，但仍然比较笼统，变化的具体情况无从得知。

吴本借助定语从句进行补译，说明日有明晦之分、月有盈亏之别，帮助读者更好地理解隐喻的具体所指。

2.……治不本四时，不知日月，不审逆从。（《素问·移精变气论》）

释义：……他们治病时，不根据四时的变化，不了解色、脉的重要，不辨别色、脉的顺逆。

李本：...[They] are unaware of [the corresponding relationship between the countenance and pulse] and the sun and the moon. [They] do not [carefully] examine the favorable and unfavorable [changes of the countenance and pulse].

威本：...It was not based upon the four seasons, there was no knowledge of sun and moon, there was no examination as to obedience or disobedience (towards the laws of nature).

文本：...The treatments were not based in the four seasons. They no longer knew of [the significance of] sun and moon. They did not recognize [whether the qi] moved contrary to or followed [its regular course].

吴本：...they do not treat according to the weather variations of the four seasons, they neglect the importance of the complexion and pulse, and do not distinguish the agreeable or adverse condition of the complexion and pulse.

本句中，"日月"用来隐喻面色和脉象的阴阳变化。"不知日月"，即不知道色脉与日月相应的变化和疾病的关系。

四个译本均将"日"和"月"直译为 the sun 和 the moon，在具体表述方面上略有不同。

威本直译为 sun and moon，文本译为 [the significance of] sun and moon，使用 significance 一词，强调其重要性。但是威本和文本均未译出"日"和"月"的内涵意义，会让读者不知所云，无法实现有效交际。

吴本意译为 the importance of the complexion and pulse，直接表述出喻义，较为贴切，但无法帮助读者建立"日月"与面色、脉象的阴阳变化之间的对应关系。

李本采用直译和意译相结合的方法详细解释"日月"，[the corresponding relationship between the countenance and pulse] and the sun and the moon，在形式上与原文有所对应，并将"日月"对应的面色和脉象诠释得较为准确，成功地表达出隐喻，便于读者理解。

（二）月经

1. 二七……月事以时下，故有子。（《素问·上古天真论》）

释义：到了十四岁时……月经按时而行，所以能够生育。

李本：At the age of fourteen... Then she begins to have menstruation and is able to conceive a baby.

威本：When she reaches her fourteenth year... Menstruation comes at regular

《黄帝内经素问》隐喻英译对比研究

times, thus the girl is able to give birth to a child.

文本：With two times seven... The monthly affair moves down in due time and, hence, [a woman] may have children.

吴本：...appears at the age of fourteen (2×7) ...her menstruation begins to appear. As all her physiological conditions being mature, she can be pregnant and bear a child.

句中"月事"为名词，隐喻女子的月经。

对于"月事"一词，李本和吴本译为名词 menstruation，意为"月经、行经"。威本译为动词 menstruate，意为"行经、月经来潮"。原文中的"月事"为名词，从形式的对应上来讲，李本和吴本的表达略胜一筹。但是，吴本随后使用独立主格结构 all her physiological conditions being mature（生理条件变得成熟）进行增译，句子略显繁琐，失去源语的凝练之美。

文本译为 the monthly affair，意为"每月的事情"，即月事。月事是一种比较隐晦的表达。自古以来，中国传统文化中对女性的认知倾向于隐忍、含蓄。the monthly affair 婉转地表达出"月事"之义，能更好地体现出女性阴柔含蓄的一面。

2. 二阳之病发心脾……女子不<u>月</u>。（《素问·阴阳别论》）

释义：胃肠有病，就会发生严重的心痹症……如果是女子的话，就会经闭不来。

李本：Diseases of double Yang (the stomach) involve the heart and the spleen, leading to...and no menstruation in women.

威本：The disease of the two Yang affects the heart and the spleen...otherwise woman will not menstruate...

文本：It is said: "Diseases in the second yang break out in the heart and in the spleen." [As a result]...females do not have their monthly [period].

吴本：The disease of second Yang indicates the disease of Yangming stomach and large intestine...and for a woman, her menstruation will stop.

句中的"二阳"即阳明，指胃和大肠二经，"不月"指月经不行。如果胃肠出现病变，病人经常会感觉二便困难，而女子则会经闭不来。此句中的"月"作动词，隐喻女子月经来潮。

从译文形式来看，原文中"不月"意为不来月经或闭经，为动词短语。威本使用动词 menstruate，意为"月经来潮，行经"，在形式上与原文较为契合。李本和吴本使用名词 menstruation，意为"月经"，未能在形式上与原文保持一致。

文本将"不月"意译为 will not have their monthly [period]，名词短语 monthly period 为"月经期"的含蓄表达。文本比较委婉隐晦地表达出古人对"不月"的认知[1]，同时使用主谓宾结构与原文形成对应，更好地表达出隐喻。

（三）其他

1. 阳气者若天与日。（《素问·生气通天论》）

释义：人体有阳气，像天上有太阳一样。

李本：Yang qi [in the human body] is just like the sun in the sky.

威本：The atmosphere of Yang is similar to Heaven and to the Sun.

文本：As for the yang qi [in man], this is like heaven and sun.

吴本：There is Yang energy in human body like there is sun in the sky.

人体之阳气，有如天上之太阳，如果太阳不能正常运行，万物就无法生存。此句中以"天"与"日"的关系隐喻"人体"与"阳气"的关系。

"若天与日"的结构为：介词"若"加上两个并列名词"天"和"日"，李本和吴本均使用名词加介词短语的形式将其分别译为 like the sun in the sky 和 like there is sun in the sky，句式稍有不同。从形式上来看，与原文不够贴合。

威本运用短语 is similar to 引出 Heaven 和 the Sun，表达人体的阳气犹如天中之日，对比鲜明，将人体和阳气的关系与"天"和"日"的关系进行关联。

文本使用介词短语 like heaven and sun，比较符合原文的表达形式，通过隐喻，使读者明白阳气对人体的重要性，犹如太阳对天的重要性。文本保留原文形式，表意明确，较好地传达原文的精髓，便于目的语读者理解。

[1] 肖卓然，贾春华.基于隐喻认知的《黄帝内经》"女子不月"探讨 [J].中医杂志，2020，24（7）：564–565.

《黄帝内经素问》隐喻英译对比研究

2. 余欲临病人，观死生，决嫌疑，欲知其要，如<u>日月</u>光。(《素问·移精变气论》)

释义：我希望遇到病人的时候，能够观察病的轻重，决断病的疑似，掌握其要领时，心中就像有日月的光亮一样豁然。

李本：I hope that, in diagnosing diseases, I can make correct prognosis, distinguish difficult and complicated [changes of the pulse] and know the key point [of treatment] as clearly as the sun and the moon.

威本：I should like to be near a sick person and to observe when death strikes. The sudden end of life fills me with curiosity and doubts. I wish to know whether the point of death can be as clearly ascertained as the light of the sun and the moon.

文本：I wish to attend a patient and when [I] observe [him to find out] whether [he must] die, or will survive, [I should like to] cast away all doubts. [I] should like to know the essentials — [they should be as clear] as the light of sun and moon.

吴本：I hope when I diagnose a patient, I can distinguish whether the disease is slight or serious, decide the doubtful point of the disease and master the essentials of the disease clearly as being illuminated by the sun and moon.

自然界中的日月之光给人间带来光明，句中以"日月光"隐喻医者掌握疾病要领时心中变得豁然开朗的状态。

三个译本都使用 sun 和 moon 表达"日"和"月"，用词上没有很大差别，但句式稍有不同。

原文中的"如日月光"用作状语，来修饰动词短语"知其要"。李本使用 as...as... 结构将"如日月光"译为 as clearly as the sun and the moon，在句式上与原文相对应，但未翻译"光"。

威本将 ascertained 放在 as...as... 结构中间，译为 as clearly ascertained as the light of the sun and the moon，使用名词 light 表达"光"的意义，在句式上与原文相对应，内容上也比较准确。

文本使用主系表结构 [they should be as clear] as the light of sun and moon 表达"如日月光"，简单明了。

吴本译为 as being illuminated by the sun and moon，动词 illuminate 本义为"用灯光照亮"，句中引申为人的思想受到启发，being illuminated 形象地

表达出医者掌握疾病要领时受到启发，变得豁然开朗的状态。

三、海

"海，天池也，以纳百川者。"（《说文解字》）先民们在观察和比较自然与物体相似性的基础上，实现了从源域到目标域的映射，从而把自然界中的海隐喻为人体的不同脏腑，使"海"成为中医学的重要概念之一。

"四海"的说法自古以来就有，不仅指具体的东海、西海、南海和北海，还用来指称海内之地，即全国各地。在联想和类比的基础上，古人逐渐认识到，自然之海能够汇聚江河之水，而人体之"海"也可以汇聚气血精髓等精微物质。与百川入海相似，气血精髓等精微物质也在人体中汇聚，所以可以对自然界之海进行多种隐喻。在《素问》中，自然之海和人体器官之间存在许多隐喻映射，主要表现在人体器官的生理功能上。另外，海还用于隐喻远大高深的医学理论。

（一）生理功能

1. 六经为川，肠胃为海，九窍为水注之气。（《素问·阴阳应象大论》）

释义：六经好像大河，肠胃好像大海，九窍好像水流。

李本：The Six-Channels act as mountains and valleys, the intestines and the stomach act as the seas.

威本：The six arteries generate streams; the bowels and the stomach generate the oceans.

文本：The six conduits are streams; the intestines and the stomach are the sea.

吴本：The six channels of a man are like rivers in circulating, and the stomach and intestine which hold the cereals are like sea that contains everything.

本句把奔流不息的"川"隐喻成人体内的六条经脉，以容纳百川的"海"隐喻可以容纳饮食水谷的肠胃。"川"意为"河流"，"海"意为"大的（器皿或容量）"。六经与肠胃的紧密联系犹如"川"和"海"的关系，六经如"川"一样滋养经过的脏腑，同时又将产生的代谢物等运送到肠胃[1]。

威本采用直译法将"川"译为 streams，将"海"译为 the oceans，使

---

[1] 郭志杰."六经为川，肠胃为海"与《伤寒论》中的下法 [D]. 北京中医药大学，2008：23-24.

用结构一致的并列句表达整句话，译文中的动词 generate 意为"产生、引起"。译文未能将"为"包含的隐喻关系表达出来，读者无法清楚地了解"川""海"和喻指对象之间的联系。

李本采用直译法将"川"译为 mountains and valleys，将"海"译为 the seas，并用 act as 引出喻指对象。act as 的意思为"充当，起……的作用"，用词较为准确恰当，将经如川、肠胃如海的关系诠释得清楚易懂。

吴本将"川"和"海"分别译为 rivers in circulating 和 sea that contains everything，侧重描述河流的循环流通和海的包容万物，形象生动，易于读者理解和接受。

文本使用 A is B 的句式，结构简单明了，将动词"为"包含的隐喻关系很好地表达出来。

2. 阳明者表也，五脏六腑之海也。（《素问·太阴阳明论》）

释义：足阳明胃经，是足太阴脾经之表，是五脏六腑的营养之海。

李本：Yangming is the exterior [of the Spleen Channel] and the sea of the Five Zang–Organs and the Six Fu–Organs.

威本：The region of the 'sunlight' in the stomach is the outer part of the spleen. The five viscera and the six hollow organs are like an ocean (a reservoir 海).

文本：As for the yang brilliance [conduit], it is the outside. It is the sea for the five depots and six palaces.

吴本：The Foot Yangming Channel of stomach is the superficies of the Foot Taiyin Channel of spleen and is also the sea of nutrition of the five solid organs and the six hollow organs.

胃能受纳水谷，供给五脏六腑营养物质，故为五脏六腑之海。本句以具有巨大包容力的"海"隐喻能够受纳水谷，为五脏六腑提供营养物质的胃。

威本将原文中的"胃经如海"错误理解为五脏六腑如海：The five viscera and the six hollow organs are like an ocean，更换了喻指对象，在句意理解上有失偏颇。

李本和文本皆采用直译法将"海"译为 the sea，表达了足阳明胃经，外合于海水，有"海"的特点，多血多气，有蓄藏容纳的功能。此译法简洁准确，使目的语读者能够体会到"胃经如海"所蕴含的中医文化特色，有较强的文化交际意义。但从整句来看，李本采用直译法，将"阳明"译为Yang-ming，未能具体指出胃经，会给读者带来些许困惑。

吴本将"海"译为 the sea of nutrition（营养之海），准确说明了"海"的具体所指。同时，吴本运用音译加意译的方法将"阳明"译为 the Foot Yangming Channel of stomach，表达出"足阳明胃经"，将"表"译为 the superficies of the Foot Taiyin Channel of spleen，清楚描述胃和脾的关系，对蕴含的医理进行详细阐述，一目了然，有利于读者的准确理解和把握。

3. 冲脉者，经脉之海也，主渗灌溪谷。（《素问·痿论》）

释义：冲脉是经脉的源泉，它能渗透灌溉分肉肌腠。

李本：Chongmai (Thoroughfare–Vessel) is the sea of the Channels. It irrigates [and nourishes] Xigu (large and small muscular interstices) and combines with Yangming [Channel] over Zongjin (sinew connected with the genitals).

文本：The thoroughfare vessel, it is the sea of the conduit vessels. It is responsible for pouring [liquid] into the ravines and valleys. It unites with the yang brilliance [conduit] at the basic sinew.

吴本：The Chong Channel is the sourse of channels, it permeates and irrigates the striae of muscles.

冲脉是十二经脉的源泉，主输送营养以渗灌滋养肌腠。冲脉贯穿全身，能统帅和调节十二经气血，可见地位的重要性。本句以"海"是生命之源的特征，隐喻冲脉能够为十二经脉输送营养物质的生理功能。

吴本采用意译法将"海"译为 the source，意思为"根源、源头"，未能表达出原文"海"的蓄藏容纳之义，在一定程度上会影响读者对"海"的理解。

李本和文本均采用直译法将"海"译为 the sea，表达出"蓄藏"之义，生动形象地诠释了喻指对象冲脉的重要地位和功能。同时，两者运用主系表结构来引出喻指对象，结构和原文基本一致，能够重现原文简洁明快的语言风格，便于读者理解。

（二）理论高深

道之大者，拟于天地，配于四海。（《素问·征四失论》）

释义：医学理论的远大，能和天地相比，能和四海相配。

李本：So profound is the theory of medicine. It is as profound as the heavens and the earth and as deep as the four great seas.

文本：The greatness of the Way it resembles [the inexhaustible space of] heaven and earth and it matches the [vastness of the] four seas.

吴本：The theory of medicine can compare favorably with heaven and earth, and match the deep sea.

本句以辽阔无比的天地和四海隐喻远大高深的医学理论。

李本使用主系表结构，简单明了，并借助 as...as... 结构表达隐喻内容，as deep as the four great seas 意为"像四海一样深奥"。但是，译文没能将"配"字表述出来。

文本和吴本均使用主谓宾结构，将"配"译为动词 match，分别译为 it matches the [vastness of the] four seas 和 it can match the deep sea。match 意为"使相配、使等同于"，用词贴切，准确表达原文中"配"的意义。vastness 侧重于描述海的巨大、广阔，而 deep 侧重于描述海之深，且 deep 本身也含有"深远、深奥"之意。将原文阐述的"医理像四海一样深奥"，用 deep 来表达，强调喻指对象"道"的特点，较为准确。

四、土

万物的生长离不开土地，土地是植物生长的基本条件之一。人们不断地观察和认识土，逐渐了解其功能特性，将土归属于五行，从而形成一个独立的概念。通过分析自然之土的功能特性和脾胃在人体内所发挥的作用，人们发现，自然之土与脾胃生理功能之间存在一系列的映射关系。自然之土的治理与脾胃治则之间也存在一系列类比映射。在《素问》中，自然之土和脾胃之间存在着诸多隐喻映射，主要表现在脾胃的生理功能、脾胃关系、外候、脉象等方面。

（一）生理功能

1. 脾脉者土也，孤脏以灌四傍者也。（《素问·玉机真脏论》）

释义：脾属土，是个独尊之脏，它的作用是滋润四旁的其他脏腑。

李本：The Spleen-Pulse pertains to Earth [in the Five-Elements]. The spleen is the solitary organ that nourishes the other four organs.

威本：The pulse of the spleen is connected with the element of the earth. The spleen is a solitary organ, but it can irrigate the four others that are nearby.

文本：The spleen [movement in the] vessels is [associated with] the soil. [The spleen] is a solitary depot serving to pour [qi] into the four sides.

吴本：The spleen associates with earth and it is a solitary viscus which has the function of moistening all around and other viscera.

万物的生长离不开土地，土地是植物生长的基本条件之一，能够为其生长提供必需的营养物质，继而为微生物、动物和人类的生存提供物质来源。本句将"脾"喻为"土"，可见脾在人体里的重要性。

李本将"土"直译为 Earth，并补译出 [in the Five-Elements]，说明土为五行之一，并使用动词短语 pertain to（属于）表达出脾属土的意义，便于读者理解。

威本使用动词短语 is connected with 引出喻指对象 the element of the earth，be connected with 意为"联系、与……相连"。原文中使用古汉语判断句式对脾进行解释，但译文未能保留原文的汉语言特色。

文本和吴本使用动词短语 is [associated with] 和 associates with 引出喻指对象 the soil 和 earth。earth 意为"陆地、泥土"，soil 意为"泥土、土地、肥料"。相比而言，soil 在意思上更为贴切，可以表达出"土"具有滋养万物之意，在内容传递方面略有优势，便于读者理解"土"的意思。另外，文本使用典型的"A is B"隐喻句式，保留了原文的语言风格，简洁明了。

2. 中央为土，病在脾，俞在脊。（《素问·金匮真言论》）

释义：中央属土，病变常发生在脾经，而表现于脊背。

李本：The center pertains to Earth [in the Wuxing (Five-Elements)] and the disorders usually involve the spleen and the Shu (Acupoint) are on the spine.

威本：In the center there is the earth; its sickness is located in the spleen and disturbances arise in the spine.

文本：The center is the soil. The diseases are in the spleen. The transporters are in the spine.

吴本：The centrality associates to earth and its condition is determined by spleen. If one's spleen energy declines, his shu-points will be hurt first. As the spleen-shu is on the spine, so the disease will occur on the spine. Although they are the shu-points of the five viscera which is being affected, but when take a step further, they will become the disease of the five viscera.

脾在五行中属土，位居中央。中央属土，病变多发生在脾。句中以自然界中土壤的特性和功能做类比，以便阐释脾胃的病理变化。

李本将"土"直译为 Earth，并补译出 [in the Wuxing (Five-Elements)]，对土的内涵进行解释说明，有利于读者理解。但遗憾的是，在表达"中央为土"时，未能保留原文的语言风格。

吴本使用动词短语 associates to（联想到）表达"为"，表意欠准确。

威本使用介词短语和 there be 句型来表达，译为 in the center there is the earth，语言简洁贴切，便于读者把握"土"在五行中的位置，随后的解释帮助读者了解脾对人体的重要性。

文本使用典型的"A is B"句式，简洁准确，同时选用名词 soil 来表达"土"。soil 意为"泥土、肥料"，说明"土"具有滋养万物之意，不仅方便目的语读者完成对"土"的意义构建，还能保留源语的语言特色。

（二）脾胃关系

四支皆禀气于胃，而不得至经，必因于脾，乃得禀也。（《素问·太阴阳明论》）

释义：四肢都受胃气的营养，但是胃气不能直达到四肢，必须经过脾的运化，水谷津液才能布达于四肢。

李本：The four limbs are nourished by Weiqi (Stomach-Qi). But Weiqi (Stomach-Qi) cannot reach them directly. So the four limbs have to depend on the spleen to provide nourishment.

威本：The four extremities are closely related to the stomach, but they cannot communicate with the stomach directly. The spleen is an essential factor and it creates the connection.

文本：All the four limbs are supplied with qi by the stomach, but [the stomach qi] is unable to reach the conduits [directly]. It is only because of the spleen that the [four limbs] get their supplies.

吴本：All the four limbs are nourished by the stomach-energy, but the stomach-energy can not reach the four limbs directly. The essence of water and cereals can only reach the four limbs after being converted by the spleen.

此句以土地对作物生长的重要性隐喻脾胃的功能。从隐喻的角度来看，补养脾胃的治则很可能来源于对土壤施肥灌溉的改土治土方法。

在表达胃和脾的关系时，原文指出"必因于脾"，强调脾功能的重要性。威本选用 essential 和 create the connection 表达脾和胃的联系。essential 意为"必不可少的"，表达出脾的功能及重要性。

李本使用动词短语 have to depend on 表达"不得不依靠"，have to 侧重指客观需要，说明四肢需要依靠脾来提供营养。

文本和吴本有异曲同工之妙，前者使用强调句型 It is... that...，并使用 only 一词表达出条件的唯一性，后者用 can only...，强调脾在运化和输布水谷、濡养机体方面发挥着至关重要的作用，表达贴切，便于读者对脾功能的准确理解和把握。

（三）外候

1. 黄欲如罗裹雄黄，不欲如黄土。（《素问·脉要精微论》）

释义：黄色应该像罗裹雄黄，黄中透红，不应像土那样黄而沉滞。

李本：...[the normal] yellow color looks like realgar wrapped in silk and should not appear like the color of earth.

威本：Yellow wants to be like the bindings of a net, put out to catch a cockbird, but yellow does not want to be like loess.

文本：A yellow [complexion] should resemble realgar wrapped up in gauze; it should not resemble clay.

吴本：...when it is yellow, it should like realgar wrapped in a piece of white thin silk in reddish-yellow, and does not like earth in yellow with residue.

句中用丝织品包裹着雄黄呈现出的黄中透红的颜色隐喻正常的面色，用"黄土"隐喻枯暗无华的面色。

关于"如黄土"，李本译为 appear like the color of earth，earth 一词没能体现出黄土的含义。

吴本译为 like earth in yellow with residue，名词 residue 意为"残渣"。该译文力图表达出面部黄色的沉滞枯暗，但用词不是特别贴切。

文本译为 resemble clay，名词 clay 意为"泥土"，与原文的"黄土"意思有些许差别，不够贴切。

威本译为 be like loess，名词 loess 意为"黄土"，句式和用词都比较准确，更便于读者理解。

2. 所谓面黑如地色者，秋气内夺，故变于色也。（《素问·脉解》）

释义：所谓面黑如炭色的，是由于秋天之气耗散内藏精华，所以面色就变黑了。

李本：The so-called blackish countenance like soil is [due to the fact that] Qiuqi (Autumn-Qi) is internally exhausted. That is why the countenance appears blackish.

文本：As for the so-called "the face is black like the color of earth," [that is to say:] The autumn qi has been lost inside. Hence, a change occurs in one's color.

吴本：The condition of black complexion like charcoal of the patient is due his quintessence has been exhausted by the autumn energy, and his complexion turns to black.

此句以"地色"隐喻因阴阳交争、精气内夺、肾虚而致的发黑面色。"面如地色"，汉语中有类似的表达，例如面如土色，形容脸色像土一样，呈灰白色，后引申为惊恐之极。

李本使用形容词 blackish（带黑色的）修饰"面"，强调出"面"的颜色，用介词短语 like soil 对面色进行进一步的描绘，基本能够忠实表达句意。

文本和吴本都选用 black 一词表达"面"色之"黑"。black 意思为"黑色的、黑人的"，不仅可以用来表达肤色，还有害怕、愤怒之意。吴本还补译出 black like charcoal，意为"炭黑色的、像炭一样黑的"，有助于读者更好地理解面部状态。

文本将"面如地色"直译为 the face is black like the color of earth，清晰描述面如土色，而且句子结构简洁，既保留原文的修辞特征，又能贴切地描述面容，更容易被读者理解和接受。

（四）脉象

脉至如颓土之状，按之不得，是肌气予不足也。（《素问·大奇论》）

释义：脉来像废土一样，重按不足，是肌肉的精气已经不足。

李本：[If] the pulse appears like decayed soil and cannot be felt it indicates insufficiency of Jiqi (Muscle-Qi).

文本：When the [movement in the] vessels arrives like loose soil {one presses it, but does not get it}.

吴本：When the coming of the pulse is like waste dust which is inadequate when by hard pressing, it shows the energy of the muscle has become insufficient.

句中以"颓土"隐喻虚大无力、精气不足、重按则无的脉象。"颓"意为"倒塌、衰败、意志消沉"，常与"废"连用构成"颓废"，意思为意志消沉，精神萎靡。

李本将"颓"译为 decayed（腐烂的，腐败的），decayed soil 可理解为腐土。根据农业常识，腐土不是一件坏事情，反而是土壤肥沃的标志之一，因此很难让读者联想到虚大无力的脉象。

吴本将"颓土"意译为 waste dust，waste 意为"废物、弃物"，dust 意为"尘土"。译文仅表达出"废、弃、无用"之义，未能表达出脉象的虚大无力。

文本将"颓土"意译为 loose soil（松散的土），意思接近原文，但亦未传递出"脉象虚大"的特点。

五、风

风是一年四季中最为常见的气候现象之一，因此人们能够普遍感知到风的存在。通过身体对风的不断体验，人们获得许多对风的认知。在对风的生理和心理体验的基础上，古人不断对比风病和自然界之风的相似性，创造性地运用自然界之风来阐释风病形成过程中人体内部的复杂机理变化。风已经不再仅仅是一个表示自然界气候因素的具体范畴，而是通过隐喻映射成为抽象的中医病因概念，从而形成一系列与风有关的隐喻。这在《素问》中的表现尤为突出。

1. 风之伤人也，或为寒热……（《素问·风论》）

释义：风邪伤害人体，有的发为寒热……

李本：Wind attack leads to either Hanre (Cold-Heat)...

文本：When wind harms a person, it may cause cold and heat...

吴本：When the wind-evil invades the body, some cause the patient to have chilliness and fever...

此句中，自然界中瞬息万变、摧折伐木的"风"被用来隐喻具有变化多端、游走不定等特征的致病因素，即"风邪"，能够"伤人"，引起人体发热、汗出、恶风等症状。"风"意为风疾、风邪。本句描述风邪伤害人体后表现出的不同症状。

李本采用直译与意译相结合的方法，将"风"译为 wind attack，生动形象地表达风邪入侵人体的状态，紧接着用动词短语 lead to 引出风邪导致的各种症状，语言简洁流畅。

吴本将"风"译为 the wind-evil，evil 意为"邪恶、灾祸"，贴切传递"风"为邪气，是不正之气的内涵，随后用动词 invade 进一步表达风邪侵袭人体，便于读者理解和接受。

文本将"风"直译为 wind，未能传递出风邪的意思。

2. 贼风数至，虚邪朝夕……（《素问·移精变气论》）

释义：贼风虚邪的不断侵袭……

李本：Besides, Zeifeng (Thief-Wind) frequently attacks and Xuxie (Deficiency-Evil) repeatedly invades...

威本：Evil influences strike from early morning until late at night...

文本：The robber wind frequently reaches [them]. The depletion evil [is present] in the morning and in the evening...

吴本：When the thief-evil invades unceasingly...

六淫之害，常于不知不觉中侵袭人体，故称"贼风"；邪气亦常乘人体之虚而入侵，故称"虚邪"。在本句中，"贼风"隐喻在不知不觉中侵袭人体的反常气候及外在致病因素。

李本采用音译加注的方法，将"贼风"译为 Zeifeng (Thief-Wind)。同时，使用动词 attack（攻击，侵袭）作为谓语，既完整保留中医学"风"的概念，又形象描绘出变化多端的外在致病因素如同窃贼一般在不知不觉中侵入人体的动态情景，使"贼风"这一抽象概念变得易于理解和接受，在语言、文化、交际三个方面均实现较为成功的转换。

威本和吴本均采用意译法，将"贼风"和"虚邪"进行合并翻译，分别译为 evil influences 和 the thief-evil，且各自使用 strike（攻击）和 invade（侵入）表达致病因素的入侵。威本用 influence 说明外界致病因素对身体的影响，但未能生动刻画出病邪乘虚而入的特点；而吴本使用 thief（贼）和 evil（邪）两个名词无法精确地传递"贼风虚邪"的含义，很可能造成读者理解困难。

文本将"贼风"直译为 robber wind，但是 robber 意为"强盗"，其行为特点与"贼"不甚相符，因此，这种译法并不贴切。

3. 故邪风之至，疾如风雨。（《素问·阴阳应象大论》）

释义：外界邪风的到来，迅猛有如疾风暴雨。

李本：The attack of Xiefeng (Evil-Wind) is as fast as gale and storm.

威本：Evil customs affect the body as much as wind and rain affect the body.

文本：The fact is, the arrival of evil wind is fast like wind and rain.

吴本：The arrival of evil-wind is like a sudden storm or tempest.

"邪风"指不正常的六气 [1]，泛指外界的致病因素 [2]。外界邪气的到来，迅猛有如疾风暴雨。此句把来势汹汹侵袭人体的邪气隐喻成迅猛的暴风雨。

李本采用音译加注的方法，将"邪风"译为 Xiefeng (Evil-Wind)。句子的表语使用 as...as... 结构，译为 as fast as gale and storm。译文既保留中医文化特色，又能还原隐喻本体的基本特征，使其与喻指对象即外界致病因素形成较好的关联性。

文本和吴本的译法较为接近，分别将"邪风"直译为 evil wind 和 evil-wind，且均使用 be 动词加表语的结构形式还原原文内容，与原句保持了形式

[1]　山东中医学院，河北医学院 . 黄帝内经校释 [M]. 北京：人民卫生出版社，1982：42.

[2]　郭霭春 . 黄帝内经素问语释 [M]. 北京：人民卫生出版社，1992：90.

上的统一。

威本将"邪风"译作 evil customs，但 custom 意为"风俗、习惯"，在意思上与"风"的概念存在较大差异，应属误译。译者由于文化背景的原因，对原句的理解出现偏差，因而无法还原隐喻内涵，也未能很好地展现原文简洁流畅的行文特点。

4. 积并则为惊，病起疾风，至如礔砺。（《素问·著至教论》）

释义：三阳之气积聚一起，就会发生惊骇，病起势如风一样迅速，病至势如霹雳一样猛烈。

李本：[When] accumulating and merging, [it causes] fright. The occurrence of diseases [is just like sudden blowing of] strong wind and [roaring of] thunder.

文本：When they have accumulated and merged, then this causes fright. The disease arises [like] swift wind; it arrives like rolling thunder.

吴本：...the accumulation of Yang causes frightening. The onset of the disease is swift like wind, and it is vigorous like the thunderbolt...

本句以人们生活中熟悉的自然现象——疾风和霹雳隐喻"三阳并至"时引发疾病的情况，迅速而激烈。

由于原文表述极为简洁，李本采用直译法，将"疾风"译作 strong wind，"礔砺"译作 thunder，且使用 sudden blowing 和 roaring 对喻指对象进行补充说明，表明疾病发作时的情况并非单纯像疾风和霹雳，而是像二者突然而至的场景，准确表达原文的内涵。缺憾是句子结构没有与原文保持一致，未能更好地还原和展现原文的语言风格。

文本同样采用直译法，将"疾风"和"礔砺"分别译作 swift wind 和 rolling thunder，且使用英语中表明喻的介词 like 引出喻指对象，句子结构与原文一致，语言简洁准确，易于理解。

吴本也使用 like 引出喻指内容，但所用的句型与文本有所不同。吴本分别使用形容词 swift（迅速的）和 vigorous（激烈的）作为表语中心词，从而强调隐喻对象的特征，更好地阐释原文内容，也更符合英语读者的阅读习惯，便于理解。但是，由于对原文句型结构做出较大调整，吴本与李本存在相似的缺憾。

六、水

水是生命之源，是世间万物赖以生存和发展不可缺少的最重要物质资源之一。自古以来，人类就对水形成了许多认识：水流不息，无处不在，能够滋养世间万物，使其生机勃勃。人类对自然界之水的流动性、润湿性、溶解性及其用途等相关知识的体察，被中医学家成功地隐喻或类比地用于说明与解释人体生理功能、病理变化以及治疗[1]。

在《素问》中，水已经不再仅仅表示自然界中的具体范畴，而是通过隐喻映射成为抽象的中医学概念，从而形成一系列与水有关的隐喻，主要体现在人体的生理功能、病理变化、脉象等方面。

（一）生理功能

1.⋯⋯诸气者皆属于肺，此四支八溪之朝夕也。（《素问·五脏生成》）

释义：⋯⋯所有的气，皆注于肺，这气血筋脉向四肢八溪的灌注就像潮水一样。

李本：...and all kinds of Qi are connected with the lung. [The Qi, blood, sinews and vessels flow into and run along] the four limbs and the Baxi (eight joints) are like morning and evening tides.

威本：...and the breath is connected with the lungs. The four limbs and their eight flexible joints are in use from early morning until late at night.

文本：...All qi is tied to the lung. This is the morning and the evening of the four limbs and the eight ravines.

吴本：...all the air in respiration lead to the lung. The air, blood, tendons and vessels are like the ebb and flow of the tide pouring to the elbows, armpits, hips, popliteal fossa and the four extremities.

朝夕，即"潮汐"的假借字[2]，言人身气血往来，如海潮之消长，早曰潮，晚曰汐[3]。句中以自然界"潮汐之往来"隐喻人体的气血筋脉向四肢八溪

[1]　贾春华.一个以水为始源域的中医概念隐喻认知系统的研究[J].北京中医药大学学报，2012，35（3）：164.

[2]　山东中医学院，河北医学院.黄帝内经校释[M].北京：人民卫生出版社，1982：70.

[3]　郭霭春.黄帝内经素问语释[M].北京：人民卫生出版社，1992：156.

灌注的状况。

李本将"朝夕"直译为 morning and evening tides，使用介词 like 引出，并在句首增译部分内容，将上文提到的"气""血""筋""脉"用作句子主语，较为准确地还原隐喻对象，帮助读者想象气血筋脉如同潮汐一般向四肢八溪灌注时的情景。

吴本采用意译法，将原文的隐喻显化，同样使用"气""血""筋""脉"作为主语，用 the ebb and flow of the tide（潮水的涨落）作为介词 like 的宾语，揭示了隐喻的内涵。与李本相比，这一译法对原文的解读和传递更为准确，但是行文不及李本简洁。

威本和文本均采用直译法，都未提及"朝夕"的喻指对象。威本对原文内涵的把握不甚到位，未能解释"朝夕"的内涵，仅仅将其理解为从早到晚（from early morning until late at night），应属误译。同样，文本也未能正确理解"朝夕"的含义，将其误译为 the morning and the evening（早晚），可能会令读者产生困惑。这两个译本在语言、交际和文化的转换上均存在一定欠缺。

2. 肾者，水脏，主津液，主卧与喘也。（《素问·逆调论》）

释义：肾是水脏，主司津液，气喘不能卧下，这是肾脏的病变。

李本：The kidney is an organ of water and governs fluids. [The disorder of the kidney] leads to inability to sleep due to panting.

威本：The water of the kidneys influences the saliva, disturbs the rest, and causes the troubled breathing.

文本：The kidneys are the depot of water; they rule the body liquids and they rule [a person's] lying down and panting.

吴本：...and kidney is a viscus of water and takes charge of the body fluid, when one has rapid respiration when lying down, it is due to the affection of the kidney.

肾主水，具有主持和调节水液代谢的功能。"肾为水脏"主要是指肾在调节体内水液平衡方面发挥着极为重要的作用。句中以水的特性隐喻肾脏的生理功能。

李本和吴本将肾脏作为句子主语，分别将"水脏"直译为 an organ of water 和 a viscus of water，较为贴切地还原隐喻对象，传递中医特色文化。下文均紧跟"主津液"，对肾脏功能进行进一步解释说明，实现原文与译文之间的最佳关联，易于读者理解。

文本同样将肾脏作为主语，采用意译法，将其译作 the depot of water。depot 意为"容器、停车场"，只能解释肾具有储水的功能，未能包含其对水液的调节作用，因此译文对原文的还原度不够。

威本将"肾者""水脏"进行合并翻译，意译为 the water of kidneys，将其用作句子主语，并以 influence 等动词作为谓语继续下文的解释。译文与原文表达的意思相去甚远，未能实现语言的转换，交际与文化的传递更无从谈及，应属误译。

3. 脾脉者土也，孤脏以灌四傍者也。（《素问·玉机真脏论》）

释义：脾属土，是个独尊之脏，它的作用是滋润四旁的其他脏腑。

李本：The Spleen-Pulse pertains to Earth [in the Five-Elements]. The spleen is the solitary organ that nourishes the other four organs.

威本：The pulse of the spleen is connected with the element of the earth. The spleen is a solitary organ, but it can irrigate the four others that are nearby.

文本：The spleen [movement in the] vessels is [associated with] the soil. [The spleen] is a solitary depot serving to pour [qi] into the four sides.

吴本：The spleen associates with earth and it is a solitary viscus which has the function of moistening all around and other viscera.

"脾属土"是土"化"、土"运"功能的类比，中医脾主运化，化生万物，维持人体所需的物质和能量[1]。句中以水之灌溉四方土地隐喻脾所具有的运化水谷、为肝心肺肾四脏输送营养物质的功能。

李本采用意译法，将"灌"译为 nourish，表明脾可对其余四脏进行滋养。译文虽未能保留原文的表达，但是利于读者理解和接受脾的重要作用及其"独尊之脏"的地位。

威本将"灌"直译为 irrigate（灌溉、冲洗）。此译法虽能还原隐喻对象，实现语言的转换，但是未能说明脾为肝、心、肺、肾四脏输送营养物质的重要功能，因而很可能对读者的理解造成偏差。

[1] 秦微，王彩霞.脾属土的文化渊源及内涵[J].中华中医药杂志，2016，31（6）：2056.

吴本也采用直译法，将"灌"译为 moisten（使湿润、滋润），与原文要表达的"滋养"之义有所差别，说明译者对原文含义的把握不甚准确。

文本将"灌"译作 serving to pour [qi]，补译出 serving 以说明"灌"是脾脏对四肢所起的作用。但是，pour 意为"灌注、倾泻"，过于简单直白，同样不利于读者深入理解原文的隐喻。

（二）病理变化

1. 目盲不可以视，耳闭不可以听，溃溃乎若坏都，汩汩乎不可止。（《素问·生气通天论》）

释义：眼睛昏蒙看不清，耳朵闭塞听不见，病势危急，正像水泽溃决，水流迅速，不可遏止，一发不可收拾。

李本：...marked by blurred vision and loss of hearing. [This disease occurs suddenly] like the overflow of a river that is impossible to be brought under control.

威本：Then the people's eyes are blinded and they cannot see. Their ears are closed and they cannot hear. They feel confused as though they were in a state of complete collapse and their will weakens continuously; this (condition) cannot be halted.

文本：The eyes are blind and cannot be used to look. The ears are closed and cannot be used to hear. [There are] kui-kui [sounds in the body] as if a city [wall] was destroyed; [there are] gu-gu [sounds in the body like rushing water that] cannot be stopped.

吴本：The disease is characterized by the syndromes of hearing nothing as if the ears are being stopped, and seeing nothing as if the eyes are dim-sighted, like the dash of water in swift and irresistible momentum which can hardly be controlled.

"溃"有横决的意思，"汩"形容水势汹涌而不可遏止。"溃溃乎"和"汩汩乎"原本用于形容水流冲决河堤，不可遏止的严峻状况，句中用其隐喻阴精耗散、阳气烦扰难以自制的病变趋势。

李本将"溃溃乎"直译为 like the overflow of a river（如同河水泛滥），使用定语从句 that is impossible to be brought under control（无法遏制）对"汩汩

乎"进行描述。译文通俗易懂，基本能表达原文意思，但是从句部分未能保留和重现原文对仗工整的语言形式，略有不足。

威本采用意译法，使用短语 as though 引导表达比喻的状语从句。但是，由于译者对原文的理解存在偏差，只将"溃溃乎"译作 in a state of complete collapse（处于完全崩溃之状态），而"汩汩乎"则未译出，语言传递不甚完整；译文句式结构也与原文完全不对应，失去了原文描写病情变化趋势的生动意境，在文化转换上有所欠缺。

文本采用音译加注法，将"溃溃乎"和"汩汩乎"分别译作 kui-kui [sounds in the body]（体内的溃溃声）和 gu-gu [sounds in the body like rushing water that]（体内如同水急速流动的汩汩声）。音译虽保留了原文的语言特色，但从加注内容来看，译者的理解明显与原文意思相去甚远，应属误译。

吴本采用意译法，分别以 the dash of water（水势汹涌）和 irresistible momentum（势不可挡）表达"溃溃乎"和"汩汩乎"，对原文的解读较为准确，但未能与原文保持语言形式的统一。

2. 其寒温未相得，如涌波之起也，时来时去，故不常在。（《素问·离合真邪论》）

释义：或寒或温，还未与正气相得，所以脉象浮大，时来时去，邪气不是留在一处。

李本：Since the cold and the warm have not interacted with each other, it fluctuates [in the vessels] and may wane and wax without fixation. Since the cold and the warm have not interacted with each other, it fluctuates [in the vessels] and may wane and wax without fixation.

威本：When the cold and the heat (the temperature of the body) are not in mutual agreement, like the rising of the bubbling waves which sometimes come and sometimes recede, then the normal temperature of the body cannot be maintained.

文本：Cold and warmth do not yet agree with each other. [The evil] will rise like breakers gushing up. At times it comes; at times it leaves. Hence, it has no regular presence [anywhere].

吴本：By this time, the evil energy which is either hot or cold, has not yet combined with the healthy energy, the pulse condition is floating and gigantic like turbulent waves, come and go without any definite position.

邪正相争，真邪尚未相合，则血脉中的邪气就像波浪一样起伏不定，时来时去，因此没有定处。此句以"涌波"的起伏不定隐喻邪气在血脉中无有定处，邪正相争，导致脉象浮大。

李本采用意译法，借助动词 fluctuate（波动，涨落）及短语 wane and wax（盈亏，兴衰）说明血脉中的邪气时来时去的活动状态。译文虽未译出原文中的"涌波"，但仍可体现其喻指对象的特征，只是略显直白，未还原出原文中的生动隐喻。

威本采用直译法，使用介词 like 引出 the rising of the bubbling waves（涌动的波浪），并运用定语从句描述其"时来时去"的特点，较为精准地表达原文隐喻的内涵。

文本同样将"涌波"直译为 breakers gushing up（碎浪涌起），接着另起一句描述"时来时去"的情景，表意较为贴切。另外，译文的句型结构与原文基本一致，较好地保留原文简洁生动的语言特色。

吴本将"涌波"直译为 turbulent waves（汹涌的波浪），实现语言转换。但是，将脉象特征译为 floating and gigantic，使用两个形容词 floating（漂浮的）和 gigantic（巨大的）对脉象特征进行描述不是十分准确，很可能会给读者造成理解困难。

3. 是人多痹气也，阳气少，阴气多，故身寒如<u>从水中出</u>。（《素问·逆调论》）

释义：这种人多有痹症，阳气少而阴气多，所以感到身体寒冷，像从水里出来一样。

李本：[These patients] have Biqi. Yangqi is insufficient while Yinqi is super-abundant. That is why they feel as cold as just getting out of cold water.

威本：In cases where man is prone to numbness in breathing（痹气），there is shortness of Yang and an abundance of Yin. Hence the body is cold as though it had come out of the water.

文本：This person has much blocked qi. [His] yang qi is diminished; [his] yin qi is present in large quantities. Hence, the body is as cold as if he had come out of water.

吴本：It is because of the patient has contracted bi-syndrome, his yang energy is deficient and his Yin energy is plenty, and his body is cold as if he has just come out from the cool water.

痹症患者阳气少而阴气多，阴胜而阳不足，阴胜而生内寒，阳虚而生外寒，故觉身寒。本句以从冷水中出来时身体感觉发冷隐喻痹症身寒之感。

李本将"水"直译为water，且根据原文含义增译形容词cold以说明水的温度，从而突出病人身体寒冷的感觉，如同从冷水中出来。译文用通俗易懂的语言较为贴切地传递原文内容，易于读者理解痹症身寒的感觉。

威本和文本的译法较为接近，二者同样都将"水"直译为water，且均使用the body（身体）作为句子的主语，表达的意思是身体冰冷如同从水中出，而原文"如从水中出"隐喻的对象应为病人的主观感受，因此，将病人作为主语更为妥当。

吴本也存在类似的问题，虽然根据原文意思增加形容词cool（凉爽的）来修饰"水"，但是程度不够，未能突出冰冷的特征。而且，吴本同样将the body当作隐喻对象，内涵传递不够准确。

4. 疾行则鸣濯濯，如囊裹浆，水之病也。（《素问·气厥论》）

释义：走得快时，可以听到肠中濯濯的水声，像皮囊里裹着浆水一样，这种病是水气形成的。

李本：...which is a disease of edema characterized by ... borborygmus in walking like water in a leather bag.

文本：If [the patient] moves quickly, then there is a [gurgling in his abdomen] sounding zho-zho and resembling [sounds generated by] a fluid in a bag. This is a water disease.

吴本：...one can hear the water moving inside when walks rapidly like water in a bay, and, to this disease, it should mainly treat the lung.

涌水之病，可有咳嗽、气喘、腹中积水、按之不坚、全身水肿等症。又肺与大肠相表里，寒邪又可由肺下移于大肠，即肠鸣频作[1]。"濯濯"，原指水激荡之声，此处指肠鸣。句中以皮囊裹着水浆发出的声音隐喻水气留居于大

---

[1] 卢芳，匡海学，刘树民. 诠释"中医之水"——水、湿、痰、饮的内涵及治疗理论 [J]. 世界中医药，2015，10（12）：1815.

肠产生的濯濯肠鸣声。

李本使用现代医学术语 borborygmus 表示肠鸣，未对"濯濯"进行翻译。但是因下文有"如囊裹浆"对肠鸣的声音予以进一步的解释说明，译文也较为通俗易懂，基本能够实现语言转换的目标，达到交际目的。

文本采用音译加注的方式，将"濯濯"译作 a [gurgling in his abdomen] sounding zho-zho，既保留原文的语言特色，又通过增译进一步解释"濯濯"所喻指的对象。

吴本采用意译法，将"濯濯"译为 the water moving inside（水在体内涌动），显然对原文的理解存在偏差。原文中的"濯濯"用于形容病人快速行走时的肠鸣之声，并非肠内确实有水涌动，因此，译文有误。

（三）脉象

1. 浑浑革至如涌泉，病进而色弊。（《素问·脉要精微论》）

释义：脉来刚硬过甚，势如涌泉，这是病情加重到了危险地步。

李本：Large pulse beating like gushing of a spring [indicates] dangerous progress of a disease.

威本：When the force of the pulse is turbid and the color disturbed like a bubbling well, it is a sign that disease has entered the body.

文本：If it is torrential and arrives urgently, like a gushing fountain, and if, in case the disease advances and the complexion is spoilt...

吴本：When the coming of the pulse is strong like water gushing from the spring，it shows the disease is turning to the worse to become dangerous.

"浑浑"，此指大脉而言。"革"，亦有版本作"革革"，即"吉吉"，形容脉来急速状 [1]。句中以泉水上涌隐喻刚硬过甚而急速之脉的感觉，易于医者把握这一微妙复杂的脉象。

李本采用直译法，将"涌泉"译作 gushing of a spring（泉水之喷涌），并且补译出动词 indicate（表明），用以衔接前后句，表明两者之间的关系，即此种脉象为病势严重且有危险的征兆。译文较为准确地体现出刚硬急速之脉的特征，保留原文形象生动的语言特点，易于读者理解。

---

[1] 山东中医学院，河北医学院.黄帝内经校释[M].北京：人民卫生出版社，1982：216.

威本将"涌泉"直译为 a bubbling well。well 作名词时通常指"水井"，而非"泉"，用于此处表意不准确。而且，译者对"浑浑"和"革革"的理解也有误，将其解读为 turbid（浑浊的）和 disturbed（错乱的），因而无法传达"涌泉"的实际特征，读者很可能会感到疑惑不解。

文本同样将"涌泉"进行直译，译为 a gushing fountain（喷涌的泉水），与原文所要表达的泉水上涌之状存在一定区别，未能对其进行准确还原。

吴本采用意译法，将"涌泉"译作 water gushing from the spring（从泉中喷涌而出的水），使用现在分词结构形象描述泉水上涌的状态，还原度较高，通俗易懂，而且句型结构也与原文保持一致，从而在语言、交际和文化方面均实现较为成功的转换。

2. 其来如水之流者，此谓太过，病在外。（《素问·玉机真脏论》）

释义：其脉来时，如水的流动，这叫作太过，主病在外。

李本：[If] the pulse comes like running of water, it is called Taiguo (excess), indicating exterior diseases.

威本：Then the pulse of the spleen beats like the unstable drifting of water, and it can be described as excessive; and disease has befallen the exterior of the body.

文本：If [the spleen movement in the vessels] comes like the flow of water, this is called "greatly excessive." The disease is in the exterior.

吴本：When the coming of the pulse is like flowing water, it is going beyond, which shows the disease is in the exterior.

本句描述了脾脉来时如水之流动的脉象，称作"太过"，主病在外。句中以"水之流动"隐喻脾之病脉的脉象。

李本将"水之流"直译为 running of water，以介词 like 引出，使用动词 come 表达"脉来"的动作，完全贴合原文内容和形式，较为准确地还原脾脉来时的脉象特征，有助于读者体会和理解脾之病脉的脉象。

文本的译法与李本较为相似，使用名词 flow 表达"流动"之义，将"水之流"译作 the flow of water，基本能传达原文的含义。但是，使用名词表达动作状态的译法不够形象生动，因而稍显逊色。

吴本使用动词现在分词结构 flowing 作为修饰语，将"水之流"译为

flowing water（流动的水）。这一译法将中心词"流"改为"水"，略偏离原文内容，未能实现原文与译文内容的完全关联。

威本将"水之流"译为 the unstable drifting of water（水的不稳定漂流）。unstable 为译者基于对原文的解读而增译的内容，但遗憾的是，这一解读并不十分准确。此外，译文使用 drifting 表达水流动的状态也不贴切，因为 drifting 侧重指物体顺水漂流，而非水的流动。可见，此译文在语言传递上不够准确，容易造成读者理解困难。

3. 脉至如喘，名曰暴厥。（《素问·大奇论》）

释义：脉来像水流般湍急的，病名叫作暴厥。

李本：[The disease with] the pulse that is surfing is called Baojue (sudden syncope)...

文本：When the [movement in the] vessels arrives as if panting, this is called "sudden recession."

吴本：When the coming of the pulse is urgent like rushing currents, it is the syncope with sudden onset.

暴厥，厥证之一，指卒然昏厥、不省人事的严重病证，其主要症状有"脉至如喘""暴厥者不知与人言""塞闭不通"[1]。"喘"指水之湍急，句中以湍急的水流隐喻发生暴厥时出现的急脉之脉象特征。

李本将"喘"译为 surfing（冲浪），与原文意思有所出入，未能准确传递原文所描述的急脉脉象，会令读者感到费解，因此不可取。

文本采用直译法，将"喘"译作 panting（喘息），且使用短语 as if 表达句中的隐喻。句子形式与原文一致，但在意思表达上存在欠缺，未能传达"喘"中包含的"如水之湍急"之义，容易造成理解偏差。

吴本采用意译法，将"喘"译作 urgent like rushing currents（湍急如激流），既准确描绘湍急的水流之特征，又准确还原暴厥时的脉象特征，便于读者把握。译文在形式上与原文对应，而且保留原文的文化意象，较为成功地完成语言、交际和文化层面的转换。

[1] 陈士玉，谢鑫.《内经》厥病考释 [J]. 中华中医药学刊，2012，30（4）：875–876.

4. 死脾脉来……如屋之漏，如水之流，曰脾死。（《素问·平人气象论》）

释义：如果脉来……如屋漏水一样地点滴无伦，如水流之速，这是死脉。

李本：Dead Spleen–Pulse is... [as dripping as] the leakage of a room and [as receding as] the running of water. This is the dead pulse of the spleen.

威本：At the point of death the pulse of the spleen moves sharply and strongly... like the leakage of a house, or even like torrents of water and then one can speak of the death of the spleen.

文本：The arrival of a dying spleen [movement in the] vessels is [as follows]: pointed and firm... like [water] dripping into a house, like the flow of water. That is called "the spleen dies".

吴本：If the coming of the pulse is wiry and hard，firm and sharp... or like the rain drops in a leaking room with uncertain intervals, or like flowing water that never comes back again，they are all the spleen pulse indicating death.

"如屋之漏"，形容脉来如屋之漏水，点滴而下，缓慢而无规律；"如水之流"，形容脉去而不至，如水之流逝。此句以屋之漏水和水之流逝隐喻脾死脉的脉象特点。

李本采用直译法，将"如屋之漏"译为 [as dripping as] the leakage of a room，"如水之流"译为 [as receding as] the running of water，并补译出 as...as... 结构、形容词 dripping（湿淋淋的）和 receding（渐渐远去的），生动描述"屋之漏"和"水之流"的状态，有助于读者把握原本非常抽象的脾死脉的脉象特征。

威本将两者分别直译为 the leakage of a house 和 torrents of water，而且使用介词 like，保留原文的语言形式。但是，使用名词 leakage（泄漏）和 torrent（奔流）作为中心词的译法较为直白，缺少"屋之漏"和"水之流"的动态特征，不利于读者理解。

文本也在直译的基础上进行补译，将"如屋之漏"和"如水之流"分别译作 like [water] dripping into a house 和 like the flow of water。前者使用 drip（滴下）的动名词结构，并补译出 water 作为逻辑主语，较为清晰地还原原文内容。后者则使用名词 flow（流动）作为中心词，未能表达出水之流逝的动态特征，在还原度上略有欠缺，形式上也与原文不甚一致。

吴本采用直译意译相结合的方法，将"如屋之漏"译为 like the rain drops in a leaking room with uncertain intervals（如同雨滴间隔不定地落在漏水的房间里），将"如水之流"译作 like flowing water that never comes back again（如同流水去而不返），详细描述屋漏时雨水点滴而下的状态和水流一去不返的情形。此译文既保留原文的形式和文化底蕴，又增加对隐喻的进一步解读，生动形象，通俗易懂，有利于中医文化的对外传播。

七、火

在人类的认识空间中，火是普遍存在的。通过观察火的性质和特点，人类逐渐加深了对火的认识，如火无质无形，火色赤，火性燥，火性动，火可烧焦他物等。古代医家在对火的性质进行体察的基础上，将对自然之"火"的认知隐喻到中医学中，形成了"火邪""火证"等概念。

在《素问》中，火的隐喻映射主要表现为天气暑热和人体的病理变化两个方面。

（一）天气暑热

1. 复则炎暑流火，湿性燥，柔脆草木焦槁……（《素问·气交变大论》）

释义：（木气受克制，则）其子气（火气）来复，那么就会炎热如火，万物湿润的变为干燥，柔嫩脆弱的草木也都焦枯……

李本：Retaliating [activity leads to] flaming summer-heat, [change of] moisture into dryness, scorching [variation] of the tender grasses and trees...

文本：When it comes to revenge, then there is flaming summerheat [as if there were] fire flowing. That which is of damp nature dries out; herbs and trees that are soft and brittle, they are scorched and wither...

吴本：As the wood energy is restricted causing the crops to become grey and white, its son energy (fire energy) will be retaliating for its mother, the weather will become as hot as fire, all the wet things will become dry, the soft and tender branches and leaves of plants will be born anew from the root...

此句描述若木气受到克制，则其子气（火气）来复，将出现的各种状况，即炎热如火，万物干燥，柔嫩脆弱的草木焦枯。句中以"流火"（炎热如火）隐喻木气受到克制时其子气（火气）来复的炎热状况。

李本将"炎暑流火"直译为 flaming summer-heat。形容词 flaming 表示炎热如火的意思，较为贴合原文，简洁明了，而且易于理解。

文本采用直译法，使用 as if 引导的状语从句对直译的内容 flaming summerheat 做进一步的解释说明。译文略显繁琐，而且 summerheat 拼写有误，应为 summer heat 或者 summer-heat。

吴本将"流火"直译为 as hot as fire，还原"火"的概念并说明其特征（hot），通俗易懂，语义贴切。缺憾是语言过于直白，不够生动形象，而且未能解释原文中"暑"的概念，形式上也未能与原文保持一致。

2. 春有惨凄残贼之胜，则夏有炎暑燔烁之复。（《素问·气交变大论》）

释义：如果春天反见寒冷伤害的金气，夏天就会有炎热如火燔烧的气候。

李本：...[if] there is harmful and impairing [Qi] in spring, there will be flaming heat in summer.

文本：If in spring there is a domination of chilling temperatures, which injures and destroys, then in summer there is a revenge [resulting in] flaming summerheat, burning, and melting.

吴本：...if the metal energy is subjugating the insufficient wood, there will be cold and destitude metal energy in spring and the son energy of the wood (fire energy) will retaliate to cause hot weather like burning fire in summer.

"炎暑燔烁"意为气候炎热，如同烈火燃烧。此句以烈火燃烧产生的强烈烧灼感隐喻夏天之炎热。

李本将"炎暑燔烁"译为 flaming heat，语言简练，成功实现语义转换，便于读者理解。但是这种译法失去了原文中隐喻的文化韵味和语言特色，在文化交际方面略有欠缺。

与李本类似，文本将其译作 flaming summerheat，但是 summerheat 的拼写有误，应为 summer-heat 或 summer heat。不同之处在于，文本紧接着使用 burning 和 melting 作为伴随状语对"燔烁"进行具体解释和描述，强调"炎暑"如同烈火燃烧产生的烧灼之感，更加形象生动。

吴本将其译作 hot weather like burning fire in summer，运用介词 like 连接"天气"与"燔烁"，使两者之间的关联性更加明确，也更易于读者理解和接受；不足之处在于译文稍显直白，未能更好地展现原文的写作风格和文化内涵。

3. 大暑流行，甚则疮疡燔灼，金烁石流。（《素问·五常政大论》）

释义：（火气当权）所以大暑流行，甚至病发疮疡、高烧。炎暑酷热的情况，好像能使金烁石流一样。

李本：...prevailing [attack of] Summer–Heat, even sores and carbuncles as scorching as burning metal and stone.

文本：Massive summerheat prevails everywhere. In severe cases, sores and ulcers [develop]. Burning [causes] metal to melt and stones to flow.

吴本：As the fire energy is in power, the great heat of summer will be prevailing, the diseases of sores and high fever may even occur. The sweltering summer heat seems capable to melt the metal and stone.

"金烁石流"形容火炎太过，可使金石熔化。本句以只有在高温情况下才能出现的"金烁石流"隐喻炎暑的酷热。

李本使用 as...as... 结构将"金烁石流"直译为 as scorching as burning metal and stone，未能与原文保持语言形式上的一致，并且误将 sores and carbuncles（疮疡）当作"金烁石流"的隐喻对象。可见，译者对原文的理解存在偏差，导致误译。

文本运用直译法，并补译出动词 causes，说明"金烁石流"现象产生的原因，将其译作一个完整的句子。译文基本能够传递原文的内容，但是并未译出其喻指的内容，即暑热，因而无法使两者之间形成符合逻辑的关联，可能导致读者误解为"金烁石流"是现实存在的情况，从而产生困惑。

吴本同样进行直译，并补译出句子主语 the sweltering summer heat，使用动词 seem 表明炎暑酷热与"金烁石流"（capable to melt the metal and stone）之间的关系。这一译法虽然行文略显繁琐，而且没有在形式上与原文保持一致，但是能够帮助读者深入理解原文内涵，有利于实现交际目标。

（二）病理变化

1. 独胜而止耳，逢风而<u>如炙如火</u>者，是人当肉烁也。（《素问·逆调论》）

释义：阳气独旺达到一定程度，生机就自行停止了。像这种四肢发热遇风邪如炙于火的病人，热邪长期存在，烁其肌肉，势必日趋干枯而消瘦。

李本：Predomination [of Yang] and stoppage of generation and growth are the reasons why [some people feel] burning hot when confronted with wind. These people gradually become emaciated.

威本：If it excels in solitude it will cease (to exist). If it meets with a wind and is affected as though it were cauterized or burnt, then man's flesh must melt (disintegrate).

文本：...{A domination that is isolated comes to a halt.} {"Encounters wind and [has a feeling] as if burned, as if [scorched by] fire" is: this person's flesh will melt away.}

吴本：Whenever the wind is encountered, the patient will be hot like being scorched, and his muscle will become emaciated gradually.

"如炙如火"，据《太素》卷十三《肉烁》校正为"如炙于火"[1]。本句隐喻人体阴虚阳亢，外遇阳邪，两阳相加，炙烤津液肌肉，逢风而发热的程度如同炙于火上。

李本采用意译法，将"如炙如火"译为 burning hot，并且增译主语 some people 和谓语 feel，以解释原文对病人主观感受的强调，但是未译出"火"的内涵，略失原文的文化韵味。

文本同样进行意译，并补译 has a feeling 充当句子的谓语，使用 as if 引出"如炙如火"（[scorched by] fire）。译文的语法存在问题，主语不明确，表语与疑似主语之间缺乏逻辑上的关联，读者理解起来会比较困难。

吴本译文比较精练，补全主语 the patient，并且将"如炙如火"译作 be hot like being scorched，含义的转换较为成功，语言简练，易于理解；缺憾是 be 动词的使用导致译文无法清晰表明"如炙如火"实际上为病人的主观感受，可能会令读者产生误解。

---

[1] 张灿玾. 黄帝内经素问语释 [M]. 济南：山东科学技术出版社，2017：252.

威本使用短语 as though 引导的状语从句来表达隐喻，但从句的主语 it 指代不明，很可能会造成读者的困惑。而医学术语 cauterized（烧灼、腐蚀），强调用化学药剂或高温烧灼伤口以止血或消毒，无法准确传递原文意思，文化层面上的转换更是无从谈起。

2. 至病之发也，如火之热，如风雨不可当也。（《素问·疟论》）

释义：疟疾发作的时候，热得像火的燃烧，寒得像风雨般不可抵御。

李本：The attack of malaria is as hot as fire and as violent as storm.

文本：When it comes to the outbreak of the disease, this is like the heat of fire, like [the coming of] wind and rain: one cannot do anything against it.

吴本：When malaria attacks, the patient can be as hot as the burning fire or as cold as the irresistible wind and rain.

句中以烈火的剧烈燃烧和暴风骤雨隐喻疟疾发作的突然性和巨大威力。

李本将"如火之热"直译为 as hot as fire，语言精练，易于理解，准确实现语言转换；但未能对烈火燃烧的状态进行描述，缺乏生动性，在语言深层含义的传递上略有欠缺。

吴本的译法与李本基本类似，同样使用 as hot as，并且增加形容词 burning 修饰 fire，突出烈火正在燃烧的状态。但是译文将 the patient（病人）作为句子主语有失妥当，与原文意思（疟疾发作时的状况）不符，属于误译，应是译者对原文理解存在偏差所致。

文本也采用直译法，将"如火之热"译作 like the heat of fire，中心词为 heat（热），意思更为贴切。主语 this 指代上文提到的疾病发作，准确实现含义转换。不足之处在于句型结构相对复杂，未能展现原文凝练而深刻的语言风格。

3. 身热如炭，颈膺如格，人迎躁盛，喘息气逆，此有余也。（《素问·奇病论》）

释义：身上发热像炭火，颈项和胸膺之间，像有东西阻隔，人迎脉噪盛，发喘，气上逆，这是有余的病象。

李本：[At the same time there are some other symptoms, such as] scorching fever, obstruction of the chest and throat, rapid pulsation of Renying pulse, panting and reverse flow of Qi, indicating excess [of Xieqi (Evil–Qi)].

文本：His body is hot like charcoal. His neck and breast are as if obstructed. [The movement in the vessels at] man's facing races and is abundant. The breath is panting and qi moves contrary [to its regular course]. {This is a surplus.}

吴本：...his body is hot like charcoal, seems to have something blocking between the neck and the chest, his Renying pulse is irritating, he has rapid breathing and adverseness of vital energy, which show the cases of having a surplus.

"身热如炭"是邪气有余的证候，句中以炭火隐喻身体发热的严重程度。

李本采用意译法，并补译出部分内容。首先以 there be 句型补译出整个句子的主干成分 there are some other symptoms，然后以短语 such as 引出下文，表明该句列举的"身热如炭"等均属于 other symptoms（其他症状）。但是将"身热如炭"意译为 scorching fever（高烧），未能充分表达隐喻高烧至"如炭"的严重程度，在意思的转换上不够全面，也未能传递原文生动形象的语言特点和文化底蕴。

文本和吴本的译法基本相同，均将"身热如炭"直译为 his body is hot like charcoal。虽然名词 charcoal 意为"木炭"，但是木炭只有在燃烧的时候才会发热，本身并不具备热的特征。因此，译文虽然语言形式上忠实于原文，但是未能准确译出原文意思，致使句子主语与其喻指内容之间缺乏逻辑上的关联，令人费解，无法有效实现交际目标。

4. 脉至如火薪然，是心精之予夺也，草干而死。（《素问·大奇论》）

释义：脉来时像火刚燃起来一样的旺盛，这是心脏的精气已经脱失的脉象，大约到冬初草枯的时候就要死亡。

李本：[If] the pulse beats like burning fire, it indicates exhaustion of Xinjing (Heart-Essence) [and the patient] will die when grasses become dry [in autumn].

文本：When the [movement in the] vessels arrives like burning fuel, [the patient] will die when the herbs dry.

吴本：When the coming of the pulse is like the beginning of the burning fire, it shows the refined energy of the heart is exhausting, the patient will die at the beginning of winter when the gasses are withered.

"然"，通"燃"，指燃烧。本句以新燃之火之不稳定性隐喻脉来其形不定，为心脏精气有脱失之象。

李本将"火"直译为 fire，将"火薪然"译为 burning fire，未能传递出"薪"的意思。burning fire 具有各方面的特征，例如灼热、旺盛、发光、飘忽不定等，读者由译文推测心脏精气脱失的脉象特征较为困难，因此无法有效实现交际目标。

吴本同样将"火"直译为 fire，与李本的区别在于用 the beginning of the burning fire 译出"火薪然"的意思，准确表达了原文内涵，能够更好地帮助读者理解此脉象所具有的旺盛而不稳定的特征，因而交际功能更强。缺点是译文使用较为复杂的长句，包含两个 when 引导的时间状语从句和 shows 的两个宾语从句，未能体现原文精练的风格特点。

文本将"火"译为 fuel（燃料），与原文内容不甚相符，burning fire 也未能准确表达"薪然"的内涵。译文语言精练，但理解存在较大偏差，而且漏译"是心精之予夺也"，因此在语言、交际和文化的转换上均相对较弱。

八、溪谷

自然界的溪和谷原本是一些常见的自然物象，被映射到人体域里，用于指代人的肢体肌肉之间相互接触的缝隙或凹陷部位。大的缝隙处称"谷"或"大谷"，小的凹陷处称"溪"或"小溪"。溪谷与人体部位之间的这种联系，反映了一种基于物理属性的相似性，即形态、走向和位置等。中医学根据穴位与溪、谷等物象在结构、位置、功能等方面的相似之处进行跨域构建，从自然域映射到人体域，形成生动易懂的隐喻概念，使得这些词语在自然物象的基础上增加了医学义项，丰富了中医学的语言表达。

《素问》中出现了以下与溪、谷相关的语句，对人体部位和经络穴位进行隐喻。

（一）人体部位

1. 溪谷属骨，皆有所起。（《素问·阴阳应象大论》）

释义：肌肉及骨骼相连属的部位，都有它们的起点。

李本：The Xigu (regions where muscles converge) were all connected with the bones with a starting point and an ending point.

威本：Just as "hollow" refers to the bones, and they all have sections which set them apart from each other.

文本：The ravines, valleys, and the joints, all have a place where they emerge.

吴本：As the Xigu (Stream Valley) points locate between the joint of bones, so they belong to the bone, they are all having their starting points and terminals.

"溪谷"（亦作"谿谷"）原指山与山之间低凹的地带，通常有小溪或河水流出。在中医学上，"溪谷"位于五体的"肉"的层次，位于肌肉交汇的部位，深入"骨"并与其相连属，浅出体表见于"皮"层的诸穴，是周身荣卫之气循行交汇的场所[1]。句中以"溪谷"隐喻这些身体部位。

李本和吴本均采用音译加注法翻译"溪谷"。音译既成功实现语言的转换，又保留了中医文化特色。但是二者的注解部分有所区别。李本将其译为regions where muscles converge（肌肉会聚之处），准确贴切地传达"溪谷"的含义。此译法语言简练，通俗易懂，是对音译内容的有效补充，便于读者理解。而吴本则使用 Stream Valley（溪谷）对"溪谷"做进一步说明，仅阐释其字面意思，未能表明其真正所指的身体部位，读者仍然无法理解"溪谷"的内涵，因而无法实现交际目标。

文本将"溪谷"直译为 the ravines 和 valleys，保留原文中的中医术语，实现语言和文化的传递，但未能解释其真正喻指的内容，即肌肉连属的部位，很可能给读者造成理解困难。

威本由于对原文解读有误，将"溪谷"直译为 hollow（凹陷、洞），并且将其与"属骨"混为一谈，属误译，语言和交际功能均无法实现，文化传递更是无从谈起。

2. 此四支八溪之朝夕也。（《素问·五脏生成》）

释义：这气血筋脉向四肢八溪的灌注就像潮水一样。

李本：[The Qi, blood, sinews and vessels flow into and run along] the four limbs and the Baxi (eight joints) are like morning and evening tides.

威本：The four limbs and their eight flexible joints are in use from early morning until late at night.

文本：This is the morning and the evening of the four limbs and the eight ra–vines.

[1] 刘斌，董福慧.《黄帝内经》"谿谷属骨"理论初探 [J]. 北京中医药，2009，28（7）：513.

吴本：The air, blood, tendons and vessels are like the ebb and flow of the tide pouring to the elbows, armpits, hips, popliteal fossa and the four extremities.

八溪，即八虚，指上肢部的肘关节、肩关节，下肢部的膝关节、髋关节，左右侧共八处。张景岳曰："八谿者，手有肘与腋，足有胯与腘，此四肢之关节，故称为谿。朝夕者，言人诸脉髓筋血气，无不由此出入，而朝夕运行不离也。"[1]

李本采用音译加注法，将"八溪"译为 the Baxi (eight joints)。音译可以部分还原中医术语，传递原文的中医文化特色。对 eight joints 注解则可以具体解释其含义，表明"溪"是对"关节"的隐喻，易于读者理解和接受。

威本将"八溪"意译为 their eight flexible joints（四肢的八个灵活关节），准确表达原文含义，通俗易懂，实现交际目的。但是，此译法未能保留和还原"溪"这一特定概念，因而在文化层面的转换上存在欠缺。

吴本同样采用意译法，将"八溪"译为 the four extremities（四肢），意思上与原文有一定差别。将数字"八"译为"四"，而且也未能保留中医术语"溪"所蕴含的文化特色，无法较好地实现交际和文化传递的目标。

文本将"八溪"译为 the eight ravines（八个峡谷），混淆了"溪"和"谷"的概念，与原文含义相去甚远，应该是由于对原文的错误解读造成的误译。

3. 冲脉者，经脉之海也，主渗灌溪谷。（《素问·痿论》）

释义：冲脉是经脉的源泉，它能渗透灌溉分肉肌腠。

李本：Chongmai (Thoroughfare–Vessel) is the sea of the Channels. It irrigates [and nourishes] Xigu (large and small muscular interstices).

文本：The thoroughfare vessel, it is the sea of the conduit vessels. It is responsible for pouring [liquid] into the ravines and valleys.

吴本：The Chong Channel is the sourse of channels，it permeates and irri-gates the striae of muscles.

对人体而言，溪指肢体筋骨、肌肉之间相互接触的罅隙、缝隙或凹陷部位。大的缝处称谷或大谷，小的凹陷处称溪或小溪。分肉之间，是溪谷会合的部位，能通行营卫，会合宗气。

---

[1] 张介宾.《类经》[M]. 北京：中医古籍出版社，2016：240.

李本采用音译加注法，将"溪谷"译为 Xigu (large and small muscular interstices)。通过音译还原"溪谷"的概念，保留文化内涵丰富的中医术语，实现语言与文化的转换。注释部分则解释说明其喻指的内容为人体的大小肌肉缝隙。译文易于读者理解，成功实现交际目标。

文本将"溪谷"直译为 the ravines and valleys（峡谷和山涧），虽然简洁明了，有助于实现语言转换，但是未能明确两者喻指的对象，很容易造成读者困惑，不利于交际目标的实现。

吴本采用意译法，将"溪谷"译为 the striae of muscles（肌肉的纹理），意思与原文相去甚远，应是理解偏差造成的误译。译文不仅无法成功传递原文的意思，而且可能造成读者误解，在语言、交际和文化的转换上均存在问题。

（二）经络穴位

人有大谷十二分，小溪三百五十四名，少十二俞。（《素问·五脏生成》）

释义：在人身上，有大谷十二处，小溪三百五十四处，那十二关还不在其内。

李本：In the human body, there are twelve Dagu (major joints) and three hundred and fifty-four Xiaoxi (Acupoints), excluding the twelve Shu (back-Shu Acupoints).

威本：Man has twelve groups of large ducts or main vessels and three hundred and sixty-four small ducts or "loh vessels"（络）, and twelve vessels of lesser importance.

文本：Man has the twelve large valleys and the 354 small ravines. {Less twelve transporters.}

吴本：There are twelve main joints in the four extremities and three hundred and fifty four small bone joints in human body, excluding the shu points in the twelve channels.

除了人体部位，溪、谷还泛指经络穴位。具体而言，谷相当于十二经脉循行的部位，溪相当于三百六十五个经穴的部位。句中以"大谷"和"小溪"隐喻人体的经络穴位。

李本采用音译加注法分别将"大谷"和"小溪"译为 Dagu (major joints)

和 Xiaoxi (Acupoints)。音译保留原文的中医术语，有利于文化的对外传播；注解部分补充说明喻指对象，即人体的经络穴位。但是，原文中的"谷"实际所指应为十二经脉循行的部位，即经络，而不是关节（joint）。因此，译文对"大谷"解释的准确性有待商榷。

文本分别将"大谷"和"小溪"直译为 large valleys 和 small ravines，保留原文的字面意思，实现语言转换；但是未能解释"谷"和"溪"在文中的真正含义，导致读者无法准确理解此处的隐喻。

威本采用直译意译相结合并辅以汉字注（解）的方法，将"大谷"译为 large ducts or main vessels（大的管道或者主要的血管），将"小溪"译为 small ducts or "loh vessels"（络）（小的管道或者小的血管）。译文与原文的内容存在较大差异，应该是由于译者未准确理解句中隐喻而造成的误译。

吴本也对原文存在误读，将"谷"和"溪"均错译成 joint（关节）。

第二节　容器隐喻及英译

容器隐喻是最典型的本体隐喻。容器是一种物质实体，既有内外和深浅，又有中心和边缘；容器具有一定的空间，可以容纳各种各样的物品；容器有充实或中空的状态；容器有门、口、孔、窗户等与外界相互交流的通道。人类从身体经验和物质体验出发，将容器的概念投射到人体以外的其他物体，如田野、丛林、房子等，甚至将一些无形和抽象的思想、情绪、事件、状态、范围等视为容器，以隐喻的方式映射到目标域，使这些抽象事物获得容器的某些形象具体的属性，形成很多隐喻概念，使人更易理解和接受[1]。莱考夫和约翰逊指出，人们把人体之外的世界视为外部世界，把自身视为独立于周围世界的实体，人们的日常活动就像进出各种容器一样，如走进教室、走出房间、进城、出城等。同时，人体本身也被视为一个具有内部空间和外部边界的容器，物质不断地进出其中，由此产生了诸如进餐、排出体内废物、呼出

[1]　谢菁.基于认知语言学的中医病因病机概念隐喻研究 [D].北京：北京中医药大学，2012：43.

空气、吸入空气等容器隐喻的表达[1]。

容器隐喻将中医理论体系中抽象的概念或范畴类比成具体的容器或者容器的通道等，使其具有一定的容积和空间，能形象地表达其功能，有助于解决中医理论在语言表达上的问题，便于人们理解。《素问》中存在着大量的容器隐喻，主要体现在身体、脏腑、门户等方面。下文将对容器隐喻进行举例说明，并对四个译本进行对比分析。

一、身体

中医学将人的身体看作体积较大的容器，将体内的一些部位或器官看作体积较小的容器，可以源源不断地与外部世界进行物质和能量交换。身体各部位和器官具有容纳具体物质或抽象概念的属性，有利于更好地阐释与理解其生理功能和病理变化。

1.膏粱之变，足生大丁，受如持虚。（《素问·生气通天论》）

释义：嗜食肥美食物的人，内多滞热，足以导致疔毒疮疡，其容易发生的程度，简直好像拿着空虚的器皿去盛东西一样。

李本：Besides, rich and greasy food tends to cause big furuncles and other diseases. Such a liability to diseases is just like to hold an empty container to receive things.

文本：In cases of changes associated with rich food, the feet generate large boils. When [the hands] receive [something] it is as if one were holding nothing.

吴本：The one who is addicted to delicious food often has stagnated heat inside and is apt to contract cellulitis and the stagnated heat stemmed from asthenia.

"受如持虚"意为好像拿着空虚的器皿去盛东西一样，句中将人体喻为空着的容器，将病邪喻为可放入器皿的东西。嗜食肥美食物的人身体易遭病邪侵袭，犹如空着的容器易装入物品一样，隐喻人体患病的容易程度。

李本采用直译法，将"受"译为receive things，"如"译为like，"持虚"译为hold an empty container，增译such a liability to diseases（这种得病的可能性）总结上句，可以准确传达原文的意思，使读者理解其中的隐喻，达到

---

[1]　Lakoff, G.& Johnson, M. *Metaphors We Live By*[M]. Chicago: University of Chicago Press, 1980: 27.

语言转换和文化交流的目的。不足之处在于 like 用作介词表示"像……"时，后面一般使用 doing 形式，因此应将 to hold 改为 holding。

吴本采用意译法解释医理，行文中使用西医术语 cellulitis（蜂窝组织炎）和 asthenia（衰弱、无力）等，虽然有一定的可读性，易于目的语读者理解，但是未译出容器隐喻，因此也就无法再现原文所描述的人体易受邪气侵袭的程度。

文本将"持虚"直译为 holding nothing。句中"虚"指空的容器，与 nothing 在意义上不对等。该译文有曲解原文之嫌，译不达意，语言转换的目标未能较好实现。

2. 仓廪不藏者，是门户不要也。水泉不止者，是膀胱不藏也。（《素问·脉要精微论》）

释义：如果肠胃不能纳藏水谷，大便不禁，这是肾虚不能禁固的关系；如果小便不禁，这是膀胱不能闭藏的关系。

李本：Failure of the Canglin (granary) to store up is due to failure of the Menhu (anus) to restrain. Incontinence of urine is due to failure of the bladder to store (urine).

威本：And when granaries and store–houses do not store provisions, it is as though doors and gateways had no meaning and importance. When water and wells do not cease to run it is as if the bladder were not able to retain liquid.

文本：When the granaries do not [keep what they] store, in this case the doors are not under control. When the water fountain does not stop, in this case the urinary bladder does not [keep what it] stores.

吴本：If the stomach and intestine of the patient can hardly hold the water and cereal with fecal incontinence, it is asthenia of kidney which fails to confine; if there is incontinence of urine, it is due to the inability of the shut and store of the bladder.

"仓廪"原指储藏米谷的仓库，此句将脾胃喻为仓廪，用以说明脾胃具有受纳水谷、运化精微的功能。"门户"指肛门，此处将肛门喻为门户，认为其与房屋的门一样具有开合功能。"要"在句中有约束、禁锢之意，说明肛门的作用。膀胱是贮存和排泄尿液的器官，句中也被隐喻成容器。

李本采用音译加注法，将"仓廪"译为 Canglin (granary)，将"门户"译为 Menhu (anus)。音译加注的形式突出中医术语，有利于中医文化的保留和传播。遗憾的是，两个注解的译法并不统一，"仓廪"为直译，"门户"为意译，易造成读者误解。如果将"仓廪"的注解译成 spleen and stomach，读者可能更容易体会其中的隐喻。

吴本采用意译法，将"仓廪"译为 the stomach and intestine，将门户译为 asthenia of kidney。直接译出喻指对象有利于实现交际目标，但是对容器隐喻采用不译的方法，无法让读者感受中医的文化特色，在文化传递上稍逊一筹。

威本和文本采用直译法将"仓廪"分别译为 granaries and store-houses 和 granaries，将"门户"分别译为 doors and gateways 和 doors，保留了容器隐喻，但是没有解释喻指对象，会给读者理解带来一定困难。

"藏"字，四个译本均译为 store，说明身体器官具有类似容器的储藏功能。此词有效地重现原文的容器隐喻，达到了语言转换和交际理解的目标。

"要"字，李本译为 restrain，文本译为 are under control，吴本译为 confine。相比而言，李本和吴本选词更为正式，虽然用词不同，但均能体现"要"具有"约束、禁锢"之意，在语言转换上区别不大。威本对原句理解出现偏差，将"要"误译为 meaning and importance，未能正确传达原文的内容。

"止"字，李本和吴本译为 incontinence，并且均将"水泉"意译为 urine，放弃了原文的隐喻，但胜在文意一目了然，有助于目的语读者理解。威本和文本将"水泉不止"分别译为 water and wells do not cease to run 和 the water fountain does not stop。直译保留了中医语言特色，若将其中隐喻稍加注解，更利于读者理解。

3. 头者，精明之府，头倾视深，精神将夺矣。（《素问·脉要精微论》）

释义：头是精明之府，如果头部侧垂，眼胞内陷，那说明精神要衰败了。

李本：The head is the house of Jingming. Drooped head and sunken eyes [are the signs] that Jingshen (Essence-Spirit) is on the verge of exhaustion.

威本：The head is the home of skill and intelligence. When man keeps the head bowed he sees only what is deep below and his vitality and spirit will be broken.

文本：As for the head, it is the palace of essence brilliance. When the head is bent and vision is in the depth, essence and spirit are about to be lost.

吴本：And the head is where the spirit locates, if the head hangs down or tilts with eyes caving in, it shows the spirit will decline soon; as the five viscera locate in the chest and abdomen...

"府"，过去指官吏办理公务的地方、高官和贵族的住宅或者官方收藏文书或财物的地方。《素问》中将人体的头、背、腰、膝、骨等部位隐喻成"府"，赋予其储藏和容纳的功能，可以理解成精神、肾、筋和髓等物质或能量的汇聚之所。

李本、威本和文本通过直译重现原文中的容器隐喻。三个译文分别将"府"译为 house、home 和 palace。这三个词都有"住宅"之义，但 house 较为中性，表示一般的建筑物；home 强调归属感，体现了头和精明、背和胸等之间的渊源，富有感情色彩；palace 常用于表示宏伟的建筑或者古代宫殿，更接近原文的"府"字。这几个词虽然侧重点不同，但是都为头、背、腰、膝和骨等身体部位圈定了住所范围，体现出这些部位储藏和容纳的功能，将容器隐喻明示给读者。

吴本使用意译法，将名词"府"转化为动词 locate（位于）。该词说明"精明"的位置，更符合英文表达，能够达到交际目的。但是没有译出体现中国文化的"府"，在文化传递上稍逊于前三个译本。

4. 开鬼门，洁净府，精以时服。（《素问·汤液醪醴论》）

释义：再想办法使汗液畅达，小便通利；注意观察病人情况，适时地给些药吃。

李本：[Besides,] [the therapeutic methods for] opening Guimen (sweat pores) and cleaning the Jingfu (the bladder) can be used [to eliminate the retention of fluid].

威本：One should restore their bodies and open the anus so that the bowels can be cleansed, and so that the secretions come at the proper time and serve the five viscera which belong to Yang, the principle of life.

文本：Open the demon gates and clean the pure palace and the essence will recover in due time.

吴本：Then, try to make the patient to perspire thoroughly, and keep his urination unobstructed, besides, give the patient, according to the condition, some medicine on due time.

"鬼门"指汗孔，"净府"指膀胱。句中将汗孔看作"门"，将膀胱视为"府"，实则是将它们隐喻成容器，赋予其容器的属性功能，能够贮存和排泄汗液、尿液。四个译本对于"鬼门"和"净府"的翻译有很大差异。

李本将"鬼门"和"净府"视为中医学术语，使用音译加注法将其译为 Guimen (sweat pores) 和 Jingfu (the bladder)，既体现中医术语特色，又直白简洁地解释其意，方便目的语读者理解。在进行注解时，李本通过意译将两个术语解释为汗孔和膀胱，一目了然，但未译出"门"和"府"蕴含的隐喻，在文化传递方面稍显不足。

文本采用逐字直译的方法将"鬼门"译为 demon gates，"净府"译为 pure palace。该译法译出"门"和"府"的概念，保留了原文的隐喻及其文化内涵。不足之处是未加解释，可能会使不熟悉中医文化的读者一头雾水，无从判断这两组词语的含义，不易达到交际目的。

威本未能准确理解"鬼门"和"净府"，将"鬼门"译为 the anus（肛门），"净府"译为 the bowels（肠），曲解了原文的意思，造成误译。

吴本通过释义将两个隐喻分别意译为 make the patient to perspire thoroughly（使病人充分出汗）和 keep his urination unobstructed（保持排尿通畅），语言地道，意思准确，易达到交际目的，但是未译出容器隐喻，在文化内涵传递方面稍显欠缺。

二、脏腑

古代解剖学尚不发达，对于古人来说，人体内部结构非常抽象。为了更好地对内脏进行建构和理解，中医学将人体内脏隐喻成容器，赋予其容器所具有的各种属性和功能。人体的内部器官被分为五脏和六腑两大类：五脏指肝、心、脾、肺、肾；六腑指胆、胃、大肠、小肠、膀胱和三焦。脏，同"藏"，为储存东西的地方；腑，同"府"，为储藏财物的地方。二字古义可通，均是具有一定存储空间的场所，能够贮存、容纳或传化物品。

1. 所谓五脏者，<u>藏</u>精气而不泻也，故满而不能实；六腑者，<u>传</u>化物而不<u>藏</u>，故实而不能满也。（《素问·五脏别论》）

释义：我们所说的五脏，它是藏精而不泻的，所以虽然常常充满，却不像肠胃那样，要由水谷充实它。至于六腑呢，它的作用是要把食物消化、吸收、输泻出去，所以虽然常常是充实的，却不能像五脏那样的被充满。

李本：The so-called Five Zang-Organs only store up Jingqi (Essence-Qi) and will not discharge it. That is why they are always Man (full) but not Shi (to be filled up). The so-called Six Fu-Organs only transport and transform food and will not store it up. That is why they are always Shi (to be filled up) but not Man (full).

威本：The so-called five viscera store up the essences of life and do not dispel them: since they must be filled they cannot be solid. The six bowels conduct and transform substance and do not store, therefore they are solid and cannot be filled.

文本：As for the so-called five depots, they store the essence qi and do not drain [it]. Hence, even if they are full, they cannot be replete. As for the six palaces, they transmit and transform things, but do not store [them]. Hence, they [may be] replete, but they cannot be full.

吴本：The function of the five solid organs is to store the essence without discharging, although they are filled often yet they are not substantialized. They are not like the stomach and intestine which are often substantialized with water and cereal. The function of the six hollow organs is to digest, absorb and transport the food, so, although they are often substantial, yet they cannot be filled like the five solid organs.

句中"藏""泻""传""满""实"等体现了五脏六腑的容器属性，是隐喻翻译的关键。对于这些词，四个译本均主要采用直译法，最大限度地保留了原文的隐喻特征。

对于"藏"字，李本和威本译为 store up，文本和吴本译为 store，形式上稍有区别，但都含有"储藏、储存"之义。译文忠实于原文，说明脏腑像容器一样具有贮藏功能。

"泻"字说明病理产物会由脏腑排出，将脏腑隐喻为能流出物质的容器。威本的 dispel 常指消除感觉，文本的 drain 常指排出液体。相比而言，李本和吴本将其译为 discharge，表示排泄，与原文更贴近。

"传"字说明物质的传送。李本和吴本将其译为 transport，表示物质的运输；威本译为 conduct，该词侧重于热或电的传导；文本译为 transmit，侧重于信号的传输。三个词相比较，transport 能够更准确地传递原文的意思。

对"满"和"实"，四个译本的译法差异较大。李本将"满"译为 Man (full)，文本译为 full，威本和吴本译为 be filled。李本将"实"译为 Shi (to be filled up)，威本译为 solid，文本译为 replete，吴本译为 be substantialized。根据原文，"满"指精气充满五脏，"实"指物质或食物充实六腑。这两个词都是较为抽象的概念，有着丰富的文化内涵，不易被目的语读者理解。相比而言，李本将其视为中医术语，使用音译加注法，既能保留中医文化特征，又能达到交际目的。

2. 脾、胃、大肠、小肠、三焦、膀胱者，仓廪之本，营之居也，名曰器……（《素问·六节藏象论》）

释义：脾、胃、大肠、小肠、三焦、膀胱都是承受和排泄水谷的，所以说它们是人体仓廪之本；水谷所化的精微，供心火以化血，所以又是产生营血的地方；由于它们都是储藏水谷的，所以名之曰器……

李本：The spleen, the stomach, the large intestine, the small intestine, the Sanjiao (triple energizer) and the bladder are the roots of granary and the location of Ying (Nutrient–Qi). These organs are called containers...

威本：In the stomach, the lower intestines, the small intestines, the three foci, the groin and the bladder, one can find the basic principle for the public granaries and the encampment of a regiment. These organs are called "vessels" ...

文本：The spleen is the basis of grain storage. It is the location of the camp [qi]. They are named containers...

吴本：The spleen is the base of storing water and cereal, it is the place where the Ying energy generates. It is called the "transfer and transform" ...

中医学认为，脾胃具有与仓廪相似的功能，即容纳和储藏，因此将"脾胃"隐喻为"仓廪"。"本"意为"基础"。李本将"仓廪之本"直译为 roots of granary（粮仓的根源），在搭配上不符合英语的表达习惯，容易引起歧义。威本译为 basic principle for the public granaries（公共谷仓的基本原理），译文偏离原文意思，无法准确传递原文的文化内涵。吴本译为 base of storing water and cereal（储存水谷的基础），文本译为 basis of grain storage（粮食储存的基础），这两种译法没有提及谷仓，而是意译出仓廪的功能，搭配较符合英语习惯，但在文化内涵的传递上存在不足。

"居"字指某物的所在，原文将"营气"这一抽象概念具体到某一范围，说明脾胃等器官有容纳营气的作用。对于"居"字，李本和文本采用直译法，将其译为 location，吴本采用意译法将其译为定语从句 the place where...。这两种译法在意义上都忠实于原文，达到了交际目的。但从形式上看，直译为 location 更加简练。由于对原文的隐喻存在理解偏差，威本将"营"误译为 encampment of a regiment（军营），在语言、文化和交际方面的效果都不理想。

句中将各种脏腑，如三焦、膀胱、大肠、小肠等，都隐喻为可以盛纳饮食水谷或代谢产物的容器，统称为"器"。李本和文本将"器"直译为 container（容器），威本直译为 vessel（器皿），用词虽不同，传达的意思和效果差别不大，均保留了原文的隐喻，易于读者产生相关的联想。吴本将其意译为 the transfer and transform，并解释了上述器官的作用，这种译法舍弃原文中"器"的字面意义及其表达的隐喻特征，突出"器"的传化功能，在语言表达上更为流畅，但在一定程度上造成了文化内涵的流失。

3. 五气入鼻，藏于心肺……五味入口，藏于肠胃，味有所藏，以养五气。（《素问·六节藏象论》）

释义：五气由鼻吸入，贮藏在心肺……五味由口进入，藏在肠胃里，它的精微可养五脏之气。

李本：When the five kinds of Qi are inhaled [into the body] through the nose and stored in the heart and the lung... When the five kinds of flavors are taken in through the mouth and stored in the intestines and the stomach, their nutrients [infuse into the Five Zang–Organs] to nourish the five kinds of Qi.

威本：The five atmospheric influences enter the nostrils and are stored by the heart and the lungs... The five flavors enter the mouth and are stored by the stomach. The flavors which are stored nourish the five atmospheric influences.

文本：The five qi enter through the nose and are stored in the heart and in the lung... The five flavors enter through the mouth and are stored in the intestines and in the stomach. When the flavors have a place where they are stored, this serves to nourish the five qi.

吴本：The five energies from heaven enter into the body through the nose and being stored in the heart and lung... The five tastes of foods from the earth enter into the body through the mouth and being stored in the stomach, when being digested, their essence will be transported and spread to nourish the energies of the five viscera.

五气经由鼻而入心肺，五味则经由口而入脾胃。"藏"字有"贮藏、蕴含、收存"之意，此处将心肺和脾胃隐喻为可以贮藏五气和五味的容器，表达"五气贮藏在心肺，五味贮藏在肠胃"之义。

四个译本均将"藏于心肺""藏于肠胃"中的"藏"字直译为 store。此译法保留了原文的文化内涵和隐喻特征，形象地说明心肺和肠胃具有类似于容器的功能，将抽象的五气和五味隐喻为可收入容器内的有形之物，有助于读者理解，达到交际目的。

对于第三个"藏"字，四个译本做了不同处理。"味有所藏"意为五味经过肠胃的消化后转化成精微。威本将其直译为 The flavors which are stored，文本译为 when the flavors have a place where they are stored，这两种译法突出了"肠胃是容器"的隐喻，但是以 flavors 作句子主语晦涩难懂，交际效果不佳。李本和吴本采用意译法，分别将其译为 nutrients 和 essence，通过前两个"藏"的翻译，读者已经可以体会到原文的隐喻内涵，此处放弃直译而改用意译，更易于读者理解。

4. 脾脏者，常著胃土之精也。（《素问·太阴阳明论》）

释义：脾脏经常贮藏胃的精气。

李本：The spleen stores the Jing (Essence) for the Stomach-Earth.

威本：The spleen, one of the viscera, manifests itself constantly in the essence (secretions) of the stomach and the soil.

文本：As for the spleen depot, it permanently stores the essence of the stomach, [i.e., of] soil.

吴本：As the spleen often activates the body fluid for the stomach and nourish the four limbs and bones of the body.

《黄帝内经素问》隐喻英译对比研究

"著"通"贮"，有"贮存"之义。此句将脾脏隐喻成具有贮藏功能的容器，可以贮藏胃的精气，并为胃行其津液。

由于文化认知的限制，威本误解了"著"的含义，将其直译为 manifest（显现），将"胃土"误译为并列短语 the stomach and the soil（胃和土），未能准确地传达原文意思，影响读者理解。

吴本采用意译的方法解释脾脏的功能，语言流畅，更易于目的语读者理解和接受，但是未译出原文中的容器隐喻，造成中医文化内涵缺失。

李本和文本将"著"直译为 store（储存），准确重现原文中的隐喻，将脾脏喻为可以贮藏"精"的器皿，引起读者对"精"这一抽象概念的想象。四个译本相比较，李本和文本更胜一筹。

5. 内舍五脏六腑，何气使然？（《素问·痹论》）

释义：痹病的病邪有内藏于五脏六腑的，这是什么气使它这样的呢？

李本：[Evil of Bi-Syndrome] is retained in the Five Zang-Organs and the Six Fu-Organs. What is the cause of it?

文本：When [the disease] proceeds into the interior and lodges in the five depots and six palaces, which qi causes that?

吴本：Some evils of the bi-disease retain in the five solid organs and the six hollow organs, what energy makes it so?

"舍"本为名词，指居住的房子，句中用作动词，意为"贮藏、容纳"。此句将人体的五脏六腑隐喻成容器，而引起疾病的各种邪气，如热气、水气等，均藏于其中。

李本和吴本将"舍"译为 retain（保持，容纳）。李本使用被动语态 be retained in，而吴本选择主动语态 retain in。从原文"何气使然"这一问句可以看出，病邪内藏于五脏六腑是"使然"，即被动，因此李本的被动译法更贴近原文，更具逻辑性。

文本采用直译法，将"舍"译为 lodge。lodge 可以用作动词，有"居住"之意，词性和意思上均与原文对等。选用 lodge 既保留原文的隐喻特征，又实现了语言转换、交际理解和文化传递等目标。

三、门户

门户是日常生活中房屋等各种建筑物的出入口，打开时可以自由进出房屋，关闭时则会影响正常出入。腠理、腧穴等经常被视为身体容器的门户。中医学将人体看作一个可以与外部世界进行物质和能量交换的容器，而腠理是肌肉和皮肤的纹理，是渗泄体液、流通气血的门户，控制着汗孔开合和汗液排泄，调节人体水液代谢和体温，具有抗御外邪内侵的功能，自然也就成为身体容器的门户。体表的孔窍也被视为脏腑容器的门户。人体的目、耳、鼻、口等器官就像自然界的孔洞一样，都是中空的，人体内部的脏腑与体表的这些器官相互对应配属。古人在对人体器官认知的基础上，通过取象比类的隐喻思维方式，将自然界中的孔窍概念映射到人体域之中。孔窍的使用充分反映出古人认知域的转移。《素问》中与门户相关的容器隐喻主要表现在腠理、孔窍和腧穴等身体门户上。

（一）腠理

腠，即肌肉的纹理；理，即皮肤的纹理。肌肉和皮肤的间隙，共称为腠理。中医学将腠理看作致病邪气侵犯人体的门户。若腠理致密，可以增强人体抵御外邪的能力，防止外邪侵袭入里。若腠理疏松或不固，风寒等外邪便会侵袭人体，引起感冒等病证；若腠理郁闭，则毛窍闭塞，肺气不宣，卫气无法外达，风寒之邪难出，导致无汗、恶寒、发热等。

1. 开阖不得，寒气从之，乃生大偻。（《素问·生气通天论》）

释义：如果腠理开阖失调，寒邪乘机侵袭，就会生成背部屈曲的大偻病。

李本：[When sweat pores] open and close abnormally, Hanqi (Cold-Qi) [will invade the body] through the sweat pores, making the body unable to straighten up.

威本：(If the atmosphere of Yang) cannot open and close (freely), the cold air will follow and the result will be a great deformity (hunchback).

文本：If opening and closing [of one's pores] are not appropriate and if cold qi follows this [opportunity to enter the body, then this] generates a severe bending [of the body].

吴本：It is normal when the skin striae of a man opens in spring and close in winter. If it does not open when it should open and does not close when it should close, it will leave the opportunity for the cold-evil to invade. When the cold-evil penetrates deep and damages the Yang energy, he may contract hunchback.

句中"开阖"指腠理的开张与闭合，通过调节开合实现抗御外邪内侵、保护人体的功能。

四个译本对体现容器隐喻特征的"开阖"均采用直译的方法，译为 open 和 close，既保留了隐喻，又简单易懂。

四个译本都对主语进行了补译。其中李本和文本将主语理解为"汗孔"，分别译为 sweat pores 和 pores。汗孔是腠理的一个主要类别，对于目的语读者来说，"汗孔"更具体，原文中的隐喻也更易理解和接受，虽然此译法导致部分文化内涵流失，但交际效果较好。

吴本将主语理解为"腠理"并直译为 skin striae。striae 为 stria 的复数形式，意为"条纹、细沟"。在意思上，striae 与中医学"腠理"的概念并不对等；在形式上吴本将 striae 视为单数，语言运用上不够严谨。此处若直接使用其单数形式 stria，能使行文更加统一。

威本将主语译为 the atmosphere of Yang，将"腠理"误解为阳气，对原文的理解出现偏差，导致误译。

2. 故风者，百病之始也，清静则肉腠闭拒，虽有大风苛毒，弗之能害。（《素问·生气通天论》）

释义：风是引起各种疾病的开端，但是，只要精神安静，意志安闲，就能使腠理闭密，阳气能够卫外，纵然有大风苛毒，也不能侵入人体。

李本：Wind is the factor responsible for various diseases. [However, if people maintain] a peaceful mood, Roucou will close up to prevent [pathogenic factors from invading the body].

威本：Thus wind is the cause of a hundred diseases. When people are quiet and clear, their skin and flesh is closed and protected.

文本：The fact is, the wind is the origin of the one hundred diseases. In case [a person is] clear and calm, the flesh and the interstice [structures] are firmly closed up and resist.

吴本：Therefore, wind is the main source of various diseases. But how can the wind-evil be resisted? The clue is to keep one's physique and spirit quiet and not being bothered by material concerns, that his Yang energy may be substantial and his striae of skin dense.

句中"肉腠闭拒"将腠理喻为可以闭合的门户，强调其抗御外邪内侵、保护人体的作用。

对于这一隐喻，李本、威本、文本以直译为主，而吴本则采用意译法。

李本将"肉腠"视为中医术语，首次出现时，采用音译加注法将其译为 Roucou (muscular interstices)。此处非首次出现，故只采用音译法，避免冗余。李本将"闭拒"译为 close up to prevent 后，又增译宾语 pathogenic factors from invading the body，使译文更为流畅。该译文既保留中医特色，又增强可读性，整体上较好地达到交际理解和文化传播的目的。

威本和文本对"肉腠"的理解不充分，分别译为 skin and flesh 和 the flesh and the interstice [structures]，虽然有一定的交际效果，但是传递的文化内涵不够准确。对于"闭拒"，二者在用词上稍有差异：威本译为 is closed and protected，强调肉腠的保护作用；文本则译为 are firmly closed up and re-sist，强调肉腠的抵御作用。二者都译出肉腠可以闭合的容器属性，保留了原文的隐喻特征。

吴本将"肉腠闭拒"意译为 striae of skin (may be) dense，并在上下文做了详细解释，读者更易理解其意思和文化内涵，但是与前三个译本相比，略显繁琐，失去原文的凝练之美。另外，striae 是 stria 的复数形式，此处被误用作单数，应该使用单数形式 stria。

3. 日西而阳气已虚，气门乃闭。（《素问·生气通天论》）

释义：到日落的时候，阳气衰退，汗孔也就随着关闭了。

李本：In the afternoon, it begins to decline and the sweat pores close up accordingly.

威本：When the sun moves toward the West Yang declines, the force of Yang becomes insubstantial and the door of the breath is then closed.

文本：When the sun is in the West, the yang qi is already depleted. The qi gates close.

吴本：The Yang energy of man... become weak in the dusk, hence–forth, the entrance of energy (the opening of sweat gland) closes in the wake of it.

对体现容器隐喻的"闭"，四个译本均采用直译法，一致选用动词 close，其中李本使用更为准确的短语 close up。通过 close，读者能够产生与门户相关的联想，体会句中蕴含的隐喻。

对另一隐喻关键词"气门"，四个译本的处理不尽相同。"气门"指汗孔，"门"体现出中医学对汗孔的隐喻，将汗孔视作身体的门户之一，指出其日西而闭的特点。

李本按照现代医学的解释，将"气门"意译为 sweat pores，意思明确，但未能体现出汗孔作为"门"的隐喻，在文化传递上有所不足。

吴本采用意译加注法，将其译为 the entrance of energy (the opening of sweat gland)。entrance 在一定程度上保留"门"的隐喻，贴近原文，注解将"气门"解释为汗孔，有利于读者的理解。但是中医学"气"的内涵较广，与英语的 energy 并不对等，此处将"气"译为 energy 并不准确。

威本将"气门"译为 the door of the breath，文本将其译为 the qi gates。door 和 gate 两词都保留了原文"门"的容器隐喻。但威本未能准确理解中医学"气"的内涵，将"气"误译为 breath，容易引起读者误解。文本则将"气"视为中医术语，直接音译为 qi，较为贴切，利于中医文化外传，但是文化差异可能会使目的语读者产生理解障碍，若此处添加注解，将会取得更好的交际效果。

4. 故风无常府，卫气之所发，必开其腠理，邪气之所合，则其府也。
（《素问·疟论》）

释义：所以风邪所侵并没有一定的地方，只要卫气与之相应，腠理开泄，邪气停留的那个地方，就是风之府。

李本：So wind does not [invades the body through] a fixated region. Thus when–ever Weiqi (Defensive–Qi) emerges, it must open Couli (muscular interstice) and gives rise to the invasion of Xieqi. This is the access [of wind to the body].

文本：Hence, the wind [that enters the body] has no permanent palace [there]. Where the guard qi is effused, the interstice structures must open. Where it joins with the evil qi [to battle], that is its palace.

吴本：Therefore, although the invading location of the evil-energy is not certain, yet, whenever the Wei-energy corresponds to it, the striae will open, the evil-energy will retains and causes disease.

句中将腠理隐喻为人体体液渗泄、气血流通的门户，具有"开""合"的功能，能够保护人体抗御外邪的侵犯。李本采用音译加注法将"腠理"译为 Couli (muscular interstice)，较好地实现语言表达、交际理解和文化传递等方面的目标。文本直译为 the interstice structures（孔隙结构）不够准确，由于文化差异，不利于目的语读者理解。吴本译为 striae，与前文相比，为求简洁省略了 skin，结合上下文来看，应该不会造成误解。三者相比，李本的交际和文化效果略胜一筹。

"府"指风邪集聚的地方，句中把抽象的"邪气"具体化，赋予其形态和贮藏之地，是一种容器隐喻。三个译本采用不同的译法。李本的 region、文本的 palace 和吴本的 location 都将"府"视为一个有形的空间，从这个角度看，三者均保留了原文的隐喻。但是三个词侧重点不同，region 指一个区域，palace 指古代的宫殿，而 location 指特定的位置。相比而言，palace 更贴近原文的"府"，即达官显贵的住所。

"则其府也"指的是邪风所在之地，三位译者对原文的理解有一定的差别。李本将其意译为 this is the access [of wind to the body]，文本直译为 that is its palace，吴本意译为 the evil-energy will retains and causes disease。李本的语言比较地道，但从意义上看，将邪气所在之地理解为风邪进入身体的通道并不准确。文本的直译保留了隐喻，比较形象。吴本对隐喻做了解释，易于理解，但语言不严谨，will retains and causes 中的语法错误影响了译文的准确性和可读性。

5. 寒则腠理闭……炅则腠理<u>开</u>，荣卫<u>通</u>，汗大<u>泄</u>，故气泄。（《素问·举痛论》）

释义：寒冷之气，能使经络凝涩……热则腠理开发，营卫之气过于疏泄，汗大出，所以说是"气泄"。

李本：[Excessive] cold leads to closure of Couli (Muscular Interstice)... [Excessive] heat leads to openness of Couli (Muscular Interstice) and the Rong (Nutrient-Qi) and Wei (Defensive-Qi), and profuse sweating. That is why it is said that Qi leaks.

《黄帝内经素问》隐喻英译对比研究

文本：When one is cold, then the interstice structures close... When one is hot, then the interstice structures open and the camp [qi] and guard [qi] pass through. Sweat flows out profusely. Hence, qi flows out.

吴本：The cold-evil causes the channel and collaterals to become rough... The heat causes the openning of the striae and the excessive excretion of the Ying and Wei energies along with the sweat. So, it is called the "excretion of the energy".

句中的"闭""开""通""泄"等词形象地说明腠理作为身体门户的作用，是体现隐喻的关键词。

李本主要采用意译法，调整原文结构，改变关键词的词性，将动词"闭""开""通""泄"译为名词。其中"闭"译为 closure，"开"和"通"均译为 openness，将"腠理开，荣卫通"两个短语合二为一，译为以 openness 为中心语的名词结构，将动词短语"汗大泄"转译为名词短语 profuse sweating（大汗）。译文符合英文的表达习惯，语言流畅地道，表述简洁清楚，并增加行文的变化。"气泄"是中医特有的表述，没有对应的英文表达，李本将其直译为 qi leaks，保留了中医文化特征。本句中，李本对同义词"开"和"通"、多义词"泄"的处理灵活恰当，成功实现了语言转换和文化传递的目标。

文本采用直译法，将"闭""开"分别译为 close 和 open，"通"译为 pass through（通过），"汗泄""气泄"中的"泄"均译为 flow out（流出）。译文虽保留了原文的隐喻，但是用词过于生硬，不够准确生动。

吴本采用意译法对医理进行解释说明，译文中仅 openning of the striae 体现了腠理的容器隐喻，"泄"字译为西医用词 excretion（排泄），译文有利于目的语读者的理解，但是在隐喻翻译和文化传递方面略逊于其他译本。

（二）孔窍

中医学认为，人体的目、耳、鼻、口等器官就像自然界的孔洞一样，都是中空的，就像人体与外界联系的门户，是阴阳二气进出人体的通道。在《素问》中，与"窍"相关的词语有九窍、七窍、上窍、下窍、空窍等。

1. 天地之间，六合之内，其气九州（九窍）、五脏、十二节，皆通乎天气。（《素问·生气通天论》）

释义：凡是天地之间，四时之内，无论是人的九窍、五脏，还是十二节，都是和自然之气相通的。

李本：[All those] within the heavens and the earth [as well as] the Liuhe (six directions) are interrelated with Tianqi (Heaven–Qi), [such as things in] the Jiuzhou (nine geographical divisions), the Jiuqiao (nine orifices in the human body), the Five Zang–Organs and the twelve Jie (joints).

威本：And between Heaven and Earth and within the six points. The (heavenly) breath prevails in the nine divisions, in the nine orifices, in the five viscera, and in the twelve joints; they are all pervaded by the breath of Heaven.

文本：Between heaven and earth and within the six [cardinal points] uniting [the world] all the qi within the nine regions, communicate with the qi of heaven.

吴本：All things on the earth and in the space communicate with the Yin and Yang energies. Human being is a small universe as human body has everything that the universe has. In the universe, there are nine states (namely Ji, Yan, Qing, Xu, Yang, Jing, Yu, Liang and Yong), and man has nine orifices (seven orifices: two ears, two eyes, two nostrils, and one mouth; two Yin orifices: external urethral orifice and the anus); there are five musical tones in the universe, man has five solid organs responsible for storing the mental activities (liver stores soul, heart stores spirit, spleen stores consciousness, lung stores inferior spirit, kidney stores will); there are twelve solar terms in the universe, and man has twelve channels. The Yin and Yang energies of human being correspond with the Yin and Yang energies of the universe, and the Yin and Yang energies of all things (including men) are communicating with that of the universe.

"窍"本义为"孔""洞"。"九窍"，指的是人体的七阳窍（眼二、耳二、鼻孔二，口一）与二阴窍（前阴一，后阴一），中医学将人体器官喻为孔洞，认为它们是人体与外界联系的门户。

四个译本中，文本对原文理解不够全面，漏译"九窍、五脏十二节"。

李本、威本和吴本均将"九窍"译为 nine orifices，实现语言对等转换，但是三个译本的具体处理方式各异，取得的效果也有所不同。

李本将"九窍"视为中医术语，将其音译为 Jiuqiao，再以加注的方法，直译为 nine orifices in the human body。这种译法能在行文中突出"九窍"概念，加注保留隐喻，能够帮助读者理解。不足之处是没有详细说明"九窍"的含义，无法帮助目的语读者深入理解其内涵。

威本将其直译为 nine orifices，行文简洁，但同样没有说明"九窍"的意思。

吴本首先将其译为 nine orifices，通过加注说明"九窍"的具体含义包括 seven orifices: two ears, two eyes, two nostrils, and one mouth; two Yin orifices: external urethral orifice and the anus。这一译法虽然稍显繁琐，但在保留隐喻的同时，提升了译文的可读性，更易于目的语读者对中医文化的理解。

2. 故清阳出上窍，浊阴出下窍。（《素问·阴阳应象大论》）

释义：所以在人体，则清阳化生之气，出于上窍，浊阴化生之气，出于下窍。

李本：Thus the Lucid–Yang moves upwards into upper orifices of the body while the Turbid–Yin moves downwards into the lower orifices of the body.

威本：The pure and lucid element of light is manifest in the upper orifices and the turbid element of darkness is manifest in the lower orifices.

文本：Hence, the clear yang exits through the upper orifices; the turbid yin exits through the lower orifices.

吴本：Yang determines the energy which is ascending, so the lucid Yang gets out from the upper orifices of a man; Yin determines the shape and is descending, so the turbid Yin gets out from the lower orifices of a man.

句中用"上窍"隐喻耳、目、口、鼻，"下窍"隐喻前后二阴。

四个译本对这两个隐喻的翻译基本一致，都采用直译法，将"上窍"译为 upper orifices，"下窍"译为 lower orifices。李本补译出定语 of the body，吴本补译出定语 of a man，比另外两个译本表述更为具体，但是并无本质区别。

直译法保留了隐喻，将耳、目、口、鼻和二阴视为身体和外界相通的孔洞，形象易懂。若脱离前后文单独使用本句，最好在两个词后加注释，分别解释 upper orifices 和 lower orifices 的具体含义，使目的语读者更容易理解。

3. 东方青色，入通于肝，开窍于目。（《素问·金匮真言论》）

释义：东方青色之气，与人身的肝相应，目是肝之窍。

李本：[For example,] the east corresponds to blue in color and is related to the liver that opens into the eyes.

威本：Green is the color of the East, it pervades the liver and lays open the eyes.

文本：The East; green–blue color. Having entered it communicates with the liver; it opens an orifice in the eyes.

吴本：Yang emerges in the east and the colour of east is green, the human liver is also green and corresponds to wood, as the energy of universe is connected with the human energy, so the east energy communicates with the liver. The liver channel gets access to the brain and connecting the eyes, so eyes are the orifices of the liver.

东方、青色、肝与目同属木，它们之间相互联系，句中的"入通""开窍"体现了这种关联。中医学认为，人体内部的脏腑都有相应的体表器官与之对应配属。其中，目与肝对应配属，目可视为肝脏容器的门户。肝出现病变可以反映在眼睛上，借助眼睛出现的异常也可以推测肝可能出现的病变。

威本和文本对原文理解出现偏差，将"东方青色"误认为"入通"和"开窍"的主语，导致误译，不利于中医文化的传播。

李本采用直译法将"入通"译为 is related to，"开窍"译为 opens into the eyes，定语从句的使用使行文逻辑清晰，简洁易懂。译文语言准确地道，达到了交际目的，open 形象地说明"窍"具有容器一样的开合属性，体现出隐喻特征，保留了文化内涵。

吴本总体上采用意译法，将"入通"译为 communicates with，将"开窍于目"变换句式，化被动为主动，译为 eyes are the orifices of the liver（眼为肝之窍），并增译出东方、青色、肝、木、目之间的联系，通过因果连词 so 加强句子之间的逻辑关系。虽然在形式上没有忠于原文，行文也较繁琐，但合理地解释了中医医理，方便读者理解句中所提事物之间的抽象关联，更好地传递中医文化。

（三）腧穴

腧穴分布于躯干，与脏腑有密切关系。中医学通常将腧穴视为气血出入之门户，是风邪入侵人体的途径。

风中五脏六腑之俞，亦为脏腑之风，各入其门户所中，则为偏风。（《素问·风论》）

释义：风邪伤于五脏六腑的腧穴，顺腧而入其脏腑，也就成为五脏六腑之风。如各随某一俞穴血气衰弱之处而侵入，偏着于一处，即为偏风。

李本：Invasion of wind into the Acupoints of the Five Zang-Organs and the Six Fu-Organs is also known as wind of the Zangfu-Organs. [When it invades the body] from any related Acupoint, it causes Pianku (paralysis).

文本：When the wind strikes the transporters of the five depots and six palaces, this, too, causes wind of the depots and palaces. In each case it enters through the respective door. Where it strikes unilateral wind results.

吴本：When the wind-evil invades into the shu-points of the five solid organs and the six hollow organs, it will become the wind of the five organs and the six hollow organs. Regardless of collateral, channel, viscus or bowel, when any of them is invaded by the wind-evil, it will become the residing of wind-evil on one side of the body.

句中把"腧穴"隐喻为门户，风邪随左侧或右侧的腧穴偏中人体，则为偏风。

李本将"门户"意译为 acupoint，和腧穴的翻译一致。该译法简单明了，易于理解，但是没有保留容器隐喻，不能突出腧穴的门户作用，在文化传递上效果不佳。

文本采用直译法，将"门户"译为 door，动词使用 enters。译文保留"门户"的隐喻，形象地说明风邪进入门户侵入人体的过程。但是，文本将"俞穴"译为 transporters，此词在西医中意为"转运蛋白"，和中医学的腧穴并不对等。通读全句后，目的语读者无法将 door 与中医学的腧穴联系在一起，晦涩难懂，不利于交际。

吴本将"门户"理解为人体的络、经、脏、腑，而非腧穴。该译文对句中隐喻的理解存在偏差，不能准确地传达原文意思。

第三节 动物隐喻及英译

动物隐喻是以各种动物及其特征为喻体，用来指称或表征需要说明或陈述的人或物[1]。自古以来，自然界中的动物与人类共同生存，共同竞争，在地球上繁衍生息。在与动物的长期相处中，人们对各种动物特性的认识不断加深，逐渐抓住动物特性与人或其他事物之间的关联性和相似性，赋予动物特性某种喻义，借助相关因素说明或描述本体的特征，由此产生了动物隐喻。

古代医家不断探索和认识医学与动物之间的关联，通过人类固有的隐喻认知把中医学和动物联系起来，利用和动物相关的词汇来表达医学概念，为构建中医隐喻提供大量喻体。

《素问》中的动物隐喻将与动物相关的词语，如动物的动作和姿态，动物的全貌、身体部位和器官，甚至动物的生活习性等，融入中医语言中，借用动物的形态、特征等来描述抽象而复杂的人体生理和病理状况。动物隐喻利用二者之间的相似性，在读者头脑中建立起一定的关联，使读者更易理解抽象而复杂的医学概念。动物隐喻主要用来表现脉象、病理变化、外候等方面。

一、脉象

1. 春日浮，如鱼之游在波……秋日下肤，蛰虫将去；冬日在骨，蛰虫周密……（《素问·脉要精微论》）

释义：春天的脉象应当浮而在外，好像是鱼游在水面上一样……秋天的脉象应当稍下于皮肤，好像昆虫将要蛰伏一样；冬天的脉象应当沉潜在骨，好像昆虫已经伏藏得很周密一样……

李本：In spring, [the pulse] is floating just like fish swimming in water... In autumn, [the pulse is beating] beneath the skin just like the insects going into hid-

---

[1] 孙毅. 认知隐喻学多维跨域研究 [M]. 北京：北京大学出版社，2013：227.

ing; In winter, [the pulse] is near the bone just like animals in hibernation...

威本：In days of Spring the pulse is superficial, like wood floating on water（浮）or like a fish that glides through the waves... In Fall days the torpid insects underneath the skin are about to come out. In Winter the torpid insects are all around the bone, quiet and delicate...

文本：On spring days, it floats at the surface, like a fish swimming in a wave... On autumn days, it descends into the skin. The hibernating creatures will soon go [into hiding]. On winter days, it is at the bones; the hibernating creatures are firmly sealed in.

吴本：The pulses are different in various seasons: in spring, the pulse is up floating like fish swimming under the water surface... In autumn，the pulse sink slightly to be under the skin like a hibernating worm entering into the hole; In winter, the pulse sinks to the bone, like a hibernating worm hiding in the hole...

句中以人们熟悉的动物——鱼和蛰虫隐喻四时脉象的特点，形象地说明脉诊的感觉和体悟。以"鱼之游在波"隐喻春脉浮而在外的特点；以"蛰虫将去"隐喻秋脉微沉，似在肤下的特点；以"蛰虫周密"隐喻冬脉沉在骨中的特点。

对于"如鱼之游在波"，李本直译为 like fish swimming in water，文本直译为 like a fish swimming in a wave。两个译本均译出基本含义，保留了动物隐喻，但是译文比较笼统，没有体现出鱼在水面游动时的轻盈和飘浮之感，目的语读者无法准确感受浮脉的特点。吴本译为 like fish swimming under the water surface，与前两个译本相比，surface 起到画龙点睛的作用，让读者体会出鱼浮游于水波表面的感觉。威本将其译为 like a fish that glides through the waves，并增译 wood floating on wate 进行对比，补充说明脉"浮"的感觉。威本将"鱼之游在波"描绘得更加细致生动，易于目的语读者抓住春脉的特点。

秋脉和冬脉均以蛰虫的活动为喻，蛰虫指藏伏土中越冬的虫。四个译本对"蛰虫"的理解不尽相同。李本将两处"蛰虫"分别译为 insects 和 animals in hibernation，文本都译为 hibernating creatures。insects、animals 和 creatures 都过于宽泛，传达的意思和原文表述有一定出入。威本的 torpid insects 和吴本的 hibernating worm 将"蛰虫"理解成蛰伏的昆虫，比较具体，更忠实于原文。遗憾的是，威本将"蛰虫"当作"秋日下肤""冬日在骨"的主语，曲解了原文，造成误译。对于秋脉和冬脉的两个动物隐喻，吴本较好地呈现原文语义，在保留隐喻的同时，更易于目的语读者理解。

2. 病肺脉来，不上不下，如循鸡羽，曰肺病。死肺脉来，如物之浮，如风吹毛，曰肺死。（《素问·平人气象论》）

释义：如脉来不上不下，如抚摩鸡毛一样，这是肺的病脉；如脉来如物之漂浮无根，如风吹动羽毛一般，这是肺的死脉。

李本：The morbid Lung-Pulse is soft at both ends, just like the feeling of a chicken feather. This is [the state of] the morbid pulse of the lung. Dead Lung-Pulse is as floating as hair blown by wind. This is the dead pulse of the lung.

威本：When man is sick the pulse of his lungs moves, but it neither rises nor falls like the wings of a chicken—and then one can speak of sick lungs. At the point of death the pulse of the lungs moves like an object that is floating and insubstantial, or like a hair blown by the wind—and then one can speak of the death of the lungs.

文本：The arrival of a diseased lung [movement in the] vessels is [as follows]: neither rising nor descending; [it feels] as if [one's fingers] passed over chicken feathers. That is called "the lung has a disease." The arrival of a dying lung [movement in the] vessels is [as follows]: resembling a floating item; it is like body hair blown by the wind . That is called "the lung dies."

吴本：When the pulse is rough like stroking the firm and sturdy feathers of a cock, it is the diseased pulse of lung; If the coming of the pulse is like weeds floating on the water or a piece of feather floating like being blown in the wind, it is the lung pulse indicating death.

句中以"循鸡羽"和"风吹毛"分别隐喻病肺脉和死肺脉的脉象特点，从而区分二者的不同之处。"循"为抚摩之意，病肺脉来，脉搏不上不下，如同抚摩鸡的羽毛。死肺脉来，轻浮而无根，如同风吹毛一样。

对于"循鸡羽"的翻译，四个译本差别较大。李本采用意译法，将"病肺脉来，不上不下"译为 The morbid Lung-Pulse is soft at both ends，将"如循鸡羽"译为 like the feeling of a chicken feather，增译 feeling 一词，指出构成隐喻双方的相似性是感觉。但是，feeling 的修饰语是 chicken feather，漏译"循"这一关键动词。原文将脉象特点隐喻为抚摩鸡羽的感觉，而译文则理解为鸡羽的感觉，在表达上存在较大差别。

文本将"不上不下"直译为 neither rising nor descending，"循鸡羽"意译为 one's fingers passed over chicken feather。但 pass over 常有"忽略"之义，若把 over 替换为 through，表示"手指穿过鸡羽"，更能贴近原文。

吴本将"不上不下"意译为脉象的感觉，但与李本相反，吴本将这种感觉理解为 rough，而非 soft。将"循鸡羽"译为 stroking the firm and sturdy feathers of a cock，并增译 firm 和 study 两个表示感觉的形容词配合 rough，形象地说明脉象特征与"循鸡羽"的共性，在保留隐喻的同时也利于读者的理解。但在美语中 cock 特指公鸡，并且有不雅的含义，改用 chicken 更为恰当。

威本未能正确理解该句的意思，将"鸡羽"误译为鸡翅，且漏译动词"循"。对于 it neither rises nor falls like the wings of a chicken 这句话，从字面上看"不上不下"与鸡翅之间没有相似性，译文晦涩，容易造成读者的误解，不利于中医文化的传播。

对于"风吹毛"的翻译，李本、威本和文本差别不大，均直译为 hair blown by the wind，保留隐喻，简单明了，易于理解。吴本将"毛"译为 feather，与 hair 相比太过具体。另外，文本增译 floating like 作为 feather 的定语。Like...a piece of feather floating like being blown in the wind 这一句中出现两个 like，表达略显繁琐。

3. 平脾脉来，和柔相离，如鸡践地……病脾病来，实而盈数，如鸡举足……死脾脉来，锐坚如乌之喙，如鸟之距……（《素问·平人气象论》）

释义：正常的脾脉来时，和柔舒缓，好像鸡足从容不迫地落地一样……脾的病脉来时，充实而数，如鸡急走之势……脾的死脉来时，如鸟的嘴、鸟的爪距一样坚硬尖锐……

李本：The normal Spleen-Pulse beats smoothly and softly as a chicken putting its claw on the ground... The morbid Spleen-Pulse is forceful and rapid like a chicken raising its claw... Dead Spleen-Pulse is as sharp and hard as the beak of a crow and the talons of a bird, [as dripping as] the leakage of a room and [as receding as] the running of water...

威本：When man is tranquil and healthy, the pulse of the spleen flows softly, coming together and falling apart like a chicken treading the earth... When man is sick, the pulse of the spleen moves fully and is large and long and slightly tense, and there is a surplus of the number of pulse beats like a chicken raising its feet... At the point of death, the pulse of the spleen moves sharply and strongly like the beak of a bird, or like the spurs of a cock...

文本：The arrival of a normal spleen [movement in the] vessels is [as follows]: harmonious, soft, and distanced, resembling chicken stepping on the earth... The arrival of a diseased spleen [movement in the] vessels is [as follows]: replete, abundant, and frequent, resembling chicken raising their legs... The arrival of a dying spleen [movement in the] vessels is [as follows]: pointed and firm, like a crow's beak, like a bird's spur...

吴本：When the coming of the spleen pulse with stomach-energy is mild but adhering with energy, likes a cock's claws falling leisurely on the ground when walking... When the coming of the pulse is substantial and rapid, like a cock running swiftly... If the coming of the pulse is wiry and hard, firm and sharp like the beak or claw of a crow...

句中以"如鸡践地""如鸡举足"和"如鸟之喙，如鸟之距"分别隐喻平脾脉、病脾脉和死脾脉的不同脉象特点。

"如鸡践地"，形容脉和缓。四个译本主要采用直译法，均保留动物隐喻。对动物主体"鸡"的翻译，吴本选用 cock，不同于其他三个译本。相比之下，chicken 泛指鸡禽，用在此处更为恰当。对动词"践地"，四个译本译法各异。李本译为 putting its claw on the ground，表达通俗直白，但是不够形象。威本的 treading 和文本的 stepping on 是同义词，表达更为地道，易于目的语读者理解。吴本译为 claws falling leisurely on the ground when walking，补译出 leisurely 和 when walking 两个状语。四个译本相比，吴本对于"践地"的处理更为生动，活灵活现地说明鸡足落地时从容不迫的感觉，给读者较强的画面感，也更容易使人理解其喻指对象的内涵，即平脾脉和柔舒缓的特点。

"如鸡举足"，"足"读"促"，有"行"的意思，指鸡行走过急，而无和缓的样子。李本、威本和文本均将"举足"理解为鸡抬起脚，并采用直译法，虽然保留动物隐喻，但是表述和原意有出入，目的语读者不易想象出鸡急走的样子。李本使用 forceful and rapid，文本使用 replete、abundant 和 frequent 形容病脾脉的特点，在一定程度上弥补了"举足"的误译，使目的语读者在通读全句后了解病脾脉的特点。威本没有正确理解数脉的含义，将"数"误解为数字的"数"，译为 number，导致整句出现误译，译文逻辑不通。吴本将"举足"意译为 running swiftly，忠实于原文，形象地说明脉来充实硬满而急数的特征。

再看"如乌之喙，如鸟之距"。喙，即鸟嘴。距，即鸟爪，指雄鸡、雉等跖后面突出像脚趾的部分，此处用来形容死脾脉锐坚而无柔和之气的特点。四个译本均采用直译法，但在用词上稍有区别。

"乌之喙"的译法基本一致。李本、文本和吴本均将"乌"译为 crow，相较于威本的 bird 更为具体；"喙"都译为 beak，并无实质区别，基本忠实原文，保留动物隐喻。

"鸟之距"，李本译为 talons，意为爪，较为准确。威本和文本没有正确理解"距"的意思，译为 spur。该词本意为马刺，可以指公鸡或雄性猎鸟用于打斗的距，用在此处不准确。吴本将"鸟"也译为 crow，把"如乌之喙，如鸟之距"合二为一译为 like the beak or claw of a crow，虽然行文上更为简洁，但在准确性上不及李本。

4. 真肺脉至，大而虚，如以毛羽中人肤……（《素问·玉机真脏论》）

释义：肺脏的真脏脉来的时候，洪大而又非常虚弱，像毛羽着人皮肤一样……

李本：The appearance of Genuine–Lung–Pulse, marked by large size and weak beating, just as stroking the skin with a feather...

威本：When the pulse of the lungs stops its large and slow beats and (sounds) as though there were hair and feathers...

文本：When a [movement of the] true [qi of the] lung arrives in the vessels, which is big and depleted, as if one touched a person's skin with fur or feathers...

吴本：When the coming of the pulse indicating the exhaustion of the lung energy is full but very feeble like a feather touching the skin of man...

"如以毛羽中人肤"，形容肺脉之浮虚无力，好像毛羽落在人的皮肤上一样轻虚。句中以"毛羽中人肤"的轻虚感觉隐喻肺的真脏脉洪大而虚软无力的脉象特点。

李本将其译为 just as stroking the skin with a feather，文本译为 as if one touched a person's skin with fur or feathers，吴本译为 like a feather touching the skin of man，三个译本均采用直译法，但在句式和用词上稍有区别。

文本增译主语 one，将"毛羽"直译为 fur（毛）和 feathers（羽）两个词，整体上较为繁琐，不如李本和吴本简洁。在动词选择上，李本的 stroke 意为轻抚，文本和吴本的 touch 意为触摸。二者相比，stroke 更加形象地描绘出羽毛的轻盈和在皮肤上一扫而过的感觉，用在此处更胜一筹。这三个译本大同小异，都较忠实地呈现原文的动物隐喻，使目的语读者通过羽毛碰触皮肤的感觉体会出抽象的脉象特点。

威本增译 sounds，将中医学用触觉感知的脉诊误认为西医学的听诊，有画蛇添足之感。另外，威本只译出"毛羽"hair and feathers，漏译"中人肤"这一动词短语，说明译者对此句的理解出现偏差，造成误译。

二、病理变化

目里微肿如卧蚕起之状，曰水。（《素问·平人气象论》）

释义：眼胞浮肿如蚕眠后之状，也是水病。

李本：Slight swelling of eyelid like silkworm indicates water [disease].

威本：When within the eye there is a minute swelling, as though a dormant silkworm were beginning to take shape, it is said to have been caused through water.

文本：When the eye lids are slightly swollen, resembling a silkworm rising from sleep, that is called: "water".

吴本：When the eyelid is swelling like the silkworm lying torpid, it is also the disease associated with water.

"目里"即上下眼睑。眼睑浮肿就像蚕眠后的样子。句中以卧蚕之状隐喻水病所表现出的眼睑浮肿的症状。四个译本均将"蚕"译为 silkworm，保留了动物隐喻，读者能够通过 silkworm 进行相关联想。除此之外，翻译的关键之处还在于蚕"卧"的形态。

李本将"卧蚕起之状"简化，仅译出 silkworm，虽取得了行文简洁的效果，但是没有将蚕的具体形态特征译出，不能完整地呈现原文的意思，不利于读者的想象。

威本中的 dormant silkworm 描绘出蚕静卧的样子，但是 beginning to take shape 是对"起之状"的逐字直译，译文的意思是"静止的蚕开始成形"。这种表述既不符合原文，也没有逻辑，若将后半句删掉效果会好一些。

文本将其译为 silkworm rising from sleep，描写出蚕刚醒的样子，富有动感，但没有译出"卧"字，与原文要表达的蚕眠之义不尽一致。

吴本将其译为 the silkworm lying torpid，"卧"译为 lying，既忠实原文又生动形象，使读者很容易想象出眼睑浮肿的症状，实现原文隐喻的目的。

三、外候

1. 青如翠羽者生，赤如鸡冠者生，黄如蟹腹者生，白如豕膏者生，黑如乌羽者生。（《素问·五脏生成》）

释义：面上的气色，如果青得像翠鸟的羽毛，那是生色；赤得像鸡冠，那是生色；黄得像蟹腹，那是生色；白得像猪脂，那是生色；黑得像乌鸦的羽毛，那是生色。

李本：[The countenance] as blue as the feathers of a kingfisher [is a] favorable [sign], [the countenance] as red as the cockscomb [is a] favorable [sign], [the countenance] as yellow as the abdomen of a crab [is a] favorable [sign], [the countenance] as white as lard [is a] favorable [sign] and [the countenance] as black as the feathers of a crow [is a] favorable [sign].

威本：When the viscera are green like the kingfisher's wings they are full of life; when they are red like a cock's comb they are full of life; when they are yellow like the belly of a crab they are full of life; when they are white like the grease of pigs they are full of life; and when they are black like the wings of a crow they are full of life.

文本：[If the complexion appears] green-blue like the feathers of the kingfisher, [the person will] survive; red like a chicken comb, [the person will] survive;

yellow like the abdomen of a crab, [the person will] survive; white like the lard of pigs, [the person will] survive; black like the feathers of a crow, [the person will] survive.

吴本：When the quintessence of the five viscera reflected on the complexion appears to be green like a bird's green feather, the patient will live; when it appears to be red like a cockscomb, the patient will live; when it appears to be yellow like the belly of a crab, the patient will live; when it appears to be white like lard, the patient will live; when it appears to be black like the feather of a crow, the patient will live.

这段话运用了诸多动物隐喻，涉及翠鸟、鸡、蟹、豕、乌鸦等动物。以人们熟悉的动物来隐喻五色之见于面，有助于学习和把握面部望诊。

四个译本均使用排比句式，在结构上忠实于原文。李本使用 as... as... 句式，威本和吴本使用了 be... like... 句式，文本采用 appear... like... 句式，喻词的使用将原文的隐喻显化，帮助读者进行联想和理解。对于体现隐喻的颜色和动物词汇，四个译本均采用直译法，仅在词语的选择上稍有差异。

"青如翠羽者"，对于颜色词"青"，李本译为 blue，威本和吴本译为 green，文本译为 green-blue。相较而言，green-blue 和翠鸟羽毛的颜色更为接近，此处文本更恰当。"翠"，鸟名，其羽毛青色，俗称翠鸟。吴本译为 bird，指意太过宽泛，而李本、威本和文本均译为 kingfisher，指代更为具体。对于"羽"，李本、文本和吴本均译为 feather，而威本将羽毛误解为翅膀，误译为 wing。相比而言，对"青如翠羽者"的翻译，文本略胜一筹。

对于"赤如鸡冠者"，李本、威本和吴本的译法区别不大，均将"鸡冠"译为 cockscomb，而文本将其译为 chicken comb。因为公鸡鸡冠更为发达，此处 cockscomb 更为贴切。

对于"黄如蟹腹者"，四个译本的区别在于"蟹腹"的译法。李本和文本译为 abdomen of a crab，而威本和吴本则译为 belly of a crab。abdomen 和 belly 都可以指动物腹部，但 abdomen 多指昆虫的腹部，此处 belly 更符合英语表达习惯。但是在原文语境下"蟹腹"指蟹黄，即雌蟹腹内的卵块，其色鲜黄嫩泽，四个译本都仅直译出"腹"，有失准确，译不达意。

对于"白如豕膏者"，豕膏，指猪的脂肪，俗称板油，其色白而明润。

李本、文本、吴本均将其译为 lard，而威本译为 grease。grease 泛指动物油脂，lard 特指猪油，相比而言，lard 更为准确。

对于"黑如乌羽者"，乌羽，指乌鸦的羽毛，其色黑而光润。李本、文本、吴本均将"乌羽"直译为 feather of a crow，忠实于原文，而威本将羽毛误解为翅膀，误译为 the wings of a crow。

本句涉及的动物隐喻虽多，但较易理解，四个译本在形式和意思上都注重与原文的对等，除威本存在个别误译之外，其他三个译本在遣词造句上都各有千秋，较好地实现了语言转换、交际理解和文化传递的目标。

2. 夫精明五色者，气之华也……白欲如鹅羽，不欲如盐。（《素问·脉要精微论》）

释义：面部的五色，是精气的外在表现……白色应该像鹅的羽毛，白而光洁，不应像盐那样的白而杂暗。

李本：Jingming (Essence–Brightness) [of the eyes] and the five colors [reflect] the splendor of Qi...[the normal] white color is like the feather of goose and should not appear like salt.

威本：Therefore, it is desirable to understand the force of the five viscera... White wants to be like the feathers of a goose and not like the color of salt.

文本：Now, the essence brilliance and the five complexions, they are the ef-fulgence of the qi... A white [complexion] should resemble goose feathers; it should not resemble salt.

吴本：The five–colour of the complexion is the outer appearance of the vital energy... When it is white, it should like the goose feather with brightness, and does not like salt which is white with mixed dark dregs.

此句对面部五色进行描述，用鹅羽的颜色隐喻五色之白色，说明白而光洁，而非盐之暗白色。鹅是人们熟悉的一种家禽，其羽毛白而有光泽，同时以盐之白色作对比，使读者更易理解和把握面部白色。

对于动物隐喻"白欲如鹅羽"，四个译本主要采用直译法，译文大同小异。四个译本都将颜色词"白"译为 white，将"鹅羽"译为 feather of goose 或者 goose feather，并无实质差别。

句中"欲"可理解为"需要、应该"。李本未将其译出，文本和吴本都译为 should，将动物隐喻准确地呈现给目的语读者，便于读者理解面色白和鹅羽颜色的相似性。威本使用逐字直译的方法，把"欲"误译为 want，整句译文读来不知所云，无法理解。

吴本采用意译和直译相结合的方法，增译状语 when it is white，并补译后置定语 with brightness 来修饰鹅羽，将鹅羽光洁的特征更为明确地传递给读者，使读者能够更准确地把握色白的程度，文化传递效果在四个译本中为最佳。

四、自然灾害

1. 其眚四维，其主败折<u>虎狼</u>，清气乃用，生政乃辱。（《素问·五常政大论》）

释义：其灾害应与东南、西北、西南、东北，其所主败坏折伤，有如虎狼之势，清冷之气也发生作用，于是生气的功能便被抑制了。

李本：[...bringing on] calamities to the four directions. [Retaliating activity of Metal–Qi] mainly impairs [animals like] tiger and wolf. [Under such a condition,] Clear–Qi [takes the advantages to] spread [while] the generating and dominating [functions of Wood–Qi] is inhibited.

文本：...Disasters occur at the four ropes. This is responsible for ruin and destruction [caused by] tiger and wolf.

吴本：Its calamities are from the four corner (southeast, northwest, southwest and northeast), and its corruption and injury are like the ferocious damage of the wild beasts of tiger and wolf. As the cool and clear weather is prevailing, the functions of the energy of generation will be subdued.

"败折"，指破坏，"其主败折虎狼"意即土运不及之年，农作物的生长受到影响，给当时以农业生产为主的人类社会造成极大的破坏，如同虎狼伤人一样。"虎狼之势"形容极凶猛的声势，此处用于隐喻土衰木盛败坏折伤的强度之大。

此句需要结合上文理解，翻译难度较大。李本、文本和吴本均将虎狼直译为 tiger and wolf，但是由于译者对整句话的理解不同，三个译本出现较大的差异。

李本补译出 retaliating activity of Metal–Qi 作句子主语，将"虎狼"作为"败折"的宾语，将其理解为金气来报复伤害虎狼等兽类。而原文是用虎狼伤人的凶猛情况来隐喻农作物受到的破坏程度，译者未能准确领会原文隐喻的含义，曲解原文意思，造成误译。

文本将虎狼造成的破坏译为 ruin and destruction [caused by] tiger and wolf，但是在增译的结构 this is responsible for 中，主语 this 指代不明，并未体现出隐喻，不利于读者理解。

吴本采用意译法，准确解释整句话的含义，指出隐喻双方分别为 its corruption and injury 和 the ferocious damage of the wild beasts of tiger and wolf，便于读者对两者产生联想。译文在内容上忠实于原文，行文流畅，同时准确地传递出原文所蕴含的中医文化。

2. 土郁之发……洪水乃从，川流漫衍，田牧土<u>驹</u>。（《素问·六元正纪大论》）

释义：土郁发作的时候……洪水于是从而泛滥，巨川奔腾四溢。大水退后，土石嵬然，形如一群放牧的马。

李本：The burst [due to] stagnation of Earth... storm falling in high [mountains] and [deep] valleys, collapse and scatter of stones, mountain torrents, overflow of rivers and lands lying waste with stones over like cattle.

文本：The outbreak of oppressed soil... This is followed by flooding. The flow of the rivers inundates [the environment], spreading everywhere. The fields and pastures [are covered with] soil colts.

吴本：In the bursting out of the suppressed earth energy... the storm breaks out from the high mountain and the deep valley to impact the sands and stones to cause floods, and the water in the river rushes on in a torrent. After the retreat of the waters, the remaining earth and stones on ground appear like horses on the pasture.

本句描述雷雨大作，山洪暴发以后的自然景象。"田牧土驹"指田地被洪水淹没，水退之后，泥土堆积成小丘，远远望去就像田野牧马的景象。句中以散牧于田野中的马群隐喻洪水退去后土石嵬然屹立的状态。

李本对原句的结构做了调整，译文呈现名词短语并列的形式，行文结构工整。同时，增译出喻指对象田野上的土石（lands lying waste with stones over），将原文隐喻显化。不足之处在于"驹"的翻译，"驹"在古汉语中多指马，将"驹"译为 cattle 不够准确。另外，喻词 like 前后结构头重脚轻，句子稍欠美感。

文本采用直译法，将"田牧"译为 the fields and pastures，将"土驹"译为 soil colts，并补译出谓语 are covered with，直译出的语言不符合英语表达习惯，而且译文没有明示出喻指对象，对于目的语读者来说理解难度较大。

吴本采用意译法，结合上下语境对此句做了解释，准确地传达出原文意思，增译出主语 the remaining earth and stones on ground、谓语 appear 以及喻词 like，将"田牧土驹"译为 horses on the pasture。appear 形象生动地描绘出洪水退去土石显露的景象，译文表达清楚，可读性强，读者能够轻而易举地体会出其中的动物隐喻，更好地理解原文的逻辑，有利于中医文化的传递。

第四节　植物隐喻及英译

植物隐喻是人们基于长期的生活经验，在思维的不断加工下，将与植物相关的文化体验逐渐上升到语言层面后形成的一种思维方式。植物隐喻是人们生活智慧和文化心理的外化符号。它体现出丰富的文化内涵，既反映了人们的信仰和文化风俗，也反映了抽象的思维活动和思维方式。植物隐喻是将植物具有的典型特征（源域）应用到人类身上（目标域）所进行的跨域投射[1]。

植物隐喻来源于人们的日常生活，是人们的生活智慧和文化心理的外化符号。它体现出丰富的文化内涵，既反映了人们的信仰和文化风俗，也反映了抽象的思维活动和思维方式。植物既可以用来隐喻人类主体，也可以用来隐喻自然界的各种客观事物。因此，植物隐喻总是基于两个最基本的隐喻，即"植物是人"和"植物是物"。每个基本隐喻包含若干个概念隐喻，而每个概念隐喻都能派生出诸多语言性隐喻，这样就形成了庞大的隐喻体系。植物

---

[1] Fauconnier, G. *Mapping in Thought and Language*[M]. Cambridge: Cambridge University Press, 1997: 18–19.

的诸多特征不仅可以投射到人类身上，也可以映射到其他事物上，用来说明事物的形状、状态、时间、空间、抽象概念等。

《素问》中植物喻体的数量也相当可观，既可以是植物的生长状态，如蕃、嫩、荣、营、枯、槁、萎、华等，也可以是整个植物或植物的构成部分，如苗、根、茎、枝、叶、刺、花、花瓣等，或者植物的果实。中国古代医家常用植物充当中医术语隐喻的喻指对象，从而形象清楚地表述中医学的理论和概念。《素问》中的植物隐喻主要用来表现脉象、病理变化、外候、大小、尺寸、形状、颜色等。

一、脉象

1. 平肺脉来，厌厌聂聂，如落榆荚，曰肺平，秋以胃气为本。（《素问·平人气象论》）

释义：正常的肺脉来时，轻浮虚软，不疾不徐，如落榆荚一般和缓，这是肺的平脉，秋时以有胃气为本。

李本：The normal Lung-Pulse beats in a floating and light way, just like the drop of an elm leaf.

威本：When man is tranquil and healthy his pulse of the lungs comes calm and peaceful. And when it is peaceful like a village, or the seeds of an elm tree...

文本：The arrival of a normal lung [movement in the] vessels is [as follows]: faded, like the murmur (of trees) resembling the falling of elm seeds.

吴本：When the coming of the lung pulse with stomach-energy which is light, floating and soft like an elm leaf blowing in wind...

"厌厌聂聂，如落榆荚"，形容正常的肺脉来时轻虚而浮的形象，就像榆荚下落一样轻浮和缓。句中以"榆荚之落"隐喻平肺脉的脉象特点，生动形象，便于学习和把握。

"榆荚"又名榆钱儿，是榆树的种子并非叶子。对于"榆荚"的翻译，四个译本皆采用直译法。李本与吴本将其误译为 an elm leaf，威本与文本表达准确，分别将其译为 the seeds of an elm tree 与 elm seeds。

肺脉的特点通过榆荚下落时轻盈舒缓的姿态表达出来。李本使用 drop（下降、下跌）表达榆荚下落的动作，并通过 in a floating and light way 描述榆荚飘落时的轻盈，让读者领会到正常肺脉轻盈的特点，句子结构紧凑，语言流畅。

吴本用 light, floating and soft 再现榆荚飘落时轻、浮、缓等特点，生动贴切。用动词 blow（吹动、刮动）体现"榆荚之落"，有效实现语言转换。威本将其意译为 when it is peaceful like a village, or the seeds of an elm tree（像村庄或榆荚一样安静祥和），无法体现"落榆荚"的轻盈动态美，不能很好地传递原文信息，且整句译文增补内容过多，略显冗余。

文本采用直译加增补的方法，译为...faded, like the murmur (of trees) resembling the falling of elm seeds（消失了，榆荚的落下好像树的低语），信息传达不够准确。"肺脉来时"与"落榆荚"是一种动态过程，侧重视觉感受，译文用...the murmur (of trees) resembling the falling of elm seeds 将视觉转换成听觉，不易体现"落榆荚"轻浮和缓的姿态。

2. 平肝脉来，软弱招招，如揭长竿末梢……病肝脉来，盈实而滑，如循长竿……（《素问·平人气象论》）

释义：肝脉来时，像举着竿子，那杆子末梢显得长而软……如果脉来盈满滑实，像抚摸长竿一样……

李本：The normal Liver-Pulse is soft and long, just like the tip of a long stick... The morbid Liver-Pulse is forceful and slippery, just like the feeling of a long pole.

威本：When man is tranquil and healthy the pulse of his liver beats softly and weakly, as if one sounded a long thin bamboo rod without a tip... When man is sick the pulse of the liver moves fully, and it is large and long and slightly tense, felt on both light and heavy pressure; but it is also slippery like the sound of many long bamboo rods strung together...

文本：The arrival of a normal liver [movement in the] vessels is [as follows]: soft and weak and waving, as if one were raising the tip of a long bamboo cane... The arrival of a diseased liver [movement in the] vessels is [as follows]: abundant, replete, and smooth, as if [one's fingers] passed along a long bamboo cane...

吴本：When the coming of the liver pulse with stomach-energy is like holding a pole with a soft and long terminal... When the pulse is substantial and slippery like stroking a headgear clipper...

句中以"揭长竿末梢"和"循长竿"隐喻"平肝脉"和"病肝脉"的不同脉象特点。"软弱招招,如揭长竿末梢",形容正常的肝脉,如长竿末梢,柔软而长。"盈实而滑,如循长竿"形容肝的病脉充实硬满而滑利,犹如以手抚摩长竿。

对于两种不同肝脉的特点"如揭长竿末梢"与"如循长竿",四个译本皆采用直译法。李本分别译为 just like the tip of a long stick(犹如长杆末梢)和 just like the feeling of a long pole(犹如长杆的感觉),虽保留原文隐喻特色,但漏译动词"揭"与"循",一方面无法有效传达出平肝脉象犹如举着长竿时,竿子末端柔软且长的触觉感受,与病肝脉象犹如用手抚摸长竿时盈满滑实的特点。另一方面,脉象特点由动态变为静态,无法有效传递两种脉象特点。

威本为 as if one sounded a long thin bamboo rod without a tip(听起来犹如一根细长而无尖的竹竿)和 like the sound of many long bamboo rods strung to-gether(犹如很多长竹竿连在一起的声音),曲解原文,造成译文与原文表达的意思相去甚远,未能实现语言的正确转换,属于误译。

文本将两处隐喻分别译为 as if one were raising the tip of a long bamboo cane(像举起地长竹竿的末梢)和 as if [one's fingers] passed along a long bam-boo cane(像手抚摸长竹竿),让抽象、模糊的脉象特点变得生动、具体,易于理解,交际效果较好。

吴本直译为 holding a pole with a soft and long terminal(拿着一根末端长且软的竿子)和 [one's fingers] passed along a long bamboo cane(手指抚摸一根长竹竿)。译文句子结构简洁,保留原文隐喻特色,但未详细译出隐喻所表达的具体脉象特点,不利于读者准确理解和把握两种脉象的特点。

3. 病肾脉来,如引葛,按之益坚,曰肾病。(《素问·平人气象论》)

释义:如果脉来形如牵引葛藤,按之更坚,这是肾的病脉。

李本:The morbid Kidney-Pulse is like drawing a piece of rattan and felt hard under pressure. This is [the state of] the morbid pulse of the kidney.

威本:When man is ill the pulse of the kidneys flows like the sound that is made by touching the stretched fibres of beans and its strength is increased; —and then one can speak of sick kidneys.

文本：The arrival of a diseased kidney [movement in the] vessels is [as follows]: as if one pulled a creeper. When one presses it, it increases in firmness. That is called "the kidneys have a disease".

吴本：When the coming of the pulse is sunken and tight, like hauling a rattan vein, it is the diseased pulse of the kidney.

葛藤是一种茎蔓生、木质藤本植物。"引葛"形容脉象坚搏牵连，如牵引葛藤一样。句中以"引葛"隐喻"病肾脉"的脉象特点。

对于"引葛"，李本直译为 drawing a piece of rattan（牵引一根藤条），文本直译为 one pulled a creeper（拉一棵藤蔓植物），吴本直译为 hauling a rattan vein（拖拉一根藤脉）。三个译本均保留了植物隐喻，分别用 rattan、creeper、rattan vein 表达葛藤，较为笼统，"葛"在英语中多用 kudzu。三个译本通过 draw、pull 和 haul 指出牵引或拖拉藤蔓需要用力，从而说明脉位低沉，需用力才能摸到，差别不大。吴本通过补充 sunken and tight 说明病肾脉沉且紧的特点，就信息传递而言，吴本在三个译本中较为出色，易于读者理解、把握该脉象的特点。

威本将"引葛"译为 the sound that is made by touching the stretched fibres of beans（犹如触摸豆类延伸的须根发出的声音），将"葛"译为 the stretched fibres of beans（豆类延伸的须根），没有正确理解葛藤的隐喻含义。此外，威本将原文"引葛"表达出的牵连、脉沉的触觉转换成听觉曲解了原文含义，造成误译，不利于中医文化的传播。

4. 真心脉至，坚而搏，如循薏苡子累累然……（《素问·玉机真脏论》）

释义：心脏的真脏脉来的时候，坚而搏指，像循摩薏苡仁那样小而坚实……

李本：The appearance of Genuine-Heart-Pulse, marked by hardness and forcefulness, just as feeling coix seed...

威本：When the pulse of the heart ceases to beat firmly and becomes weary like the seeds of "Job's tears" (coixlachryma)...

文本：When a [movement of the] true [qi of the] heart arrives in the vessels, which beats and is firm and strong together, as if [one's fingers] passed along [a line of] seeds...

吴本：When the pulse indicating the exhaustion of the heart-energy is firm and hitting the fingers like touching the Job's-tears which are tiny and firm...

"薏苡子"，形如珠子而稍长，俗称为薏苡珠子。"如循薏苡子"，形容脉象短实而坚，如以手抚摸薏苡珠子一样。句中以抚摩薏苡子所带来的短实、坚硬连续不断的感觉隐喻心的真脏脉坚硬而搏指的脉象特点。

李本将"如循薏苡子"直译为 just as feeling coix seed，威本采用直译加注法译为 like the seeds of "Job's tears" (coixlachryma)，吴本直译为 like touching the Job's-tears。coix seed 与 the seeds of "Job's tears" 是对于薏苡子的两种不同称呼，实际指同一种事物。李本行文简洁，能够完整呈现原文的意思，便于读者理解。

威本以加注的方法给出薏苡仁的拉丁语名称，信息传递准确。但威本漏译"循"，不利于读者将该处植物隐喻与脉象产生关联。此外，句中"累累然"意为连续成串，并非劳累之意，威本误译为 weary，给读者造成理解障碍。

吴本译为 Job's-tears，通常不使用连词符，整体上欠准确。

文本译为 [a line of] seeds，译文较笼统，未译出"薏苡仁"及其特点，仅用一个模糊的词汇 seeds 来表达，未能表达出真脏脉如薏苡仁"坚硬而搏指"的脉象特点，译不达意，故无法有效实现交际目标。

5. 脉至如散叶，是肝气予虚也，木叶落而死。（《素问·大奇论》）

释义：脉来时像散叶一样，这是肝气虚极的脉象，大约到树木叶落的时候，就要死亡。

李本：[If] the pulse is like falling leaves, it indicates deficiency of Ganqi (Liver-Qi) [and the patient] will die when leaves of trees have fallen.

文本：When the [movement in the] vessels arrives like scattered leaves, [the patient] will die when the leaves of the trees fall.

吴本：When the coming of the pulse is like overgrowing thorns, it is the pulse condition of extreme asthenic of the liver energy, the patient will die at the time when the leaves are falling.

"散叶"指落叶。本句以"散落的树叶"隐喻浮泛无根、飘虚缓散的脉象。对于"脉至如散叶"，三个译本皆采用直译法，但选词各不相同。

李本将"散叶"译为 falling leaves，蕴含着一种动态、轻盈无力、浮泛无根的姿态。译文忠实于原文，语言表述准确。读者可以借助形象生动的描述理解该脉象的动态特点。

文本译为 scattered leaves（散落的叶子），是一种静态描述，枯叶散落在地上，体现不出浮泛的状态。枯叶在地的静态画面，不能有效地传达"肝气虚极"浮泛无力的脉象特点。

吴本译为 overgrowing thorns（过度生长或疯狂生长的荆棘），与原文意思相差较远，不能体现"散叶"时那种轻盈无力的状态，也与"肝气虚极"的脉象不符。故吴本既未实现语言的有效转换，也未实现交际理解和文化传递的目标。

二、病理变化

1. 化气不政，生气独治，云物飞动，草木不宁，甚而摇落……（《素问·气交变大论》）

释义：这是土气不能行其政令，木气独胜的现象，因此，风气就更猖獗起来，使天上的云物飞扬，地上的草木动摇不定，甚至枝叶摇落……

李本：[Since the Earth] fails to transform Qi and the generating Qi [of Wood] is predominant, clouds are flying, things are fluctuating, grasses and trees are unstable. [Under serious condition, grasses and trees] are broken...

文本：The policy of the qi of transformation is not enacted; the qi of generation governs alone. [As a result,] cloudy things fly by. Herbs and trees are kept in constant motion. In severe cases, they are shaken and fall down...

吴本：These are the phenomena when the earth energy fails to implement its decree and the wood energy is overabundant solely. So, the wind energy will be running wildly, causing the clouds flying in the sky, the grasses and woods on earth swaying, and the leaves and branches falling down...

句中的"化气"指土气，"生气"指木气。此处以"草木不宁，甚而摇落"隐喻"化气不政，生气独治"所导致的结果，生动形象地说明疾病的病理变化。

三个译本均采用直译法，保留"草木不宁"中的植物隐喻，但译文内容存在一定的差异。李本将"草木"译为 grasses and trees，泛指生长于大地的草和树，用词简单明了，具有代表性。"不宁"译为 unstable，为读者营造出草木在猖獗的大风中备受蹂躏、无法保持稳定姿态的画面感，生动形象，易于理解。

文本将"草木"译为 herbs and trees，由于 herbs 主要指香草、草药，导致将草的范围缩小。此外，"不宁"译为 in constant motion，虽然表达出草木处于不断运动的状态，但往往带有位置的变化，与实际不符，也无法表现草木因狂风摧残而被迫摇摆的姿态，故该译文不妥。

吴本将"草木"译为 the grasses and woods on earth，其中 woods 多指代树林、森林或木头，不如 trees 涵盖范围更全面。另外，将"不宁"译为 swaying，指缓慢地摇动，无法体现狂风肆虐时草木无法保持独立而被迫摇摆的姿态。

"甚而摇落"是草木摇摆不定的结果，风力强劲、程度严重时，会出现枝叶摇落的情况。李本与文本采用直译加增补的方法，分别补充 under serious condition 与 in severe cases 来说明情形的严重。李本译为 are broken（被折断、被损坏），符合原文意思。吴本译为 they are shaken and fall down，强调严重情形下草木被摇晃而倒落在地，与原文"草木动摇不定，甚至枝叶摇落"相比，程度上有所加重。吴本采用直译法，将其作为 cause 的结果状语之一，译为 the leaves and branches falling down，意思与原文一致，采用 falling 表达枝叶摇落时的状态，生动形象。

2. 振拉飘扬，则苍干散落，其眚四维……（《素问·五常政大论》）

释义：土衰木盛，所以暴风骤起，草木摇折，随之干枯散落，其灾害应与东南、西北、西南、东北。

李本：[If] the shaking, breaking and flying [Qi of Wood-Motion is severe], [it will lead to] dryness and desolation [due to retaliation of Metal-Qi, bringing on] calamities to the four directions.

文本：If there is shaking and pulling, whirling and surging, then aging and drying, dispersion and falling to the ground [appear in revenge]. Disasters occur at the four ropes.

吴本：As the earth energy is deficient, and the wood energy is prosperous, the gale will blow all of a sudden, the grasses and woods will be swaying and broken to become withered and falling. Its calamities are from the four corner (southeast, north-west, southwest and northeast).

"苍干散落"意为"草木摇折，干枯散落"。句中以此隐喻"土衰木盛"导致的结果。

"苍干散落"，暗含着主体"草木"，在翻译时应当译出其中的植物隐喻，以便于读者理解。李本将其直译为 dryness and desolation，传达出"干燥"和"荒芜"的信息，与原文"草木摇折，随之干枯散落"的意思存在差距。而且"苍干散落"的主体"草木"未能译出，令读者难以与草木摇折、干枯散落的场景建立联系。

文本采用直译法，将"苍干散落"译为 aging and drying, dispersion and falling to the ground，意思为"苍老""干燥""散布"和"落地"，由于未能准确领会原文隐喻的含义，译文较生硬。此外，文本也未能将"草木"译出，进一步给读者带来阅读障碍。

吴本意译为 the grasses and woods will be swaying and broken to become withered and falling，将"苍干散落"的主体"草木"译出，能够让读者知晓植物隐喻的主体。草木由于摇摆、折断导致枯萎、掉落，从而明确"土衰木盛"导致"苍干散落"的因果关系，能够有效地传递信息。

三、外候

1. 五脏之气，故色见青如草兹者死，黄如枳实者死……（《素问·五脏生成》）

释义：五脏荣于面上的气色，表现出的青黑色像死草一样，那是死征；表现出黄色像枳实一样，那是死征……

李本：The countenance as blue as dead grass [is a] fatal [sign], [the counte-nance] as yellow as the seed of the trifoliate orange [is a] fatal [sign]...

威本：When their color is green like grass they are without life; when their color is yellow like that of oranges they are without life...

文本：{The qi of the five depots}. Hence, if the complexion appears green-blue like young grasses, death [is imminent]; yellow like hovenia-fruit, death [is imminent]...

吴本：When the quintessence of the five viscera reflected on the complexion appears to be green and black like the dead grass in dark, the patient will die; when it appears to be yellow like the fruit of unriped citron, the patient will die...

本句运用"草兹"和"枳实"等隐喻五脏之气外现于面的五色，为面部望诊提供重要参考依据。

四个译本均通过使用喻词将原文中的隐喻显化，便于读者进行联想和理解。李本使用 as...as... 句式，威本使用 be...like... 句式，文本采用 appear...like... 句式，吴本使用 appear to be 将句中隐喻体现出来。此外，四个译本均直译句中体现隐喻的颜色和植物，但由于理解不同，各译本之间存在一定差异。

对于"青如草兹"的翻译，其中颜色词"青"，李本译为 blue，威本译为 green，文本译为 green–blue，吴本译为 green and black。"青"用来形容枯死的青草的颜色，青中带有枯黑，故文本、吴本与枯草的颜色较为接近。"草兹"指枯死的青草，四个译本稍有差异。李本译为 dead grass，与原文保持一致，威本译为 grass 不准确，文本将"草兹"误解为小草，故误译为 young grasses，吴本译为 the dead grass in dark（黑暗中的枯草），不易理解。比较而言，对"青如草兹"的翻译，李本较接近原文。

对于"黄如枳实"，四个译本的区别在于"枳实"的译法。"枳实"是芸香科植物酸橙或甜橙的干燥幼果，其色黑黄不泽。李本译为 the seed of the trifoliate orange，将"枳实"误解为枳的种子，因此出现误译。威本译为 yellow like that of oranges，过于宽泛、笼统，译不达意。文本译为 hovenia–fruit，意为枳椇，又名拐枣、金果梨，与枳实为完全不同的事物。吴本译为 the fruit of unriped citron，与"枳实"较为接近，由于"枳实"为干燥的果实，若再添加 dried 则更为准确。另外，unriped 为拼写错误，正确形式应该为 unripe。

2. 生于脾，如以缟裹栝楼实。（《素问·五脏生成》）

释义：脾脏有生气的色泽，就像白绢裹着瓜蒌实一样。

李本：[if] the spleen [is full of] vitality, [the countenance looks] like thin white silk wrapped with the seeds of Chinese trichosanthes.

威本：The color of life displayed by the stomach is like the juniper berry colored lining of a white silk robe.

文本：If [the complexion] is generated by the spleen, it resembles a gua–lou fruit wrapped up in white silk.

吴本：The colour of vitality of spleen is like trichosanthes seed (reddish-yellow) wrapped in white thin silk.

"栝楼实"为多年生葫芦科植物栝蒌的果实，色正黄，可入药。句中运用植物"栝蒌"隐喻五脏之气外现的颜色，这对于面部望诊具有重要意义。

对于植物隐喻"如以缟裹栝楼实"，四个译本采用的翻译方法不尽相同，且在语言转化和文化传递方面存在较大差异。"缟"指白绢，是一种白色的薄型丝织品，李本为 thin white silk，文本为 white silk，吴本为 white thin silk，三个译本大同小异，无实质差别。威本为 a white silk robe（白色丝绸长袍），增加 robe 属于赘余。

对于"栝楼实"的翻译，四个译本各不相同。李本与吴本分别译为 the seeds of Chinese trichosanthes 和 trichosanthes seed (reddish-yellow)，由于理解偏差，两个译本都将"栝楼实"误解为栝楼的种子，因此均出现误译。吴本加注的内容，表明了栝楼实的颜色，就交际而言，起到了辅助理解的作用。威本直译为 juniper berry（杜松子），与"栝楼实"实质上为两种不同的事物，未能实现语言的有效转换。文本采用音译和意译结合法，译为 gua-lou fruit，有益于中华文化的输出。就信息传递的准确性而言，文本略胜一筹。

四、大小

1. 刺手太阴阳明，出血如大豆，立已。（《素问·刺热》）

释义：治法当刺手太阴和手阳明两经，刺出豆大的血滴病就好了。

李本：[It can be treated by] needling Hand-Taiyin and Hand-Yangming. [It is usually] cured immediately after letting out a drop of blood as large as a grain of soybean.

威本：(Then) one should apply acupuncture to the hands at the region of the great Yin and the "sunlight", and the blood will gush forth as though a large vessel had been placed there.

文本：Pierce the hand major yin and [hand] yang brilliance [conduits]. [Let] blood in the size of a large bean come out. [The disease] comes to an end immediately.

吴本：In treating, it should prick the Hand Taiyin and Hand Yangming channels. The disease will be cured when blood drops of pea size occur after pricking.

句中以"大豆"隐喻针刺"手太阴"和"手阳明"两经时血滴的大小，对针刺放血量的要求贴近日常生活而且易于操作，只需刺出"大豆大小的血滴"即可。

李本将"出血如大豆"直译为 letting out a drop of blood as large as a grain of soybean，保留植物隐喻，既译出了滴血量的大小，又运用 as...as... 结构将植物隐喻进行明示，生动形象，便于读者理解。

威本将"出血如大豆"意译为 the blood will gush forth as though a large vessel had been placed there，其中 gush forth 意为"涌出"，说明出血速度快，出血量大，这与原文刺出如豆大的血滴相差很大，曲解了原文，造成误译。此外，译文没有保留植物隐喻，且采用意译 as though a large vessel had been placed there，整句读来令人不知所云，无法理解。

文本将句中隐喻直译为 [Let] blood in the size of a large bean out，保留植物隐喻，通过使用 in the size of 将出血量的大小准确地传递给读者，便于读者理解大豆与出血量之间的相似性。

吴本将植物隐喻直译为 blood drops of pea size occur，将说明出血量大小的隐喻"大豆"误译为 pea（豌豆），没有准确传递原文信息。

总体而言，李本与文本在形式和内容上都注重与原文的对等，较好地实现了语言转换、交际理解和文化传递的目标。

2. 以四乌鲗骨一藘茹二物并合之，丸以雀卵，大如<u>小豆</u>。（《素问·腹中论》）

释义：用四分乌鲗骨，一分藘茹，两种药合并，用雀卵和为丸，制成如小豆大小的丸药。

李本：Cuttlefish bone and Lüru (also known as Qiancao, Herba Rubiae, Indian madder), with the ratio of 4：1, are mixed up with bird eggs and made into pills as large as a red bean.

文本：Take four black cuttlefish bones and one [measure/root of] madder, combine these two items and form pills in the size of small beans using sparrow eggs.

吴本：Combine four portions of cuttle-bone and one portion of rubia root and prepare them with the bird's egg to form pills in the size of a red bean.

小豆，指赤小豆，色红形长圆。此句以"小豆"隐喻丸药的大小。

对于"大如小豆"的翻译，李本为 as large as a red bean，文本为 in the size of small beans，吴本为 in the size of a red bean。三个译本均采用直译法，但在选词和句式上略有不同。

李本使用 as large as，文本与吴本使用 in the size of（大小为），将植物隐喻进行明示，都便于读者理解该处隐喻用来说明药丸的大小，区别不大。

李本与吴本将"小豆"直译为 a red bean（红豆）。就文化对等而言，red bean 在西方文化中是集合名词，泛指带有红色外衣的豆类，其中包括颗粒较大的 red kidney bean（红芸豆，大红豆）以及 Honduran red beans（洪都拉斯红豆）等。原文中所说的"小豆"指赤小豆，别名米豆、饭豆，在英语中通常用 red rice bean 来指代。由于文化差异，李本与吴本会令目的语读者感到困惑。

文本译为 small beans，由于未能正确理解原文，译文比较笼统，没有实现隐喻的有效转换，不利于跨文化交际。

3. 刺解脉，在郄中结络如黍米，刺之血射以黑，见赤血而已。（《素问·刺腰痛》）

释义：治疗时，应刺解脉。解脉在郄中部分，取络脉结如黍米大即是。刺的时候有黑血射出，等到血色变赤为止。

李本：[It can be treated by] needling the stagnant point, like a grain of the broomcorn millet, in Xizhong (Weizhong, BL 40) on the Collateral of Jiemai...

文本：Pierce the separator vessel where there is, in the cleft, a knotted network [vessel] resembling a millet grain...

吴本：When treating, prick the Untied Channel... The knot of the Untied Channel is on the juncture of collaterals in a size of a glutinous millet.

"黍"是一年生草本植物，其子实熟后有黏性，是中国古代的主要粮食及酿造作物，列为五谷之一。句中以"黍米"隐喻郄中结络的大小。

李本将"黍米"直译为 a grain of the broomcorn millet，以介词 like 引出，在句中做状语，说明郄中结络的大小，与原文内容一致，便于读者进行想象和理解。

文本将"黍米"译为 a millet grain（小米粒），由于理解偏差，译文中的事物与原文不对等。millet 指"小米、稷、黍类"等，虽然在外观上与"黍米"一样都呈鲜黄色，颗粒状，但 millet 的颗粒比"黍米"要小。此外，文本使用 resembling 表达结络似"黍米"，往往侧重于各个方面的相似性，而原文主要以"黍米"隐喻大小，故该词欠妥当。

吴本将"黍米"意译为 a glutinous millet，准确翻译出"黍米"的本质特征，即与小米相比，"黍米"除颗粒略大外，还带有黏性。此外，吴本使用 in a size of 可以体现出在大小方面的隐喻，便于读者准确理解和把握"郄中结络"的大小。

五、尺寸

刺手中指次指爪甲上，去端如韭叶各一痏。（《素问·缪刺论》）

释义：应当刺手中指旁次指上，距离爪甲约韭菜叶那样宽处的关冲穴，左右各刺一次。

李本：[It can be treated by] needling [the region] above the nail of the fourth finger, [the distance about the width of] one leaf of Chinese chive to the angle of the nail once respectively.

文本：Pierce the finger next to the middle finger above the nail, generating one wound each [the width of] one leek leaf away from the [finger] tip.

吴本：When treating prick the Guanchong point (SJ. 1) which is in the distance of the Chinese chive leaves beside the nail on the tip of the finger next to the small finger, prick once each on the left and right side.

此句介绍针刺时的取穴位置，以"韭叶"隐喻针刺穴位与爪甲之间的宽度。

对于植物隐喻"如韭叶"的翻译，李本与文本采用直译加注法，分别译为 [the distance about the width of] one leaf of Chinese chive 和 [the width of] one leek leaf。通过增补内容说明"韭叶"代表针刺穴位与爪甲之间的距离，便于读者理解。

李本将"韭叶"译为 one leaf of Chinese chive，其中 Chinese chive 指"韭菜"在英语中已被广泛接受。文本将"韭叶"译为 one leek leaf，实际上，

leek 指韭葱，与中国文化中的"韭菜"差异较大。韭葱的叶子与大蒜的叶子相似，叶宽条形，略对褶，背面呈龙骨状。与韭葱相比，韭菜叶较窄较细，叶片扁平呈带状。就此处以"韭叶"隐喻尺寸而言，李本表达准确，在实现隐喻语言转换的同时，有利于输出中华文化。

吴本采用意译法，将"如韭叶"译为 in the distance of the Chinese chive leaves。与李本相同，吴本也将"韭菜"译为 Chinese chive，便于目的语读者根据韭菜叶的宽度进行联想，进而准确把握针刺穴位与爪甲之间的宽度。但吴本使用 in the distance of 表示距离，语言不够规范。

六、形状

太虚深玄，气犹麻散，微见而隐，色黑微黄，怫之先兆也。（《素问·六元正纪大论》）

释义：水郁发作的时令，是在军火与相火当令的前后，而天色高远，微黄色黑，其气如散麻一样，稍微看到而又隐约不清，则是郁积将发的先兆。

李本：[During this period of time,] the sky looks profound and dark, Qi appears like scattered hemp, slightly visible but unclear, dark and slightly yellow. [These are] the indications of impending burst.

文本：When the Great Void is deep dark, when the [cloud] qi resembles powdered hemp, which is hardly visible, and when its color is black and slightly yellow, these are the first signs of harrassed [water qi ready to break out].

吴本：When the sky is high and far with yellowish-dark energy like disorderly fibre which can be dimly seen, they are the omens of the bursting of the suppressed water energy.

"麻"本质上是"一种植物纤维"。"麻散"，指散乱如麻。句中以"麻散"隐喻天空中云气的隐约不清。

对于"气犹麻散"的翻译，李本直译为 like scattered hemp（散乱的麻），使用喻词 like 将隐喻显化。scattered 可以传递给读者一种散乱、无序的状态。hemp 既可以指草本植物麻，也可以指该植物的茎皮纤维，根据语境此处指后者。李本译为 scattered hemp，忠实于原文，完成了语言和文化有效的转换。

文本将"散麻"译为 powdered hemp（粉末状的麻），是对原文的误读，造成误译，给读者造成理解障碍。

吴本将植物隐喻意译为 disorderly fibre，通过 disorderly 将无序凌乱的状态表达出来，fibre 通常指纤维，将"散麻"凌乱无序，若隐若现的特征直接、明确地传递给读者，便于读者更准确地把握云气隐约不清的状态，信息传递效果较好。

七、颜色

先视身之赤如小豆者尽取之。（《素问·刺疟》）

释义：若先见皮肤上发出赤小豆般的红点，应该都用针刺去。

李本：[If] hemorrhagic spots like red beans on the body [of the patients] are found before [needling], they must be pricked with needles to let out blood.

文本：In cases where an initial observation shows that the body is red like small beans, take the [blood] entirely.

吴本：When there is some red points like adzuk beans appear on the skin, it should be prickd to cause them vanish.

本句中的"赤如小豆"是以赤小豆的颜色隐喻患者身上出血点的颜色。

对于句中的植物隐喻"赤如小豆"，李本直译为 like red beans，通过喻词 like 将隐喻显化。李本将"小豆"译为 red beans（红豆），在英语中对应为多种表皮为红色的豆类。就文化对等而言，译文与原文不对等。但就此处通过植物隐喻来说明患者身上出血点的颜色而言，虽然英语中有多种 red beans，但其产生的颜色关联与原文大体一致，在一定程度上有助于读者的想象和理解。

文本直译为 red like small beans，将"小豆"字对字翻译为 small beans，仅侧重豆子的大小，不能体现豆子的颜色，不利于读者想象，因此传递的信息不准确。

吴本采用意译法，将句中植物隐喻译为 like adzuk beans appear on the skin。将"小豆"直译为 adzuk beans（红豆、赤豆），正确拼写应为 adzuki beans。此处"小豆"指赤小豆，与赤豆虽外观相似，但仍有区别。赤豆外观为短圆柱形，呈暗棕红色，有光泽，而赤小豆外观为长圆形而稍扁，表面颜色为紫红色，通常无光泽或微有光泽。此处植物隐喻旨在说明出血点的颜色。

吴本将"小豆"误译为 adzuk beans（赤豆），但由于两者颜色较为接近，便于读者进行颜色的联想。吴本增加 appear on the skin，有助于读者将此处隐喻理解为皮肤上出现的赤小豆般的红点。

小　结

本章介绍《素问》中有关自然、容器、动物、植物等本体隐喻的用法，并对四个译本进行对比分析。由于文化背景和学术背景有所不同，译者在译法选择、内容侧重点和语言运用等方面风格各异，译本呈现出不同的特色。

在《素问》中，自然隐喻主要涉及天地、日月、海、土、风、水、火和溪谷等方面。李本对中医思维和哲学思想的把握程度较高，对原文的解读比较准确，根据语言、交际、文化目标实现的具体需要采用直译、意译或音译加注等不同方法，译文的内容和形式基本做到忠实于原文。其中，音译加注法使用频率较高，也比较有特色。例如，将"邪风"译作 Xiefeng (Evil-wind)，保留中医术语和源语特色，有利于中医文化的对外输出。吴本对自然隐喻的理解比较到位，更侧重交际目标的实现，译文中多采用意译法，并常常根据需要进行补译和增译；缺点是行文时常略显繁琐，句式复杂，无法呈现原文语言简洁的特点。文本和威本较为类似，更重视对原文语言的还原程度，因此多使用直译的方法。例如，二者均将"川"译作 streams，将"天地"译作 heaven and earth（Heaven and Earth）等，最大限度地实现语言转换，还原隐喻对象的特征。缺点是译文过于简单直白，有时出现释义不明、译不达意等现象。

容器隐喻主要表现在身体、脏腑、腠理、孔窍、腧穴等人体门户上。对于容器隐喻，李本以直译为主，配合意译和音译加注的方法，译文语言准确，同时凸显文化特色。威本和文本主要采用直译法保持语言的原汁原味，但是由于文化差异，有时对中医文化和容器隐喻的理解不到位，译文出现了误译或译不达意的情况。吴本主要采用意译法，使用通俗的语言解释医理，可读性较强，但是过多的解释和改写导致行文略显冗长繁琐，失去原文语言的凝练之美。

　　动物隐喻主要用来表现脉象、病理变化、外候等。动物隐喻例句中大多出现了喻词"如"，喻指对象较为明显。李本、威本和文本多采用直译法，吴本多采用意译法，表述虽稍有区别，但都能较准确地传递原文信息，并保留其文化内涵。对于没有出现喻词的动物隐喻，李本通常采用意译和直译结合的方法，内容上基本忠实于原文，用词直白，表达相对准确。威本、文本常使用逐字直译的方法，虽在用词上颇为讲究，但译文有时不符合中医医理和逻辑，易造成误解。吴本通常会明示句中的喻指对象，便于读者体会喻指对象和动物特征的相似性，取得较好的效果。

　　植物隐喻大致分为两类：关于植物的生长状态和关于整个植物或植物的构成部分。对于植物隐喻的翻译，从总体翻译方法和翻译效果而言，李本与文本以直译法为主，根据不同的译文内容适当进行增补，目的是为更好地传播中医文化。相比而言，李本在语言结构与文体上基本与原文保持一致，译文贴切，语言表达流畅，但也存在少量误译。文本在语言结构上与原文相似，但存在逐字翻译的现象，译文稍显呆板，而且多处存在语言错误。威本较多地采用意译、直译加增补的方法，目的是为增强译文的可读性和读者的接受度，但有时译文略显拖沓，而且对源语文化的保留较少。吴本以读者为导向，增补内容较多，但表达有些通俗化，不注重语言表达的规范性，而且词汇、句法方面的错误较多，容易给读者造成理解困难。

　　综上所述，李本对原文中本体隐喻的理解相对更为全面和深入，多采用直译、直译与意译相结合、音译加注等译法，较为准确地传递本体隐喻的内容；译文侧重文化转换目标的实现和读者的接受性；形式和文体风格与原文较为一致，语言准确流畅、通俗易懂，句式简洁精练。在四个译本中，李本在译法选择、文化目标及交际目标的实现、原文语言风格传递等方面都略胜一筹。

第六章　结构隐喻及英译

　　结构隐喻指以一种结构清晰的概念来建构另一种结构模糊的概念，使两种概念相互叠加，从而能够将谈论某一概念各方面特征的词语用于谈论另一个概念。一般而言，源域中已知的、具体的或较为熟悉的概念被用于类比目标域中未知的、抽象的或相对陌生的概念。结构隐喻中两个概念的认知域有所不同，但其结构能够保持一致，即它们各自的构成成分之间存在着一种规律性的对应关系。源域为目标域进行框架构建提供了必要的基础，这些框架能够决定人们思考和讨论目标域时所指代的实体和活动，进而制约人们的行为或开展活动的方式。

　　《素问》中存在大量的结构隐喻。它以阴阳学说、精气学说、藏象学说作为理论基础，并以这些学说蕴含的隐喻思维去发掘、整理和提高以前的医疗经验和医学知识，为中医学的形成和不断发展做出了巨大贡献。其中阴阳学说、精气学说、藏象学说等都表现出明显的结构隐喻的特点，说明古代医家已经能够非常娴熟地运用隐喻理论来建构和诠释中医学基础理论。此外，治疗疾病犹如战争的隐喻思维在该书的战争隐喻中得到具体体现。

第一节　阴阳相关隐喻及英译

　　阴阳思想萌芽于殷周之际，是《黄帝内经》的理论根基，也是中医学形成和发展的理论基础之一。最初，阴阳概念的建立是基于古人对自然和地理现象的认知。后来，古人基于阴阳属性与向阳、背阳事物之间的相似性，运用隐喻的思维方式不断泛化阴阳概念。以阴阳作为隐喻对象的事物是对阴阳意义范畴的投射。古代医家将阴阳的相对属性推广到医学领域，探索和说明生命的起源、人体的生理功能和病理变化，指导疾病的诊断、质量与预防，对中医学理论体系的逐渐形成与不断发展，产生了非常重要的影响[1]。

阴阳学说认为，宇宙空间中任何具有相互关联而又相互对立关系的事物或现象，或同一事物内部相互对立的两个方面，都可以通过阴阳来概括和分析其各自的属性。阴阳关系主要通过隐喻的认知方式建构而成，具体表现在阴阳对立制约、阴阳互根互用、阴阳消长平衡和阴阳转化等几个方面。阴阳学说在中医学中的应用十分广泛，《素问》中不但将阴阳分类的方法用于概括天地、人体脏腑内外，而且用来探索人体生命的本源，阐释人体的组织结构、生理功能及病理变化，指导疾病的诊断和治疗。

一、阴阳隐喻

阴阳最初指太阳的向背。后来，古人以隐喻的方式认识到，世间万物与自然界昼夜的光线明暗转换关系之间存在着巨大的相似性，于是将与朝向太阳的事物有相似性的范畴归为阳，将与背对太阳的事物有相似性的范畴归为阴。这样，阴阳概念被用于说明宇宙中具有对立统一关系的事物或现象，或同一事物内部的两个方面。在《素问》中，阴阳被用于隐喻天地、日月、四时、自然规律和脉象等。

（一）天地

1. 余闻天为阳，地为阴。（《素问·阴阳离合论》）

释义：我听说天是属阳的，地是属阴的。

李本：I have heard that the heavens pertain to Yang while the earth to Yin.

威本：It is said that Heaven was created by Yang (the male principle of light and life), and that the Earth was created by Yin (the female principle of darkness and death).

文本：I have heard: heaven is yang, the earth is yin.

吴本：I was told that the heaven is Yang and the earth is Yin.

[1] 兰凤利. 中医古典文献中"阴阳"的源流与翻译 [J]. 中国翻译，2007（4）：69.

古人认为，天在上，天气轻清、上浮为阳；地在下，地气重浊、下沉为阴，根据两者的相似性进行类比推理，使其抽象化，故以阴阳隐喻天地。

对于句中"阴阳"隐喻的翻译，李本、文本、吴本均采用音译法，译为 Yin 和 Yang，但在原文信息传递方面各有不同。李本通过使用动词词组pertain to（属于）向读者传递出"阴""阳"分别为地和天的属性，在一定程度上增加了交际的有效性。文本与吴本仅使用音译，对读者而言难以产生译文与原文在意义上的推理和关联，不利于有效交际。

威本采用音译加注法，通过补充 the male principle of light and life 与 the female principle of darkness and death 具体说明天地的属性特点，有效地表达出阴阳在句中的隐喻含义，这不仅可以有效传播中医文化，而且可以加强目的语读者对原文的理解，提高接受度。

2. 寒暑燥湿风火，天之阴阳也……木火土金水火，地之阴阳也……（《素问·天元纪大论》）

释义：寒、暑、燥、湿、风、火是天的阴阳……木、火、土、金、水、火是地的阴阳……

李本：Cold, Summer-Heat, Dryness, Dampness, Wind and Fire represent Yin and Yang of the heavens... Wood, Fire, Earth, Metal and Water stand for Yin and Yang of the earth...

文本：Cold, summerheat, dryness, dampness, wind, and fire, these are the yin and yang of heaven... Wood, fire, soil, metal, water, these are the yin and yang of the earth...

吴本：The cold, heat, dryness, wetness, wind and fire are the Yin and Yang of heaven... When the Yin and Yang of heaven and that of earth combine...

句中指出，天气的阴阳变化表现为寒、暑、燥、湿、风、火等形式，地气的阴阳具体表现为木、火、土、金、水、火等形式。由此可见，阴阳不仅用于隐喻天地，还用于隐喻天气和地气的各种阴阳变化。

三个译本均采用音译法，将"阴阳"译为 (the) Yin and Yang of (the) heaven。其中李本选用动词 represent 更好地体现出"寒、暑、燥、湿、风、火"所代表的天之阴阳属性。对于"木、火、土、金、水、火"用 stand for 引出，明确体现了地之阴阳的隐喻关系，有利于读者正确理解阴阳在不同语境中的具体含义。

文本和吴本分别使用 these are... 和 are... 来说明"寒、暑、燥、湿、风、火"与"木、火、土、金、水、火"是天气、地气的不同表现形式，但未能译出"阴阳"在句中的隐喻关系。

3. 天有阴阳，地亦有阴阳。（《素问·天元纪大论》）

释义：天有阴阳，地也有阴阳。

李本：[There are] Yin and Yang in both the heavens and the earth.

文本：Heaven has yin and yang; the earth has yin and yang, too.

吴本：There are Yin and Yang in the six kinds of weather in heaven, and there are Yin and Yang in the five elements of earth.

此句意在说明，以天地而论，则天阳而地阴，而天地之中，又各有阴阳。这是阴阳可分的具体体现，用来说明天地自身的不同方面。

对于句中隐喻，三个译本均采用音译法，保留了中医学特有的概念"阴阳"。通过李本与文本的语境可以感知"阴阳"是处于同一事物内部的两个方面，但对目的语读者而言通过音译找不到理解"阴阳"的线索，不能有效理解该词，故达不到相应的认知和理解。

吴本采用音译并适当增补 in the six kinds of weather 与 in the five elements，给目的语读者提供了一定的信息线索，便于读者进一步理解译文所要传达的信息。读者通过语境可以感知"阴阳"在不同范畴内所代指的相关事物有所不同，其含义相对具体化。

（二）日月

日为阳，月为阴。（《素问·阴阳离合论》）

释义：日是属阳的，月是属阴的。

李本：The sun belongs to Yang while the moon to Yin.

威本：The sun represents Yang and the moon represents Yin.

文本：The sun is yang; the moon is yin.

吴本：The sun is Yang and the moon is Yin.

日出则天亮，日光普照大地，温煦世间万物，也给人类带来光明与温暖；月出则天黑，月光朦胧晦暗，让人产生寒凉、孤寂的感觉。基于对"日月"这些特征的认知，古人将"日月"与"阴阳属性"关联起来，用"阴阳"隐喻"日月"。

四个译本均采用音译法，保留中医文化负载词"阴阳"。但在"阴阳"隐喻日月属性方面，各译本存在一定差异。李本借助动词词组 belongs to（属于）清晰地体现出日月的不同属性，便于读者准确把握日月不同的属性特点。威本使用 represent（代表、象征）在一定程度上传达出"阴阳"的隐喻含义。文本与吴本在采用音译的同时忽略了原文"阴阳"的隐喻含义，不利于信息的有效传递。

总体而言，四个译本均保留了源语的文化特色，但在语言的有效转换、隐喻关系的表达方面，李本比威本略胜一筹。

（三）四时

天以阳生阴长，地以阳杀阴藏。（《素问·天元纪大论》）

释义：天是以阳生阴长的，地是以阳杀阴藏的。

李本：[In] the heavens, Yang [manages] germination and Yin governs growth; [on] the earth, Yang [manages] killing and Yin [controls] storage.

文本：Heaven employs yang [qi] to generate, yin [qi] to stimulate growth. Earth employs yang [qi] to kill, yin [qi] to store.

吴本：In heaven, the Yang generates and the Yin promotes growing, on earth, the Yang restrains and the Yin stores.

春夏为天之阴阳，主生主长。秋冬为地之阴阳，主杀主藏。春夏温暖，万物勃发，秋冬寒冷，万物萧瑟，这与日月给人带来的感觉相似。古人对四季特征的认知使得阴阳获得新意，阴阳被用来隐喻一年之中的春夏秋冬。

李本与吴本采用音译法，同时保留了中医文化特色和句中的隐喻含义。李本增加表示"管理、控制"意义的动词 manages、governs 以及 controls 表明主谓关系，句子表达完整。吴本使用及物动词 generates（产生）、restrains（控制）以及 stores（贮藏）表明主谓关系，但因缺乏宾语，导致句意表达不够完整，达不到有效交流的目的。

文本采用音译加注法，增加 qi 来表明"阴阳"为"阴气"和"阳气"。实际上，句中"阴阳"被用来隐喻四季而非"阴气"和"阳气"，故译文欠妥当，未能实现有效交际。

（四）自然规律

1.上古之人，其知道者，法于阴阳，和于术数。（《素问·上古天真论》）

释义：上古时代的人，他们大都懂得养生的道理，效法天地变化的规律，知道调养精气的方法。

李本：The sages in ancient times who knew the Dao (the tenets for cultivating health) followed [the rules of] Yin and Yang and adjusted Shushu(the ways to cultivate health).

威本：In ancient times those people who understood Tao [the way of self cultivation] patterned themselves upon the Yin and the Yang [the two principles in nature] and they lived in harmony with the arts of divination.

文本：The people of high antiquity, those who knew the Way, they modeled [their behavior] on yin and yang and they complied with the arts and the calculations.

吴本：Those who knew the way of keeping a good health in ancient times always kept in their behavior in daily life in accordance with the nature. They followed the principle of Yin and Yang and kept in conformity with the art of prophecy based on the interaction of Yin and Yang. They were able to modulate their daily life in harmony with the way of recuperating the essence and vital energy.

上古时期，懂得养生之道的人，深谙天地阴阳和自然变化的规律，并努力去加以适应。句中以"阴阳"隐喻"天地自然变化的规律"。

李本与威本均采用音译加注法翻译句中"阴阳"。李本译为 [the rules of] Yin and Yang，保留源语隐喻，译文简洁，通过增补译文 [the rules of]（……的规律），便于读者产生语义关联。威本译为 the Yin and the Yang [the two principles in nature]，通过增补"两个自然法则"向读者传递出"阴阳"隐喻为自然变化规律的具体含义。

文本采用音译法，未能传递出"阴阳"在语境中的具体含义，对目的语读者而言接受度不高。

吴本则采用音译与意译结合法，将"阴阳"译为 the principle of Yin and Yang，表达出"天地自然变化的规律"之隐喻义。此外，吴本尽可能多地提供语境信息帮助读者理解，导致译文冗长，失去原文的凝练之美。

2. 上古有真人者，提挈天地，把握阴阳，呼吸精气。（《素问·上古天真论》）

释义：上古时代有一种人叫作真人，他能把握住自然的变化，掌握阴阳消长的规律，吐故纳新以养精气。

李本：There were so-called Zhenren (immortal beings) in ancient times [who could] grasp the law of nature. They followed the principles of Yin and Yang, inhaling fresh air.

威本：In ancient times there were so-called Spiritual Men（真人）；they mastered the Universe and controlled Yin and Yang [the two principles in nature]. They breathed the essence of life.

文本：In high antiquity there were true men. They upheld [the patterns of] heaven and earth and they grasped [the regularity of] yin and yang. They exhaled and inhaled essence qi.

吴本：In ancient times, some people who were very good at preserving their health, reaching the level of being a "perfect man". All their behaviours adapted to the change of nature quite at ease, they could master the law of the wax and wane of Ying and Yang. They respired the refined energy.

上古真人善于掌握天地阴阳变化规律，努力使自己的精神和形体适应大自然的要求，从而达到养生的目的。句中以"阴阳"隐喻天地自然运动和变化的规律。

李本与吴本采用音译与意译结合法，将"阴阳"分别译为 the principles of Yin and Yang（阴阳的法则）和 the law of the wax and wane of Ying and Yang（阴阳消长的规律）。但吴本将"阴"的音译误拼为 Ying，而且 wax and wane 通常用作动词词组表达"盈亏、兴衰成败"，改为名词词组 waxing and waning，表达"此消彼长"较为恰当。除此之外，两个译本保留隐喻表达，通过意译将"阴阳"蕴含的"自然变化或自然规律"之义表达出来，有效实现语言与文化的双层转换。

威本与文本采用音译加注法，将"阴阳"分别译为 Yin and Yang [the two principles in nature] 和 [the regularity of] yin and yang。两个译本分别增加"自然中的法则"与"规律性"，意在说明"阴阳"在句中代表着客观规律，加注内容能够帮助读者理解"阴阳"的含义。

3. 夫四时阴阳者，万物之根本也。（《素问·四气调神大论》）

释义：所以四时阴阳的变化，是万物生长收藏的根本。

李本：[The changes of] Yin and Yang in the four seasons are the roots of all the things [in nature].

威本：Thus the interaction of the four seasons and the interaction of Yin and Yang [the two principles in nature] is the foundation of everything in creation.

文本：Now, the yin and yang [qi] of the four seasons, they constitute root and basis of the myriad beings.

吴本：The energies of all things on earth are born in spring, grow in summer, yield in autumn and hide in winter, they are all promoted by the law of variation of Yin and Yang energies of the four seasons. So Yin and Yang energies of the four seasons are the root-energies of birth and growth of all things.

"四时阴阳"，指春温、夏热、秋凉、冬寒的四季变化和一年之中阴阳变化的规律。句中以"阴阳"隐喻四时变化的规律。

李本、威本、文本采用音译加注法，在保留隐喻表达的同时，尽可能为读者的理解提供线索。李本将"阴阳"译为 [The changes of] Yin and Yang（阴阳的变化），通过语境读者可以领会"阴阳"在句中被隐喻为自然规律。威本译为 the interaction of Yin and Yang [the two principles in nature]，增补"自然中的两种法则"说明阴阳的隐喻义，便于读者理解。文本译为 the yin and yang [qi]（阴气、阳气），增补内容未能忠实于原文，增补 qi 是对该处"阴阳"含义的误解，未能实现信息的正确转换。

吴本采用音译与意译结合法，将"阴阳"译为 the law of variation of Yin and Yang energies，通过使用 law 表达出阴阳变化是一种客观规律，补充 energies（能量）将"阴阳"的抽象意义具体化，对于目的语读者而言易于理解。

4. 阴阳者，天地之道也，万物之纲纪……（《素问·阴阳应象大论》）

释义：阴阳的道理，是宇宙的普遍规律，是一切事物的纲领……

李本：Yin and Yang serve as the Dao (law) of the heavens and the earth, the fundamental principle of all things...

威本：The principle of Yin and Yang [the male and female elements in nature] is the basic principle of the entire universe. It is the principle of everything in creation...

文本：As for yin and yang, they are the Way of heaven and earth, the fundamental principles [governing] the myriad beings...

吴本：Yin and Yang are the ways of heaven and earth. As the birth, growth, developement, harvesting and storing of all things are all carried out according to the rule of growth and decline of Yin and Yang, so, Yin and Yang are the guiding principles of all things...

阴阳普遍存在于天地自然之中，其对立统一是自然界的基本规律，是宇宙万物发生、发展、变化及消亡的本原和起点，也是千变万化的各种运动现象的原动力。句中以"阴阳"隐喻自然界的规律。

李本、文本、吴本均采用音译法，将"阴阳"译为 Yin and Yang。李本通过语境中的 Dao (law) 帮助读者理解此处隐喻的具体含义，在实现有效交际的同时保留隐喻形式，有利于中医文化的对外传播。文本与吴本虽然保留了隐喻特色，但在目的语读者不了解源语文化的情况下，很难将"阴阳"与其隐喻义"自然界的规律"对等起来。

威本采用音译加注法，将"阴阳"译为 The principle of Yin and Yang 并补译出 [the male and female elements in nature]，通过注释说明"阴阳"为自然界中对立属性的事物。威本在保留源语文化的同时也考虑到读者对译文的接受度，能够有效进行信息传递。

（五）脉象

所谓**阴阳**者，去者为**阴**，至者为**阳**；静者为**阴**，动者为**阳**……（《素问·阴阳别论》）

释义：所谓脉象的阴阳，脉往叫作阴，脉来叫作阳，脉静叫作阴，脉动叫作阳……

李本：The Yin and Yang [pulses can be defined in this way], the receding [pulse] is Yin and the coming [pulse] is Yang. The quiet [pulse] is Yin while the throbbing [pulse] is Yang...

威本：It is said about Yin and Yang that those who kill are influenced by Yin, those who reach the highest good are influenced by Yang. Those who are peaceful and quiet are influenced by Yin, and those who are active are influenced by Yang...

文本：As for the so-called yin and yang [associations], that which leaves is yin; that which arrives is yang. That which is quiet is yin; that which moves is yang...

吴本：In distinguishing the Yin, Yang from the pulse condition, all the going, calm and slow pulses belong to Yin, and all the coming, mobile and rapid pulses belong to Yang...

"去"和"至"指以脉搏之落起分阴阳，"静"和"动"指以脉搏之气势分阴阳。句中以"阴阳"分别隐喻各种不同的脉象。

句中多处出现关于"阴""阳"的表达，四个译本中，除第一处"阴阳"的译法存在较明显的区别外，其他几处均采用音译法。第一处"阴阳"隐喻的翻译成功与否，对交际而言影响较大。李本与文本采用音译加注法，补充必要的信息，以增进读者的理解。李本译为 the Yin and Yang [pulses can be defined in this way]（脉象可以这种方式定义），增补内容有利于读者理解此处阴阳的含义，即以阴阳来描述不同的脉象，此外也为读者理解句中其余两处"阴""阳"的隐喻义做好铺垫。文本译为 yin and yang [associations] 传达出"所谓阴阳的联想"之意，此处阴阳并非联想，而是以隐喻的方式描述两种相对的脉象。比较而言，李本更准确，有利于顺利实现交际。

威本对于句中隐喻完全采用音译法，保留源语隐喻和语言特色。但译文中使用被动结构 are influenced by（受……影响）说明不同的脉象由"阴""阳"造成，是对原文的误读，不利于有效交际。

对于句中隐喻，吴本采用音译与意译结合法，并通过增补 in distinguishing 来说明"阴阳"是用来区分不同的脉象，并分别把具有"阴""阳"特点的脉象归纳在一起译出，译文简洁，便于读者通过对比把握具有不同特点的脉象。

第二节　精气相关隐喻及英译

　　精和气是中医学的两个基本概念，具有丰富的内涵和外延。从认知语言学的角度来看，精气概念系统是古人以隐喻的认知方式对周围世界进行类比思考而形成的。从认知规律来看，人类的认知过程实际上是进行类比思考的过程，而作为认知成果的概念通常是以类为单位进行存放。古人对精和气的认知亦是如此。在中医学的悠久历史中，精气概念一直贯穿始终，并且不断丰富、演化和拓展，逐渐形成系统的精气理论，同时通过隐喻的方式衍生出许多与精气相关的词汇。

　　《黄帝内经》主要研究人体生理病理规律，在哲学精气学说的基础上，加上古人对人类自身繁衍的观察和体悟，建立了中医学的精气神学说。该学说认为"精"是人体的本原，并且把"精"和"气"进行了划分，使它们各自具有了不同的内涵，同时也对"神"进行论述，建立了科学的"精气神"理论。[1]"精气"的内涵可概括为：①指宇宙万物本原之精气，概念内涵同气；②指自然界之清气；③指人体中的精；④指人体之气，包括正气；⑤指人体中精与气的合称。[2]

　　在《素问》中，"精"出现的频率很高。精的隐喻，是一种从自然域到人体域的认知转化，是从物态到功能态的组合。《素问》中与"精"相关的隐喻主要表现在自然之精和人体之精两大方面。

　　在《素问》中，"气"的概念使用范围很广，是《素问》中的重要概念之一，可以说是这一中医典籍的哲学和医学理论的基石。气的隐喻，实际上是一种从自然域到人体域的认知转化，一种从物态到功能态的组合。《素问》中与"气"相关的隐喻主要表现在自然之气和人体之气两大方面。

　　本节选取《素问》原文中有关"精气"的结构隐喻内容，对四个译本的

---

[1]　郭海，龚婕宁.对《内经》精气神理论的思考 [J].中国中医基础医学杂志，2009，15（5）：327–329.

[2]　孙广仁.《内经》中有关精气理论的几个核心概念的辨析 [J].北京中医药大学学报，2007，30（4）：224.

翻译方法和特点进行对比研究与分析。

一、自然之精

《素问》中，自然之精为"精"自然域的原型所指，如构成万物的灵气、物质精华、日月星辰等。

1. ……提挈天地，把握阴阳，呼吸<u>精气</u>，独立守神，肌肉若一。（《素问·上古天真论》）

释义：……他能把握住自然的变化，掌握阴阳消长的规律，吐故纳新以养精气，超然独立，精神内守，使他的身体好像和精神结合为一。

李本：...[who could] grasp the law of nature. They followed the principles of Yin and Yang, inhaling fresh air, cultivating their spirit and keeping their muscles integrated.

威本：...they mastered the Universe and controlled Yin and Yang [the two principles in nature]. They breathed the essence of life, they were independent in preserving their spirit, and their muscles and flesh remained unchanged.

文本：...They upheld [the patterns of] heaven and earth and they grasped [the regularity of] yin and yang. They exhaled and inhaled essence qi. They stood for themselves and guarded their spirit.

吴本：...All their behaviours adapted to the change of nature quite at ease, they could master the law of the wax and wane of Ying and Yang. They respired the refined energy, guarding the spirit independently and thus their muscles would be an integrated whole.

句中"呼吸精气"，指呼吸清新的空气，意在强调真人善于选择环境，吸收最精纯的清气，调节呼吸运动，以达到养生之目的。此处以"精气"隐喻精纯的空气。

对于"精气"的理解，四个译本各不相同。李本将其意译为 fresh air（新鲜空气），准确传递其内涵意义，顺利实现交际。

威本将"精气"意译为 the essence of life（生命的精华），将句中"精气"误解为人体之精，未能忠实传递原文内容。同时，威本将"呼吸精气"译为 breathed the essence of life，令读者不知所云。

本句中"呼吸精气"是隐喻的说法，文本未能准确把握此处"精气"的准确含义，将其译为 essence qi 欠妥当。

吴本将"精气"意译为 the refined energy（精炼的能量），误解了"精气"在本句中的含义。故造成对原文的误译，不利于实现有效交际。

2. 天有精，地有形，天有八纪，地有五里，故能为万物之父母。（《素问·阴阳应象大论》）

释义：天有精气，地有行质；天有八节的气序，地有五方的布局。因此，天地能成为万物生长的根本。

李本：So the heavens has Jing (Essence-Qi) and the earth has forms. The heavens demonstrates the eight solar terms and the earth displays the rules of Wuxing (Five-Elements). That is why [the heavens and the earth are regarded as] the parents (source) of all things.

威本：In Heaven there are ethereal spirits; upon earth there is form and shape. In Heaven there are eight regulators; upon earth there are five principles; and by means of these all living creatures can be transformed into parents.

文本：The fact is, heaven has the essence; the earth has the physical appearance. Heaven has the eight arrangements; the earth has the five structures. Hence, [heaven and earth] can be father and mother of the myriad beings.

吴本：The reason of the heaven and earth can be the parents of all things is that the heaven has its invisible refined energy and the earth has its visible substance. The heaven has eight weather terms..., and the earth has the distribution of five elements to be the guiding principle to breed all things.

"精"，指清轻之气。古人认为，天有精气，地有形质，因此可以成为宇宙万物生成的根本。句中"精"指构成宇宙万物的灵气，专指气中的精粹部分，是构成人类的本原。以此隐喻天地合二为一成为万物的根本。

李本采用音译加注的方法，将"精"译为 Jing (Essence-Qi)。通过音译保留中医文化特色，加注 Essence-Qi（精华之气），便于目的语读者更好地理解"精"的内涵，以实现有效交际。

威本将"精"意译为 ethereal spirits（超凡的精神），对于本句隐喻存在误读，与其原义"气中的精粹部分"不符，令读者费解。此外，"天有精，地有形，天有八纪，地有五里"，意在说明天地为万物之根本，而威本误译为 ...by means of these all living creatures can be transformed into parents（通过该方式，所有生物都可转化为父母），造成信息传递错误，不利于实现有效交际。

文本将"精"直译为 the essence，与"精"在句中意思接近，但未译出此处的"精"是"气中的精粹部分"，译文意思模糊，逊色于李本。此外，"精"的直译造成文化空缺，不利于中医文化的对外传播。

吴本将"精"意译为 invisible refined energy（无形的精炼能量）。该译文指人体的"水谷精微"较为恰当，但用在此处指构成宇宙万物的灵气和气中的精粹部分欠妥当，不利于目的语读者理解源语的内涵。

3. 地者，所以载生成之形类也。虚者，所以列应天之精气也。形精之动，犹根本之于枝叶也。（《素问·五运行大论》）

释义：大地是负载它所生成的有形物类的，天空是分布日月五星的。大地上的物类与天空上日月五星的运动，好像根本与枝叶一样密切。

李本：So the earth supports all the things with forms. And the sky is distributed with [the stars that] reflect the Jingqi (Essence) of the heavens. The motion of the forms [on the earth] and the Essence [in the heavens] are just like the root and twigs [of a tree].

文本：The earth is [the foundation] which carries all physical appearances that come to life and reach maturity. The [Great] Void is that by which the essence qi corresponding to heaven are arranged in order. The movements of physical appearance [in relation to] essence [qi] resemble the relationship of root and base with branches and leaves.

吴本：The earth is loading all the visible things. The sun, moon and the five stars are spreading in heaven. All things on earth and the movements of sun, moon and the five stars in the sky are related with each other closely like the trunk of a tree connecting its branches and leaves.

句中"精"指日月五星。"应天之精气"，指日月五星等是感受天体之精气而形成的。大地载运各类有形的物质，太空布列受天之精气的星象。地之形质与天之精气的运动，就像根本和枝叶的关系。句中将"有形物类"与"日月五星"联系起来，并以树木根本与枝叶的关系来隐喻二者之间的相互作用。

李本采用意译法，并通过增补译法，将"精"译为 [the stars that] reflect the Jingqi (Essence) of the heavens（受天体之精气而形成的星体），将"应天之精"准确表达出来，但"精"不仅指"星"还指"日月"等，应当一并译出。

文本将"精"直译为 the essence qi，未能考虑到"精"的语境含义，并非所有的"精"都有"精气"之意。句中"精"指日月五星，由于误译，译文所传达的信息会令读者感到茫然。

吴本采用意译法，将"精"译为 the sun, moon and the five stars，表达出"精"的具体内涵意义。译文虽未保留原文的语言特征，但信息表达充分，有助于提高读者对译文的接受度。

二、人体之精

《素问》中的"人体之精"主要表现为气、血、神、津液、脏腑之精、水谷精微、生殖之精等。

（一）气

1. 和于阴阳，调于四时，去世离俗，积精全神。（《素问·上古天真论》）

释义：能够符合于阴阳的变化，适应四时气候的递迁，避开世俗的纷杂，聚精会神。

李本：Abiding by [the changes of] Yin and Yang, adapting [themselves] to the changes of seasons, abandoning secular desires, avoiding distraction and roaming around on the earth and in the heavens.

威本：They lived in accord with Yin and Yang, and in harmony with the four seasons. They departed from this world and retired from mundane affairs; they saved their energies, and preserved their spirits completely.

文本：They adapted themselves to [the regularity] of yin and yang and they lived in harmony with the four seasons. They left the world and they departed from the common. They accumulated essence and preserved their spirit.

吴本：They could keep their behaviours and minds to fit the law of the wax and wane of Yin and Yang and the sequent weather changes of the seasons. They were able to maintain their primordial energy concentratively by freeing themselves from wordly turmoil so as they could keep their physique strong, their spirit abundant, and their ears and eyes acute.

句中"精"指精气。"积精全神",指积蓄精气,集中精神。中古至人深谙养生之道,能够把握阴阳的变化,远离世俗的干扰,积蓄精气,集中精神,从而达到延长寿命和强身健体的目的。

对于"积精全神"的理解,威本、文本与原文含义较为接近。威本采用直译法,将"精"理解为"精力或精神",而非"精气",故将其译为...saved their energies, and preserved their spirits completely(节约他们的精力并完全保存精神),译文将"精"译为精力,也未能兼顾"集中精神"的含义。文本将"精"直译为essence(精华),须增加qi才能表达句中"精"指精气的含义。此外,文本将"去世离俗"译作...left the world and they departed from the common(离开这个世界,与世俗告别)属于误译,会令读者感到困惑。

李本采用意译法,译为avoiding distraction and roaming。将此处的"精"与"神"结合在一起理解为"避免干扰、集中注意力",仍未将"精气"的含义准确表达出来。

吴本采用意译,对于此处隐喻的翻译以释义为主,将"积精全神"译为...maintain their primordial energy concentratively by freeing themselves from wordly turmoil so as they could keep their physique strong, their spirit abundant, and their ears and eyes acute. 吴本对"精"的意译,存在过度翻译。与原文对照,译文显得过于拖沓,用词繁琐,失去原文的凝练之美。

2. 以长为短,以白为黑,如是则精衰矣。(《素问·脉要精微论》)

释义:如果长短不分,黑白颠倒,就证明精气衰败了。

李本:[If the eyes] take long as short and white as black, [it is a sign that] Jing (Essence) is declining.

威本:When they mistake a long pulse for a short one and when they mistake white for black or commit similar errors, then it is a sign that their skill has deteriorated.

文本:If long is regard as short, if white is regard as black, in this case the essence has decreased.

吴本:If one can no more distinguish the length and the black and white, his vital energy has already been exhausted.

句中"精"指精气，是人体生长发育及各种功能活动的物质基础。本句以"精"隐喻构成人体的基本物质。

李本采用音译加注法，将"精"译为 Jing (Essence)，既有利于中医文化的对外传播，又能达到有效交际的目的。但此处"精"指精气，若在译文的基础上改为 Jing (Essence-qi) 则更能够准确地体现原文的意思。

文本采用意译法，将"精"译为 essence（精华）。该译法的优点在于，向目的语读者传达出该物质的内涵，便于理解，从而顺利实现交际目标。但句中"精"指精气，文本将其仅译作 essence 则过于笼统。

吴本将"精"意译为 vital energy（生命能量、元气），在一定程度上易于目的语读者理解"精"之所指，便于信息传递。

威本将"精"意译为 skill（技能），意义偏离原文。由于误译导致信息传递错误，无法实现有效交际。

3. 邪气盛则实，精气夺则虚。（《素问·通评虚实论》）

释义：邪气盛，就是实证，正气被伤，就是虚证。

李本：Predomination of Xieqi (Evil-Qi) is called Shi (Excess) and insufficiency of Jingqi (Essence-Qi) is called Xu (Deficiency).

威本：When harmful influences are plentiful then we can speak of fullness; when the essences are decreased we can speak of emptiness.

文本：When evil qi abounds, then [this is] repletion. When the essence qi is lost, then [this is] depletion.

吴本：When the evil-energy is overabundant, it is sthenia, when the healthy-energy is injured, it is asthenia.

"精气"，指人体之正气；"邪气"，指风寒暑湿之邪。句中"精气"与"邪气"形成对比，揭示中医虚实症状的病因，即精气不足则为虚，邪气盛于人身则为实。

李本采用音译加注法，将"精气"译为 Jingqi (Essence-Qi)，essence 对人体之正气进行扩充解释。这种译法既保留中医术语的特色，又清楚地对"精气"的隐喻义进行解释说明，较为完整。但是，essence 意为"精华、精髓、本质"，因此，Essence-Qi 意为"精华之气"，与原文所要表达的"人体之正气"的意义并不完全相符。

文本将"精气"译为 the essence qi，威本则将其译为 the essences。文本采用音译保留原文中的"气"，以 essence 作为其修饰语进行解释，实现语言转换；而威本将 essence 用作可数名词，未能实现语言的转换。但是，这两个版本的译法对"精"的理解与李本基本相同，都与原文要表达的意义存在一定偏差。

与以上三个译本不同，吴本采用意译法，将"精气"译为 the healthy-energy，与 the evil-energy 形成对比，较为准确地传递原文的意义。但是该译法未能完整保留中医文化特有的概念"精气"，因而在文化层面的转换上稍显不足。

4.……以从为逆，正气内乱，与精相薄。（《素问·四时刺逆从论》）

释义：以顺为逆，就会使正气内乱，邪气和真气相搏击。

李本：...violation instead of following [the changes of Qi in the four seasons] leads to internal disorder of Zhengqi (Healthy–Qi) and conflict between [Xieqi (Evil–Qi)] and Jing (Essence).

文本：...and if one considers compliance as opposition, [then] the proper qi is in disorder internally and strikes at the essence.

吴本：...taking the agreeable condition as the adverse condition, it will cause the healthy energy to become confused inside, and the evil–energy to combat with the healthy energy.

本句解释的是针刺时应懂得四时经气所在部位以及疾病发生的原因，如若不然，将会造成内在的正气逆乱，邪气与正气相迫而生大病的后果。句中"精"喻指人体的正气，与邪气相对。

李本采用音译加注法，将"精"译为 Jing (Essence)，虽然达到了既保留中医专有词汇又补充说明其具体意义的目的，但是在对"精"的意义理解上存在偏差，也未能在形式上做到与前文的 Xieqi (Evil-Qi)（邪气）相统一。

文本将"精"直译为 the essence，与李本的理解较为相似，也存在一定偏差，未能译出其隐喻的对象，即人体之正气。

吴本采用意译法，将"精"译为 the healthy energy，与 the evil-energy 形成对应，较为准确地表达正气与邪气相搏的意义。略有遗憾的是，该译法虽有助于读者理解原文，却无法完整地保留和传递中医学中极为重要且抽象的概念"气"，未能完全实现文化阐释功能。

（二）血

……**精不足者，补之以味。**（《素问·阴阳应象大论》）

释义：精气不足的，应用甘温药温补其气。

李本：...and insufficiency of Jing (Essence) [should be treated by] nourishing [therapy with tonic] herbs.

威本：...and if the spiritual essence is not able to bring improvement to a patient, the five flavors must be applied.

文本：...When the essence has insufficiencies, supplement it with flavor.

吴本：...Deficiency of essence shows the decline of Yin, it should be replenished by qifen drugs.

句中"精"指阴血、精血，若阴精不足，则要用厚味之品加以滋补。

四个译本均用 essence 表达"精"的概念。

李本采用音译加注法，将"精"译为 Jing (Essence)，虽保留了中医术语的特色，但并未传达出"精血"之隐喻义，不利于读者理解，无法实现对中医文化精髓的成功转换。

文本和吴本均采用直译法，分别将"精"译作 the essence 和 essence，语言上实现转换。遗憾的是，与李本一样，这两个译本都未能准确清晰地说明其隐喻义，造成译不达意。从句式上看，文本的表达更为简洁，而吴本的句型更符合目的语读者的语言习惯，词汇也更为丰富，只是主从句之间缺少连词，存在语法错误。

威本将"精"译为 the spiritual essence（精神实质），显然对原文理解存在偏差而造成误译，无法实现交际目标，文化层面的转换也无从谈及。

（三）神

1. 精神不进，志意不治，故病不可愈。（《素问·汤液醪醴论》）

释义：如果病人的神气已经衰微，病人的志意已经散乱，那病是不会好的。

李本：Declination of Jingshen (Essence and Spirit) and distraction of Yizhi

《黄帝内经素问》隐喻英译对比研究

(mind) make it difficult to treat diseases.

威本：If man's vitality and energy do not propel his own will his disease cannot be cured.

文本：When essence spirit fails to enter and when the mind is in disorder, a disease cannot be healed.

吴本：If the spirit and the energy of the patient are disappearing, his will and consciousness are dispersing, the disease can by no means be cured.

此句强调精神志意的重要性，句中"精"指精神，神气，与现代汉语中的"精神"意义较为接近。因此，"精神不进，志意不治"，是指精神衰微，志意散乱不定。

李本采用音译加注法，将"精神"译为 Jingshen (Essence and Spirit)，注解中的 essence and spirit 实为直译，虽实现语言转换，但对其解读不够准确，因而出现译不达意。

文本将"精神"直译为 essence spirit，但与李本不同的是，文本使用 essence 修饰中心词 spirit，这与原文中"精神"的含义不完全符合。

威本采用意译法，将"精"译为 man's vitality and energy，并将其作为 if 条件状语从句的主语，将 his own will 作为谓语动词 propel 的宾语，该从句表达的意思是"精神不进"造成"志意不治"，偏离了原文的内涵意义。

吴本亦采用意译法，将"精神"译作 the spirit and the energy，不仅准确传达原文意思，而且与下文的 will and consciousness 保持形式统一，在较大程度上保留原文的语言风格。

2. 惊而夺精，汗出于心。（《素问·经脉别论》）

释义：受惊而影响精神的时候，由于心气受伤而汗出于心。

李本：Fright depletes Jing (Essence) and leads to sweating from the heart.

威本：When man is shocked and startled he does violence to his spirit and vitality, and perspiration is produced by the heart.

文本：When one was frightened and has lost essence, the [resulting] sweat originates from the heart.

吴本：When one is frightened, his heart will certainly be hurt.

句中"精"亦指精神，神气。受惊会影响精神，此时，会出现由于心气受伤而引起汗出于心的情形。

李本采用音译加注法，将"精"译为 Jing (Essence)，实现语言转换的目标。但 essence 未能解释出其喻指的确切意义，会造成读者理解困难，影响交际目标的实现。

与李本类似，文本将"精"直译为 essence，同样可能因为过于简单直白而致使读者无法正确把握其在句中的含义，从而影响对句意的理解。

威本采用意译法，将"精"译作 spirit and vitality，较准确地实现意义转换，相对而言，该译法更易于读者理解和接受。缺憾是译文中未能保留中医文化中"精"的抽象概念，翻译的文化阐释功能较弱。

吴本对本句进行删译，对原文中"精"和"汗"两个概念均未进行翻译和解释，只强调"惊"（when one is frightened）可能会影响（hurt）"心"（heart），因此在语言和文化的转换上都有所欠缺。

（四）津液

1. 饮入于胃，游溢精气，上输于脾；脾气散精……水精四布，五经并行。（《素问·经脉别论》）

释义：水液进入胃里，放散精气，上行输送到脾脏；脾脏散布精华……这样，气化水行，散布于周身皮毛，流行在五脏经脉里。

李本：When water is taken into the stomach, the Jingqi (Essence–Qi) is distributed around and is transported to the spleen. The spleen distributes Jing (Essence)... [In this way,] the Jing (Essence) of water is distributed all through the body and into the five Channels.

威本：Drink enters the stomach, flows and overflows into the secretions, its essence ascends and is introduced into the spleen. The spleen distributes its secretions... The liquid secretions are spread in four (directions) and united in the five passages (arteries 经).

文本：Beverages enter the stomach. Overflowing essence qi is transported upward to the spleen. The spleen qi spreads the essence... The essence of water is spread to the four [cardinal points], it moves through all the five conduits simultaneously.

吴本：When the water enters the stomach, it evaporates the refined energy

《黄帝内经素问》隐喻英译对比研究

and spread it to the spleen above. And the spleen spreads the essence... In this way, with the production, circulation activity of the vital energy and the promotion of the water, the refined energy spreads to the skin and hair of the whole body, they circulate in the channels of the five viscera.

"游溢精气"中的"精气"是对"水汽"的隐喻;"脾气散精"中的"精"是对"水谷精微"的隐喻;"水精"是对"水液"或者"津液"的隐喻。

李本使用音译加注法将"精气"译为 Jingqi (Essence-Qi),将"精"译为 Jing (Essence),将"水精"译为 Jing (Essence) of water。音译保留了源语的隐喻特色,注解使目的语读者对于"精"有更准确的理解,有利于中医文化的对外传播。

文本在熟悉源语文化的前提下,将句中三处"精"皆意译为 essence,这与李本一致,能够有效进行信息传递和语言交际,但在文化传递上略逊于李本。

吴本将"精气"和"水精"皆译作 the refined energy(精炼的能量),以 energy 来隐喻中医文化中的"精""气",利于信息传递,但忽略了文化交际。

威本采用意译法,将"精气"译为 its essence,此处 its 指代上一句中的 water,即 water's essence 或 essence of water;将"精"译为 water's secretions (分泌物);将"水精"译为 liquid secretions(水液分泌物)。secretion 在隐喻功能上难以传递"气"的信息,liquid(water's)secretions 更让目的语读者难以理解源语的内涵。

2. 风客淫气,精乃亡,邪伤肝也。(《素问·生气通天论》)

释义:风邪侵入人体,渐渐侵害元气,精血就要损耗,这是由于邪气伤害肝脏的缘故。

李本:When wind attacks the body, [it gradually] damages Qi and exhausts Jing (Essence). [This is because of] the impairment of the liver by Xie (Evil).

威本:If the wind enters the body and exhausts man's breath, then his essence will be lost and the evil influences will injure his liver.

文本:When wind settles [in the body] and encroaches upon the [proper] qi, then the essence vanishes,and the evil harms the liver.

吴本:Owning to the wind associates with the liver (liver correspond to the wind and wood), when one is hurt by excessive wind-evil, the essence of life and blood will suffer severe damage. As blood is stored in the liver, the wind-evil will hurt the liver too.

句中"精"是对"精血"的隐喻，亦称为"阴精"，与阳气相对而言。

吴本将"精"意译为 the essence of life and blood，具体又准确地向目的语读者传达出此处"精"应为"精血"之意，但表述过于复杂难以彰显源语文字的简洁之美，无法做到形义兼顾。

李本依旧采用直译加注法，将"精"译为 Jing (Essence)；威本和文本皆采用意译法将"精"译为 essence。三个译本虽然在一定程度上保留原文的隐喻，但在信息传递上都不如吴本到位。

另外，受译者自身对源语文字和文化的领悟所限，威本、文本和吴本皆对该句中"邪伤肝也"的翻译出现误译，主要是对"也"的理解出现偏差。"也"在此处实为句末语气词，表示陈述或解释语气。威本和文本中使用 and 构成并列句，无法表达"精乃亡"的原因。吴本虽将原因译出，但使用副词 too 来翻译句末语气词"也"实属误译。李本采用增补译法，既说明"精乃亡"的原因又兼顾文字表达的简洁，在这方面李本胜于其他三个译本。

3. 开鬼门，洁净府，精以时服。(《素问·汤液醪醴论》)

释义：然后用缪刺方法，使他的形体恢复起来。再想法使汗液畅达，小便通利；则孤精得以被按时而制服。

李本：[Besides,] [the therapeutic methods for] opening Guimen (sweat pores) and cleaning the Jingfu (the bladder) can be used [to eliminate the retention of fluid].

威本：One should restore their bodies and open the anus so that the bowels can be cleansed, and so that the secretions come at the proper time and serve the five viscera which belong to Yang, the principle of life.

文本：Open the demon gates and clean the pure palace and the essence will recover in due time.

吴本：Then, try to make the patient to perspire thoroughly, and keep his urination unobstructed, besides, give the patient, according to the condition, some medicine on due time.

句中"精"意为"孤精",也就是积液、积水。

吴本对原文存在误解,将"精"理解为"药",误译为 medicine,妨碍了信息的正确传递,无法达到有效交际。

威本采用意译法,将"精"译为 the secretions(分泌物),显然没有完全理解原文。后半句中,威本误解源语中的"服",将其理解为"服务",译为serve,这导致后半句的误译,也无法实现有效交际。

文本将"精"意译为 essence,在信息传递上过于笼统,不能使目的语读者真正理解此处的"精"是"孤精"之意,该译文不能准确地进行信息传递。

李本对"精"进行意译,译为 the retention of fluid(积液、积水),正确地理解此句中"精"的内涵。"孤精"为"无气之精",实为病气。李本译法将源语信息向目的语读者进行准确传递,为四者中的最佳译文。

(五)脏腑之精

1. 五阳已布,疏涤五脏,故精自生,形自盛……(《素问·汤液醪醴论》)

释义:待五脏阳气输布了,五脏郁积荡涤了,那么精气自然会产生,形体自然会强盛……

李本:[In this way,] the Jing (Essence) will flow normally, the Yang in the Five Zang-Organs will distribute smoothly and [the stagnation in] the Five Zang-Organs will be cleansed. [Consequently,] the Jing (Essence) is produced automatically, the body becomes strong again...

威本:One should put in order the five viscera which were remiss and cleanse and purify them. Then the secretions are certain to produce life, and the body contains flourishing bones and flesh without further help...

文本:When the five yang [qi] have spread [everywhere], this clears the five depots and opens the passage through them. Hence essence is generated by itself and the physical appearance will be marked by itself by abundance [again]...

吴本:When the Yang-energy in the five viscera of the patient being spread, the stagnations in the five viscera being cleared, his essence and energy will be sure to regenerate, his body will certain become strong...

本句中,"精"为脏腑之精气,也称后天之精,由水谷精气和自然界之清气而化生。句中"精"隐喻脏腑之精气。

李本仍旧采用音译加注法，将"精"译为 Jing (Essence)，很好地保留了中医术语特色，但若目的语读者对中医文化的了解不够，那么该译法很难让读者精确理解此"精"乃"脏腑之精"之意。李本对"五阳已布，疏涤五脏"进行增补翻译，即 [In this way,] the Jing (Essence) will flow normally，在一定程度上弥补了对"精"翻译的不足，使信息传递的准确性得以提高。

文本采用意译法，将"精"译为 essence，只注重信息传递，而放弃了文化传递。文本将"自成"译作 generated by itself，从遣词上看，文本的 by oneself（单独地、独自地）略逊于李本的 automatically（自动地）。此外，文本对"五阳已布，疏涤五脏"的翻译不如李本精准。在句式上，文本使用时间状语从句 When the five yang [qi] have spread [everywhere]，并且对"阳"进行增补翻译，译作 yang [qi]，但是后半句 this clears the five depots and opens the passage through them 中，由于 this 和 them 指代不明确，影响了信息的准确传递。

吴本将"精"进行意译加补译，译作 essence and energy，在某种程度上可以使目的语读者更好地理解"脏腑之精气"的含义。

威本采用意译法，将"精"译作 secretions（分泌物）。虽然在西医中有术语 secretion，但在两种医学文化中，"分泌"与"精气"并不一致，此译文难以准确传递信息。

2. 东方青色……藏精于肝；南方赤色……藏精于心。（《素问·金匮真言论》）

释义：东方青色……精华藏于肝脏；南方赤色……精华藏在心。

李本：[For example,] the east corresponds to blue in color... stores Jing (Essence). The south is related to red in colors... [The heart]...stores Jing...

威本：Green is the color of the East, ...retains the essential substances within the liver. Red is the color of the South, and retains the essential substances within the heart...

文本：The East; green–blue color. Having entered it communicates with the liver...The South; red color. Having entered it communicates with the heart...

吴本：Yang emerges in the east and the colour of east is green...The Yin essence is stored in the liver where the soul lies. The colour of the south is red... The energies of the five viscera are dominated by the heart...

句中多次提到"精",均指五脏之精气。

李本和文本皆沿用自身惯用的翻译方法,行文简洁,信息传递准确。

威本仍采用意译法,没有沿用 secretions(分泌物),改用 the essential substances(基础物质)。在信息传递精准度上明显提高,但对中医术语"精"的文化内涵传递较少。

吴本从阴阳归属上对"精"进行增补,采用音译加意译法,将其译为 Yin essence,在一定程度上提高了中医文化外传和翻译的精准度。随后的几处译文,仍采用 essence,与文本的翻译一致。

(六)水谷精微

1. 食气入胃,散精于肝,淫气于筋。食气入胃,浊气归心,淫精于脉。(《素问·经脉别论》)

释义:食物进入胃里,经过消化一部分精微输散到肝脏,濡润着周身的筋络;另一部分谷气注入到胃,化生精微之气,注入于心,再浸淫到血脉里去。

李本:When food is taken into the stomach, Jing (nutrient substance) is transported to the liver to nourish the sinews. When food is taken into the stomach, Zhuoqi (Turbid–Qi) is transported to the heart to nourish vessels.

威本:Food enters the stomach; its essence is then distributed into the liver and its vital force flows over into the muscles. Food enters the stomach; its putrid gases are sent up to the heart and its essence overflows into the pulse.

文本:The qi of food enters the stomach. [The stomach] spreads essence to the liver. Excessive qi [flows] into the sinews. The qi of food enters the stomach. The turbid qi turns to the heart. Excessive essence [flows] into the vessels.

吴本:When the food enters into the stomach, after being digested,part of it which is the refined substance is transported to the liver to moisture the tendons of the whole body. Another part of it which is the essential substance from cereals is poured into the spleen and being soaked into the channel and blood.

本句中,"精"指水谷精微。

李本采用音译加注法,将其译为 Jing (nutrient substance),音译保留了原文隐喻，注解采用意译，解释此处的"精"为"水谷精微"，译作 nutrient substance（营养物质），把源语中"精"的文化信息和语义信息准确地传递到目的语。译文采用排比句式，较好地保留了源语行文之美。

吴本将"精"进行意译，一处译作 the refined substance，另一处译作 the essential substance。refined 意为"凝练的"，essential 意为"根本的、必须的"，二者意义上稍有差别，但都能传递"水谷精微"由水谷化生而来，是人体所必须的"精微物质"和"根本物质"等基本信息。substance（物质），从微观上说明"精"的细微特征。

威本和文本都将"精"笼统地意译为 essence，无论在信息传递的准确性上还是对源语文化的保留与传递上，都逊于李本和吴本。

2. 人所以汗出者，皆生于谷，谷生于精。（《素问·评热病论》）

释义：人体所以出汗，是由于水谷入胃，化生精微。

李本：Sweating comes from Jing (Essence) transformed from food.

威本：The life of all those people who perspire springs from grain, and grain is produced from (pure) essence.

文本：That because of which sweat leaves man is generated by grain; grain generates essence.

吴本：The sweat is stemmed from water and cereals which arc converted into refined energy for nourishing the whole body, when the refined energy of water and cereals is excreted to the surface of skin, it is sweat.

句中"精"指水谷所化的精气，即水谷精微。水谷精气旺盛，胜过邪气而汗出。因此，句中使用"精"隐喻"汗液"。

李本采用音译加注，将"精"译为 Jing (Essence)，保留源语隐喻，整个句式以简单句加分词定语形式呈现，简洁明了，既准确传递信息又兼顾源语的凝练之美。

吴本采用意译法，将"精"译为 refined energy，也能表达出汗液乃由水谷提供的能量（energy）化生而来，"凝练"后，其中一部分为"汗"。虽能准确传递源语信息，但从句式结构上看，吴本过于繁杂，略逊于李本。

文本依然采用意译法，将其译为 essence，在此不做赘述。

威本运用意译加增补的方法，将其译作 (pure) essence。pure（纯净的）

对"精"在意思表达上作用不大，略显赘余。此外，威本没有准确理解"谷生于精"中介词"于"的意思，将该句误译为 Grain is produced from (pure) essence（水谷源于精微），显然是对中医理论的误解。

（七）生殖之精

1. 二八，（肾气盛），天癸至，精气溢（泻），阴阳和，故能有子。(《素问·上古天真论》)

释义：（男子）到了十六岁时，天癸发育成熟，精气充满，男女交合，所以有子。

李本：At the age of sixteen, as Shenqi (Kidney-Qi) is abundant and Tiangui occurs, he begins to experience spermatic emission. If he has copulated with a woman at this period, he can have a baby.

威本：When he is sixteen years of age the emanations of his testicles become abundant and he begins to secrete semen. He has an abundance of semen which he seeks to dispel; and if at this point the male and the female element unite in harmony, a child can be conceived.

文本：With two times eight, the qi of the kidneys abounds; the heavengui arrives and the essence qi flows away. Yin and yang find harmony. Hence, he can have children.

吴本：His kidney energy becomes prosperous by the age of sixteen (2×8). he it is filled with vital energy and is able to let out sperm. If he conducts sexual intercourse with a woman, he might have a child.

句中使用"精气"隐喻精液。

李本和吴本采用意译法，将"精"译作 sperm（精子、精液）；威本采用意译法，译作 semen（精子、精液）。两者差别不大，注重信息传递，但忽略了文化传递。

文本使用意译加直译法，将"精"译作 essence qi。这在很大程度上保留源语的隐喻，有利于中医文化外传，但 essence qi（精气）并不能完全替代原文"精气"，因此，在信息传递准确性上欠佳。

此外，由于受自身中文水平所限，威本和文本都未能正确理解"阴阳和"实为"男女交合"之义，分别将"和"直译为 unite in harmony 和 find harmony，表意不准确。而李本和吴本熟悉中国文化，汉语功底深厚，分别将"阴阳和"意译为 he has copulated with a woman 和 he conducts sexual intercourse，表达出"男女交合"之内涵意义。

2. 此虽有子，男子不过尽八八，女子不过尽七七，而天地之精气皆竭矣。（《素问·上古天真论》）

释义：这种人虽然能够生育，但在一般情况下，男子不超过六十四岁，女子不超过四十九岁，到这个岁数，男女的精气都竭尽了。

李本：[Although] these [old people] still can bear children, [they lose such an ability at the age of] sixty-four in men and forty-nine in women.

威本：Yet if they children, their sons will not exceed their sixty-fourth year and their daughters will not exceed their forty-ninth year, because at that time the essence of Heaven and Earth will be exhausted.

文本：Although [someone] has children, males do not exceed the end reached at eight times eight and females do not exceed the end reached at seven times seven, when the essence qi of heaven and earth are all exhausted.

吴本：Nevertheless, for a man, the age for having a child can not exceed sixty four (8×8), and for a woman, can not exceed the age of forty nine (7×7). When the essence and vital energy of a man or woman being exhausted, it is also impossible for them to have any child.

句中的"天地精气"，指男女的生殖之精，以"天地之精气"隐喻男女生殖之精。

吴本采用意译法，将"天地之精气"译作 the essence and vital energy of a man or woman，说明译者真正理解了源语中的隐喻所指，"天地"隐喻"男女"，故译作 man or woman，但该译法不能体现源语"天地"隐喻之美；"精气"隐喻"生殖之精"，意译为 the essence and vital energy（精华和生命能量），在准确传递源语信息层面稍有欠缺。

威本采用意译加直译法，将"天地之精气"译作 the essence of Heaven and Earth，意译将"精"的含义准确传递到目的语中，"精气"实为"精"，故译作 essence；将"天地"直译为 Heaven and Earth 保留了源语隐喻之美。

文本采用意译加直译法，"天地之精气"译作 the essence qi of Heaven and

Earth，在文字表述上跟源语一致，同样也保留源语"天地"之隐喻功能。因为此处"精气"实为男女生殖之"精"，所以 essence qi 在表述上不如威本简洁。

李本漏译"而天地之精气皆竭矣"。

三、自然之气

《素问》中的自然之气主要表现为阳气和阴气、天气和地气、以及人气等。

（一）阳气、阴气

积阳为天，积阴为地……阳化气，阴成形。（《素问·阴阳应象大论》）

释义：从阴阳变化来看，清阳之气，积聚上升，就成为天；浊阴之气，凝聚下降，就成为地……阳易动散，故能化气，阴易凝敛，故能成形。

李本：The [lucid] Yang [rises and] accumulates to form the heavens and the [turbid] Yin [descends and] accumulates to constitute the earth... Yang transforms Qi while Yin constitutes form.

威本：Heaven was created by an accumulation of Yang, the element of light; Earth was created by an accumulation of Yin, the element of darkness... Yang causes evaporation and Yin gives shape to things.

文本：The accumulation of yang, that is heaven; the accumulation of yin, that is the earth... Yang transforms qi, yin completes physical appearance.

吴本：Heaven situates on up above, it is the accumulation of lucid Yang above; earth situates in down below, it is the accumulation of turbid Yin below... Yang has the function of activating the vital energy, and Yin has the function of shaping up the bodies of all things.

"阳化气"中的"气"隐喻一切易动散之物。

李本和文本都使用音译法，将"阳化气"译作 Yang transforms qi。音译 qi 保留源语隐喻和中医术语的特色，但"气"在中医文化中概念范畴非常广，泛指一切无形、易动散之物，因此，单纯的音译很难让目的语读者领悟"气"为何物。

吴本使用意译法，将"阳化气"译作 Yang has the function of activating the vital energy。使用 the vital energy（生命能量）翻译源语中的"气"，在一

定程度上易于目的语读者理解"气"之所指，便于信息传递。但吴本在遣词造句上过于繁琐，远不及李本和文本简洁凝练，不利于中医文化的外传。

威本采用音译加意译法，将"阳化气"译作 Yang causes evaporation。在信息传递层面，evaporation（蒸发、气化）使"阳化气"的语义信息在目的语中得以传递，也容易被目的语读者理解和接受。但是，evaporation（蒸发、气化）无法涵盖中医文化中的"气"，这在一定程度上妨碍文化传递和信息传递。

（二）天气、地气

地气上为云，天气下为雨；雨出地气，云出天气。（《素问·阴阳应象大论》）

释义：地气上升就成为云，天气下降就变成雨；雨虽是天气下降，却是地气所化；云虽是成于地气，却赖天气的蒸发。

李本：Diqi (Earth-Qi) rises to become clouds and Tianqi (Heaven-Qi) descends to produce rain. Rain results from Diqi while clouds originate from Tianqi.

威本：When the vapors of the earth ascend they create clouds, and when the vapors of Heaven descend they create rain. Thus rain appears to be the climate of the earth and clouds appear to be the climate of Heaven.

文本：The qi of the earth rises and turns into clouds; the qi of heaven descends and becomes rain. Rain originates from the qi of the earth; clouds originate from the qi of heaven.

吴本：The earth energy ascends to become cloud by the evapouration of heaven energy. The heaven energy becomes rain when it descends. Thus, although the rain falls from heaven, yet it is transformed by the earth energy; although the cloud is formed from the earth energy, yet it depends on the evaporation by the heaven energy, and these are the relations of mutual functions of Yin and Yang.

句中"地气"为地之阴气，"阳气"为天之阳气，二者为相对概念。

李本采用音译加注法，将"地气"译为 Diqi (Earth-Qi)，将"天气"译为 Tianqi (Heaven-Qi)。音译 Diqi 和 Tianqi 体现了中医术语的特点，有利于中医文化外译、外传，直译 Earth-Qi 和 Heaven-Qi 能较好地保留源语隐喻。然而，"地气"和"天气"为中医文化中特有的术语，当目的语读者不了解源语文化时，Earth-Qi 和 Heaven-Qi 很难将源语信息对等地传递到目的语中。

文本采用意译法，将"地气"和"天气"分别译为 The qi of the earth 和 the qi of heaven。从信息传递角度来看，文本译法跟李本相似，但从术语的表述特点来看，文本表述略显口语化。

吴本采用意译法，将"地气"和"天气"分别译为 the earth energy 和 the heaven energy。energy（能量、精力、活力）虽然不完全等同于"气"，但 energy 能把中医文化中"气"的概念以隐喻的形式在目的语中表述清楚，有利于目的语读者领会"气"的概念。

威本采用意译法，将第一分句中的"地气"和"天气"分别译为 the vapors of the earth 和 the vapors of Heaven。vapor（蒸汽、水蒸气）确实含有云雨两种自然现象，但在文化层面上，vapor 完全不等同于中医学中的"气"，在内涵上远比"气"少得多。在翻译第二分句时，将其中的"地气"和"天气"分别译为 the climate of the earth 和 the climate of Heaven。climate（气候、风气）在概念上与"气"相去太远，仅仅把"气"禁锢在气候学层面，造成文化和信息传递的欠缺。

（三）人气

夫人生于地，悬命于天，天地合气，命之曰人。（《素问·宝命全形论》）

释义：人虽然是生活在地上，但也丝毫离不开天，天地之气相合，才产生了人。

李本：Man is born on the earth and is endowed with life by the heavens. [Owing to] the integration of the Tianqi and Diqi, man comes into existence.

威本：Man draws life from Earth, but his fate depends upon Heaven. Heaven and Earth unite to bestow life-giving vigor as well as destiny upon man. When heaven and earth combine their qi, that is called "Man".

文本：Now, man receives his life from the earth; his fate depends on heaven. When the energies of heaven and earth are combining, it produces man. Heaven and earth combine [their] qi, separating it into the nine fields and dividing it into the four seasons.

吴本：Although man lives on earth, but his life can by no means divorce from heaven. When the energies of heaven and earth are combining, it produces man.

"天地合气"，也就是，地气和天气结合。天地之气是万物生成的本原，正是在天地之气的孕育和滋养中，人气才得以形成。

李本采用音译法，将"天地合气"译为 the integration of the Tianqi and Diqi。音译 Tianqi 和 Diqi 能很好地保留源语隐喻和内涵，但从信息传递上看，此种译法很难让目的语读者真正理解"天地之气"的含义，更难理解以"天地之气"隐喻"人气"。

威本采用直译加音译，将其译作 heaven and earth combine their qi，音译 qi 保留源语文化，使"气"的概念完整外传。同李本一样，目的语读者也很难理解此处"气"的真正内涵。

文本和吴本译法一致，都采用意译法将其译作 the energies of heaven and earth are combining。此处的"天地合气"造就的是"人"，而"人"不能简单地归类于"自然现象"，故以 energy（能量）隐喻"人气"，目的语读者能够理解源语所指，较好地进行信息传递，达到交际目的。

四、人体之气

《素问》中的人体之气主要表现为先天之气、五脏之气、经络之气和营卫之气。

（一）先天之气、后天之气

1. 丈夫八岁，<u>肾气</u>实，发长齿更。二八，（<u>肾气</u>盛），天癸至……（《素问·上古天真论》）

释义：男子八岁时，肾气盛，头发长长，牙齿更换。到了十六岁时，天癸发育成熟……

李本：For a man, at the age of eight, his Shenqi (Kidney-Qi) becomes prosperous and his teeth begin to change... At the age of sixteen, as Shenqi (Kidney-Qi) is abundant and Tiangui occurs...

威本：When a boy is eight years old the emanations of his testes (kidneys 肾) are fully developed; his hair grows longer and he begins to change his teeth... When he is sixteen years of age the emanations of his testicles become abundant and he begins to secrete semen...

文本：In a male, at the age of eight, the qi of the kidneys is replete; his hair grows and the [initial] teeth are substituted... With two times eight, the qi of the kidneys abounds; the heaven gui arrives...

吴本：For a man, his kidney energy becomes prosperous by the age of eight. By then, his hair developer and his permanent teeth emerge...His kidney energy becomes prosperous by the age of sixteen (2×8)...

肾藏精，主生长，发育。"肾气"属先天之气，是人类得以繁衍生息的精微物质。

李本采用音译加注法，将"肾气"译作 Shenqi (Kidney-Qi)。音译保留了源语术语特色，将中医特有术语"肾气"传递到目的语。李本使用西医术语 kidney（肾脏）翻译中医学中的"肾"，虽然在两种文化中，"肾"的概念并不一致，但采用标准的西医解剖术语来翻译中医文化中的"肾"可以将中医文化很好地外传，目的语读者接受度更高。

文本采直译法，将"肾气"译作 the qi of the kidneys。此译法在文化保留上虽不如李本到位，但能将信息准确传递到目的语。从术语表达层面来看，kidney-qi 比 the qi of the kidneys 更显规范。

吴本采用直译加意译法，将"肾气"译作 kidney energy。"肾"的译法跟李本和文本一致，"气"依旧沿用 energy。

威本采用意译加注法，将"肾气"译作 the emanations of his testes /testicles (kidneys 肾)。testicle（睾丸）源于希腊语 testis（睾丸），emanation 意为"散发出的稀薄物质"，两者结合将此处"肾气"所指传递到位，采用 kidney 加汉字"肾"进行注解，很好地保留了源语文化。

此外，在西医中，肾并非生殖器官，故李本、文本和吴本译法很难让目的语读者理解"肾气"与"有子"之间的联系，而威本译文易于让目的语读者理解两者的联系。

2. 真气从之，精神内守，病安从来。（《素问·上古天真论》）

释义：真气深藏，精神守持于内而不耗散，这样，疾病从哪里来呢？

李本：[In this way] Zhenqi in the body will be in harmony, Jingshen (Essence-Spirit) will remain inside, and diseases will have no way to occur.

威本：The true vital force accompanied them always; their vital (original) spirit was preserved within; thus, how could illness come to them?

文本：The true qi follows [these states]. When essence and spirit are guarded internally, where could a disease come from?

吴本：The true energy will come in the wake of it. When one concentrates his spirit internally and keeps a sound mind, how can any illness occur?

此句中的"真气"即是"元气"，是生命之气的根本。元气是由先天之气和后天之气及自然界之清气结合而成，是维持人体生命活动的基本物质与原动力。

李本使用音译法，将"真气"译作 Zhenqi，此种译法旨在促进中医文化外传，在一定程度上会使目的语读者难以理解"真气"的概念与内涵。

吴本、威本和文本都采用直译法，将"真气"中的"真"译作 true（真正的）。这种译法实际上很难向目的语读者传递"真气"之含义。在对"气"进行翻译时，文本音译 qi 在文化保留和信息传递层面上优于威本和吴本。吴本和威本均采用意译，体现隐喻所指，威本的 the vital force（生命之力）比吴本的 energy（能量；精力）在信息传递上更加准确，从而利于读者理解"真气"。

3. 气味合而服之，以补精益气。（《素问·脏气法时论》）

释义：将谷果肉菜的气味合而服食，可以补精养气。

李本：Harmonic mixture of proper flavors can supplement Jing (Essence) and nourish Qi.

威本：Their flavors, tastes and smells unite and conform to each other in order to supply the beneficial essence (of life).

文本：When they are consumed in [appropriate] combinations of their qi and flavors, they serve to supplement the essence and to enrich the qi.

吴本：When one takes the tastes of the cereal, fruit, meat and vegetable in combination, it can invigorate the essence and nourish the vital energy.

句中的"气"指后天之气，即饮食水谷化生的精微物质。

对于"补精益气"的翻译，李本、文本和吴本均采用直译加音译，分别译为 nourish Qi、enrich the qi 和 nourish the vital energy。"益"，意为"增加，使健壮充实"。nourish（滋养、使健壮）与 enrich（使充实、使富足）在意思上非常接近，在此均能将"益"的含义以隐喻的方式得以准确传递。在对"气"进行翻译时，吴本的意译 the vital energy（生命能量）将"气"之所指传递到目的语中，便于读者理解，但从文化保留和信息传递层面上看，吴本的意译不及李本和文本的音译。

威本采用直译加意译，笼统地将"补精益气"译为 supply the beneficial essence (of life)。supply（补充、提供）不能同时涵盖源语中的"补""益"动作行为；"精"和"气"同为中医理论中的"精微"，相似又有一定差异，essence（精华）难以同时涵盖"精""气"的内涵，因此，该译法不能准确地传递源语信息。在术语表述上，源语中的"补精益气"是一个并列关系的短语，因此威本的译法在此逊于其余三者。

（二）五脏之气

1. 天气通于肺，地气通于嗌，风气通于肝，雷气通于心，谷气通于脾，雨气通于肾。（《素问·阴阳应象大论》）

释义：天气与肺相通，地气与咽相通，风气与肝相通，雷气与心相通，谷气与脾相通，雨气与肾相通。

李本：Tianqi (Heaven–Qi) communicates with the lung, Diqi (Earth–Qi) communicates with the pharynx, Fengqi (Wind–Qi) communicates with the liver, Leiqi (Thunder–Qi) communicates with the heart, Guqi (Grain–Qi) communicates with the spleen and Yuqi (Rain–Qi) communicates with the kidney.

威本：The heavenly climate circulates within the lungs; the climate of the earth circulates within the throat; the wind circulates within the liver, thunder penetrates the heart; the air of a ravine penetrates the stomach; the rain penetrates the kidneys.

文本：The qi of heaven communicates with the lung; the qi of the earth communicates with the throat; the qi of the wind communicates with the liver; the qi of thunder communicates with the heart; the qi of valleys communicates with the spleen; the qi of rain communicates with the kidneys.

吴本：The lung situates on the upper part of the body and takes charge of respiration, so the heaven energy communicates with the lung, the larygopharynx is the exit of the stomach which receives the cereals, so the earth energy communicates with the larygopharynx, As the wind energy produces the liver wood, so the wind energy corresponds with the liver; as the heart associates with the fire, and the thunder also associates with the fire, since like draws to like, so the thunder energy plays a part in the heart; the spleen takes charge of transporting and digesting the cereals, so, the energy of essential substance from cereal communicates with the spleen; the kidney is a solid organ of water, so the rain energy can moisten the kid–ney.

天气、地气、风气、雷气、谷气、雨气等分别与肺、咽、肝、心、脾、肾等相通应。

对于中医文化中的这几种特殊之气，李本依然采用音译加注的办法，这在中医文化外传和术语翻译工整方面确实优于其他三本，但在语义和信息传递上则稍显不足。

威本采用直译加意译的方法，将"天气"和"地气"分别译为 the heavenly climate 和 the climate of the earth。直译 heavenly 和 earth 保留源语文化特色，但是以 climate（气候）来隐喻"气"不利于源语信息的传递。威本分别将"风气""雷气"和"雨气"直译为 wind、thunder 和 rain，从信息对应上看，此三种自然现象与源语中的"风气""雷气"和"雨气"差距太大，有损中医文化中"气"概念的外传。此外，威本和文本都误解"谷气"之"谷"的所指，误将此处的"水谷"理解为"山谷"，分别译为 ravine（山涧、峡谷）和 valley（山谷、流域），此为其中医文化底蕴不足所致。

吴本依旧采用直译加意译，在此不再赘述。吴本对"气"和"脏"相应的原因进行增补，此法虽然使行文复杂，失去了源语凝练之美，但通过增补法帮助目的语读者更好地理解"气脏相应"，有利于语义传递和文化外传。

2. 天食人以五气……五气入鼻……五味入口……以养五气。（《素问·六节藏象论》）

释义：天供给人们五气……五气由鼻吸入……五味由口进入……它的精微可养五脏之气。

李本：The heavens provide man with five kinds of Qi... When the five kinds of Qi are inhaled [into the body] through the nose... When the five kinds of flavors are taken in through the mouth... their nutrients [infuse into the Five Zang–Organs] to nourish the five kinds of Qi.

威本：Man receives the five atmospheric influences as food from Heaven... The five atmospheric influences enter the nostrils... The five flavors enter the mouth... The flavors which are stored nourish the five atmospheric influences.

文本：Heaven feeds man with the five qi... The five qi enter through the nose... The five flavors enter through the mouth... this serves to nourish the five qi.

吴本：The heaven provides the human being with five energies... The five energies from heaven enter into the body through the nose... The five tastes of foods from the earth enter into the body through the mouth... their essence will be transported and spread to nourish the energies of the five viscera.

句中有三处"五气"，前两处"五气"有两解，其一解为：臊、焦、香、腥、腐；其二解为：风、暑、湿、燥、寒。第三处"五气"为"脏腑之气"。

李本和文本采用直译加音译法，将三处"五气"采用统一译法，李本使用 five kinds of Qi（五种气），文本使用 five qi（五气）。这两种翻译差别不大。在对"气"的翻译上，两个译本均能保留源语文化与隐喻，相比之下，文本表述更符合术语翻译的规范，李本采用 kind（种类）一词意在强调"五气"的类别。从信息传递角度来看，李本和文本将三处"五气"均用同一表述，会使目的语读者难以理解第三处"五气"乃"脏腑之气"，显然不利于信息准确传递和文化交际。

威本采用意译法，将此三处"五气"均译作 five atmospheric influences（五种大气影响）。如果仅从隐喻角度来看，atmospheric influences 确实能很好地传递前两处"五气"的信息，但用 atmospheric influence 来隐喻"五脏之气"对信息传递造成一定影响，导致目的语读者对该处"五气"产生误解。

吴本采用直译加意译的方法，将前两处"五气"译作 the five energies from heaven，并采用加注的方法，解释"五气"与"五脏"相应；将第三处"五气"译作 the energies of the five viscera（五脏之气）。此法在信息传递上优于其余三个译本，以 energy 隐喻"气"也容易让目的语读者理解"气"的内涵，信息传递到位。但从行文来看，表述繁琐，易懂却尽失源语简洁之美。

（三）经络之气

五脏之间、五脏与其他组织器官之间依靠经络来连接。气不仅储藏于脏腑之中，而且还在经络之中运行，成为经络之气。对于经络之气，《素问》也有很多例证。

1. 上盛则气高，下盛则气胀，代则气衰，细则气少。（《素问·脉要精微论》）

释义：若见上部脉盛，是病气塞于胸；若见下部脉盛，是病气胀于腹；代脉是病气衰；细脉是病气少。

李本：Vigorous [beating of the pulse at] the upper [indicates] shortness of breath; vigorous [beating of the pulse at] the lower [indicates] distension; Dai (slow irregular and intermittent pulse) [indicates] decline of Qi; thin pulse [indicates] shortage of Qi.

威本：When the upper pulse is abundant then its impulse is strong; when the lower pulse is abundant then it indicates flatulence. When the pulse is irregular and tremulous and the beats occur at irregular intervals（代）, then the impulse of life fades; when the pulse is slender[smaller than feeble, but still perceptible, thin like a silk thread（细）], then the impulse of life is small.

文本：If it is abundant above, then the qi is [situated] high [in the body]. If it is abundant below, then this is a distension [because of] qi. If it is intermittent, then the qi is decreased.

吴本：If the pulse for the upper of the body is over-abundant, it shows the evil-energy is stagnated in the chest, if the pulse for the lower part of the body is overabundant, it shows the evil-energy is expanding in the abdomen; the intermittent pulse shows the debility of the energy, the thready pulse shows the patient to have less evil-energy.

本句讲述了脉诊的各种脉象，指出不同脉象的经气运行情况，如：大脉为邪气方张，代脉为元气衰弱，细脉为正气衰少，涩脉为血少气滞等。

对本句中"气"的翻译，李本和文本皆采用音译法，译作 qi，保留了中医术语的特色。从原文来看，"代则气衰，细则气少"中的"气"应为"正气"；"上盛则气高，下盛则气胀"中的"气"应为"邪气"。故李本和文本的

《黄帝内经素问》隐喻英译对比研究

音译难以将"气"的真正内涵传递到目的语，有损信息传递的准确性。

吴本采用意译法，将文中的气译为 vital energy（生命能量）或者 evil energy（邪恶的能量）。吴本译法对原文中的"气"表述具体，有利于目的语读者领悟此处"气"的内涵，在信息传递准确性上，吴本优于李本和文本。

威本对原文中"气"的理解有欠缺，将其意译为 pulse（脉冲）或者 impulse（脉冲）。pulse 和 impulse 对原文中的"脉"表述具体，但以此译"气"似有不妥，也不利于信息传递。

2. 脉气流经，**经气**归于肺，肺朝百脉，输精于皮毛。(《素问·经脉别论》)

释义：脉气流行在经络里，而上归于肺，肺在会合百脉以后，就把精气输送到皮毛。

李本：Maiqi (Vessel-Qi) flows in the Channels and Jingqi (Channel-Qi) flows to the lung. The lung is connected with all the vessels and transports Jing (Essence) to the skin and hair.

威本：The force of the pulse flows into the arteries（经）and the force of the arteries ascends into the lungs; the lungs send it into all the pulses（百脉）, which then transport its essence to the skin and the body hair.

文本：The qi in the vessels flows through the conduits. The qi in the conduits turns to the lung. The lung invites the one hundred vessels to have an audience with it. They transport essence to the skin and the body hair.

吴本：The channel-energy circulates in the channels and goes up to the lung. After the various channel-energies being converged in the lung, they are transported to the skin and hair.

血气流行在经脉之中，而到达于肺，肺又将血气输送到全身百脉中去，最后把精气输送到皮毛。此处的"气"为气血，"脉气"和"经气"应为对流经不同身体部位的气血的称谓。

李本采用音译加注法，将"脉气"和"经气"分别译为 Maiqi (Vessel-Qi) 和 Jingqi (Channel-Qi)。这有利于中医文化的外传和中医术语的规范。文本采用音译加注法，将"脉气"和"经气"分别译为 qi in the vessels 和 qi in the conduits。conduit 和 channel 都有"沟渠"之意，以此隐喻"经脉"，两种译法都能将源语信息准确传递到目的语。文本不重术语翻译规范，偏重于信息传递。

吴本采用意译法，将两者皆译作 channel-energy，信息传递准确，保留源语的隐喻，但在文化传递上略逊于李本。

威本采用意译法，将"脉气"和"经气"分别译为 the force of the pulse（脉搏之力）和 the force of the arteries（动脉之力）。虽然 pulse 和 artery 不完全对等于中医学中的"脉"和"经"，但这两种译法能将源语信息传递到位。

（四）营卫之气

1. 荣者，水谷之精气也……卫者，水谷之悍气也。（《素问·痹论》）

释义：荣是水谷所化成的精气……卫是水谷所化成的悍气。

李本：Rong (Nutrient-Qi) is the essential nutrient of water and food... Wei (Defensive-Qi) is the Hanqi (Swift-Qi) of water and food.

文本：The camp [qi], that is the essence qi of water and grain... The guard qi, that is the violent qi of water and grain.

吴本：The Rong energy is a refined energy which is transformed from water and cereals... The Wei-energy is the rough energy which is transformed from water and cereals.

"荣"，通"营"，"荣气"即"营气"。"营气"是水谷化生的精气；"卫"即"卫气"，是水谷所化的悍气。

李本采用音译加注法，将"荣"和"卫"分别译为 Rong (Nutrient-Qi) 和 Wei (Defensive-Qi)。Rong 和 Wei 体现中医术语的特点，注解中将"荣卫"直译为 nutrient（营养的、滋养的）和 defensive（防御的、自卫的），很好地保留原文隐喻；qi 保证了中医文化外传。李本对"荣卫"的翻译达到了文化及信息传递和术语翻译规范的要求。

吴本采用音译加意译法，将"荣""卫"译作 Rong energy 和 Wei energy。音译 rong 和 wei 能保证中医术语特征，但有碍信息传递，使目的语读者难解"荣""卫"的本意。

文本采用意译加音译，将"荣"和"卫"译作 camp qi 和 guard qi。guard（卫兵、守卫）不及李本所用 defensive（自卫的）准确，李本所用 defensive

《黄帝内经素问》隐喻英译对比研究

更能体现"卫气"的自发卫外功能，并非简单的守卫之功。文本误解了通假字"荣"，将"营养"之"营"理解为"宿营"之"营"，导致对"营气"误译。

2. 以从为逆，荣卫散乱，真气已失，邪独内著……（《素问·离合真邪论》）

释义：使顺证变成逆证，以致病人荣卫散乱，正气消耗，邪气旺盛……

李本：Taking Cong (favorable) as Ni (unfavorable) will cause disorder of Rong (Nutrient-Qi) and (Defensive-Qi), loss of Zhenqi and retention of Xie (Evil) in the body...

威本：Instead of bringing about compliance they bring about resistance. Blood and vital substances become scattered and spoiled, the normal constitution becomes completely lost and evil influences alone reign inside the body...

文本：He considers compliance to be opposition, causing camp and guard [qi] to disperse in disorder. The true qi has been lost already, while the evil [qi] alone remains attached internally...

吴本：In this way, the case of a favourable prognosis will become a case of an unfavourable prognosis, the Rong-energy and the Wei-energy of the patient will be confusing, his healthy-energy will be exhausting, and the evil-energy will become prosperous...

句中"荣卫"指"荣气"和"卫气"。

李本、文本和吴本沿用各自对此术语的一贯译法，分别将"荣卫"译为 Rong (Nutrient-Qi) and (Defensive-Qi)、camp and guard [qi] 和 the Rong-energy and the Wei-energy，此处不再赘述。

威本采用意译法，将"荣卫"译作 Blood and vital substances（血液和生命物质）。该译法能简单地表述"荣"的信息，但无法表达"卫"的信息，导致信息传递不对等。此外，单纯意译保留了源语隐喻所指，却忽视了源语文化外译和术语翻译的规范，有碍信息传递和文化交际。

第三节　脏腑相关隐喻及英译

"藏"，指藏于人体内的脏腑，包括五脏、六腑和奇恒之腑。由于五脏是人体最重要的脏腑器官，因此"藏"实际上是指以五脏为中心的五个生理病理系统。"象"相当于隐喻中的相似性，具体而言，是指脏腑与自然界或脏腑与社会中的事物及现象之间的相似性，即这五个系统的外在表现。通过隐喻的方法，可以使自然界或社会中与脏腑具有相似性的事物或现象的一部分意义投射到该脏腑之上，从而形成脏腑的特性。"藏象"实现了形与象的有机结合，充分反映出中医学对人体生理病理活动的认知方法。

总之，藏象学说是古代医家在长期的生活、医疗实践中，以古代解剖知识为基础，运用整体观察、取象比类等方法，观察脏腑反映于外的各种征象，经过不断的概括、抽象、推理，逐渐归纳而成。换言之，藏象理论是古人在客观所见与主观推理相结合的基础上构建起来的理论体系。在这一构建过程中，隐喻的思维方式起到了非常重要的推动作用。

1. 心者，君主之官也，神明出焉。（《素问·灵兰秘典论》）

释义：在人体内，心的重要性就好比君主，人们的聪明智慧都是从心生出来的。

李本：The heart is the organ [similar to] a monarch and is responsible for Shenming (mental activity or thinking).

威本：The heart is like the minister of the monarch who excels through insight and understanding.

文本：The heart is the official functioning as ruler. Spirit brilliance originates in it.

吴本：The heart is the supreme commander or the monarch of the human body, it dominates the spirit, ideology and thought of man.

这是一个十分典型的隐喻，心被隐喻成"君主之官"。君主是一国之首，主宰和控制着国家的一切。中医学认为，心是五脏六腑中最为重要的脏器，

《黄帝内经素问》隐喻英译对比研究

既能够统摄五脏六腑，又能配合其他脏腑的功能活动，对人的生命活动至关重要。另一方面，五脏六腑都要保护心，使其免受外界的干扰。因此，如果把人体看作国家，那么心即为至高无上的"国王"，是"君主之官"。

李本将原文句中隐喻做了显性处理，借助 similar to 将"心"类比为 monarch，强调心作为君主的主导地位。另外，李本采用直译加注法，将"神明"译为 Shenming (mental activity or thinking)，易于读者理解接受，同时还很好地保留了源语特色。

威本将该句译为 The heart is like the minister of the monarch who excels through insight and understanding（心脏就像帝王的大臣一样有敏锐的洞察力和理解力）。对该隐喻理解出现了偏差，错误地将"心"译为 minister（大臣），没有准确表达"心"这一脏器如君主一样的作用；同时，该译本也未能译出"神明出焉"的源语内涵，将其理解为 excels through insight and understanding（有敏锐的洞察力和观察力），这样会使读者无法准确理解心脏的功能。

文本基于忠实原文的原则，将"君主之官"译为 the official functioning as ruler，较好地保留了原文喻体；将"神明"译为 spirit brilliance，诠释出"心"的重要作用。

吴本采用直译法，译出"心"这一脏器的君主地位，同时增译 the human body，使用动词 dominate（支配、控制）表现出"心"在人体内的重要作用。这种直译加增译的方法，可以让读者更好地理解"心为君主"这一隐喻。将"神明"译为 spirit, ideology and thought，较为完整地阐释出"心"的职能作用。

2. 肺者，相傅之官，治节出焉。（《素问·灵兰秘典论》）

释义：肺好像是宰相，主一身之气，人体内外上下的活动，都需要它来调节。

李本：The lung is the organ [similar to] a prime minister and is responsible for Zhijie (management).

威本：The lungs are the symbol of the interpretation and conduct of the official jurisdiction and regulation.

文本：The lung is the official functioning as chancellor and mentor. Order and moderation originate in it.

吴本：The lung governs the various vessels and regulates the energy of the whole body, like a prime minister assisting the king to reign the country.

"傅"为辅助的意思，"相"即为宰相。句中以"相傅之官"隐喻肺，把肺比喻成朝廷中的宰相，具有辅佐君主的职能，用来说明肺具有辅助心脏的功能。

李本、吴本都将"相傅"译为 prime minister，文本将其译为 chancellor and mentor。"相傅"与 prime minister 或 chancellor 的职能和作用相类似，通过 prime minister 或 chancellor，目的语读者也能理解"相傅"的含义，产生类似的认知体验。用译语形象代替源语形象，在一定程度上较好地传达了源语的文化内涵。

威本没有直接翻译"相傅"，而是采用意译法，将该句译为 The lungs are the symbol of the interpretation and conduct of the official jurisdiction and regulation，阐述了"肺"的功能。这样易于目的语读者理解，但缺失了源语文化的特色 [1]。

吴本将"相傅"译为 a prime minister assisting the king to reign the country 较为准确，使用 assist 传递出肺具有"相傅"一样的职能。同时，用 govern the various vessels 和 regulate the energy of the whole body 两个动词短语说明肺的功能，即朝百脉和主治节。

3. 肝者，将军之官，谋虑出焉。（《素问·灵兰秘典论》）

释义：肝譬如将军，一切策略和智谋考虑，都产生于肝。

李本：The liver is the organ [similar to] a general and is responsible for strategy.

威本：The liver has the functions of a military leader who excels in his strategic planning.

文本：The liver is the official functioning as general. Planning and deliberation originate in it.

吴本：The liver is a vigorous viscera, its emotion is anger, it is like a general who is valiant and resourceful.

[1]　罗茜.《黄帝内经·素问》隐喻翻译对比研究 [J]. 海外英语，2017（24）：120.

将军，在古时为高级武官，性刚强而勇猛，负责统率全军。肝属风木，性动而急，恰如将军之勇。此处将肝喻为"将军之官"，用将军刚强急躁的性格来形容肝的生理特征。

李本和吴本分别用 similar to 和 like 将句中的隐喻显化。李本完整地译出原文，将"肝者，将军之官"直译为 The liver is the organ [similar to] a general，但未能具体指出"肝"与"将军"的共通之处。而吴本用 vigorous、anger 和 valiant 这几个词指出肝的"刚""怒""勇"，体现出"肝"与"将军"的共通之处。

威本把"将军"译为 a military leader（军事领导），未能准确体现"将军"一词的含义，不能准确地表达出肝的作用。

文本将"肝"译为 the official functioning as general，直接将"肝"比作"具有将军职能的官员"，较为忠实地体现了源文化的内涵。但美中不足的是，文本并未指出"肝"与"将军"的共通之处。

4. 胆者，中正之官，决断出焉。（《素问·灵兰秘典论》）

释义：胆是清虚的脏器，具有决断的能力。

李本：The gallbladder is the organ [similar to] an official of justice and is responsible for making decision.

威本：The gall bladder occupies the position of an important and upright official who excels through his decisions and judgment.

文本：The gallbladder is the official functioning as rectifier. Decisions and judgments originate in it.

吴本：The gallbladder is like an impartial judge who makes one to judge what is right and what is wrong.

胆除了具有贮藏和排泄胆汁的功能，还具有决断的功能，句中将胆喻为"中正之官"。中正之官，说明胆主决断的作用，不偏不倚，公正、果敢。将"胆"与"中正之官"进行类比，旨在进一步强调胆的这一功能。

李本和吴本分别用 similar to 和 be like 两个短语将原句中的隐喻做了显性处理，将"中正之官"分别译为 an official of justice 和 an impartial judge。"中正之官"是一种官职，显然李本将其译为 official（官员），较吴本中的 judge（法官）更为准确。

文本用 the official functioning as rectifier 对"中正之官"进行解释，并用 rectifier（改正者、矫正者）补译出了"中正之官"的职能，但 rectifier 强调的是"改正错误"，无法使读者更好地理解"胆"作为"中正之官"主决断的功能。

威本采用意译法将"中正之官"译为 occupies the position of an important and upright official。important 表示"重要的"，upright 表示"诚实的"，这两个形容词仅能使读者了解到这一官职很重要，且官居此位的官员都很诚实，但无法使读者准确理解其职能的真正内涵。

5. 膻中者，臣使之官，喜乐出焉。（《素问·灵兰秘典论》）

释义：膻中像个内臣，君主的喜乐，都由它透露。

李本：The pericardium is the organ [similar to] an envoy and is responsible for happiness and joy.

威本：The middle of the thorax (the part between the breasts) is like the official of the center who guides the subjects in their joys and pleasures.

文本：The danzhong is the official functioning as minister and envoy. Joy and happiness originate in it.

吴本：The Tan Zhong (indicating the pericadium here) is like a butler of the king who can transmit the joyfulness of the heart through it.

句中将膻中比喻为"臣使之官"。五脏六腑之中并无膻中，通常认为是心包。心包既对心脏具有保护功能，又会接受和执行心脏的命令，就像君主身边忠实的臣使，可代君受罚，苦其所苦，亦可传布心志之喜，乐其所乐，行使臣使之官的职能。

威本将"膻中"译为 the middle of the thorax (the part between the breasts)，把"膻中"理解为"膻中穴"是有失偏颇的。此处"膻中"应指"心包"。"心包"在英文中对应词汇为 pericardium，所以李本和吴本将其译为 pericardium 较为准确。

吴本中将"臣使之官"译为 butler（男仆），与"臣使"一词所表达的释义是有区别的，不能完整诠释"臣使"一词所表述的内涵[1]。

---

[1] 张焱，张丽，黄雯琴等.《黄帝内经》脏腑认知隐喻翻译研究（之二）[J]. 语文学刊（外语教育教学），2015（08）：4.

文本采用音译法，将"膻中"译为 danzhong，较好地保留了源语特色。将"臣使之官"译为 the official functioning as minister and envoy，用 minister（大臣）和 envoy（使者）两个词来表述"臣使"，能使读者更好地理解膻中的功能，即作为臣使，传达心志之喜。

6. 脾胃者，仓廪之官，五味出焉。（《素问·灵兰秘典论》）

释义：脾胃受纳水谷，好像仓库，五味化作人体的营养，是由它那儿产生的。

李本：The spleen and stomach are the organs [similar to] a granary official and are responsible for [digestion, absorption and transportation of] the five flavors.

威本：The stomach acts as the official of the public granaries and grants the five tastes.

文本：The spleen and the stomach are the officials responsible for grain storage. The five flavors originate from them.

吴本：The spleen is like an officer who is in charge of the granary, it takes charge of the digesting, absorbing, spreading and storing of the essence of food.

句中将脾胃喻为"仓廪之官"，仓廪是指贮存谷物的仓库。脾胃具有受纳水谷、运化精微、供应人体需要的各种物质的功能，行使了"仓廪之官"的职能。

李本、吴本分别使用 similar to 和 be like 显化处理原文中的隐喻，将"仓廪之官"分别译为 a granary official 和 an officer who is in charge of the granary，使读者更容易理解和接受"仓廪之官"主管粮仓的职能，从而更好地理解"脾胃"的受纳功能。

文本采用通俗易懂的语言将"仓廪之官"直译为 the officials responsible for grain storage，简洁明了地解释出"脾胃"的"仓廪"职能。

威本将"仓廪之官"译为 the official of the public granaries，译出了脾胃的"仓廪"功能，但在翻译"脾胃"时，只译出了胃 stomach，却漏译了脾 spleen，会使读者对"脾胃"的理解出现偏差。

7. 大肠者，传道之官，变化出焉。（《素问·灵兰秘典论》）

释义：大肠主管输送，食物的消化、吸收、排泄过程是在它那儿最后完成的。

李本：The large intestine is the organ [similar to] an official in charge of trans-portation and is responsible for Bianhua (change and transformation).

威本：The lower intestines are like the officials who propagate the Right Way of Living, and they generate evolution and change.

文本：The large intestine is the official functioning as transmitter along the Way. Changes and transformations originate in it.

吴本：The large intestine is the route for transmitting the drosses, it transforms the drosses into faeces and then excretes them to the outside of the body.

大肠为六腑之一，主要功能是传导水谷糟粕。饮食经小肠消化吸收后，其糟粕部分下输大肠，由大肠继续吸收浊中之清，其余的形成粪便。在大肠之气的作用下，将粪便传送至大肠末端，并排出体外，故句中将大肠喻为"传道之官"。

李本和文本分别将"传道之官"译为 an official in charge of transportation 和 the official functioning as transmitter along the Way，transportation（运输）和 transmitter（传输者）两词较好地表达出大肠的传导作用。

威本由于受其自身文化背景影响，将"传道之官"错误地译为 the officials who propagate the Right Way of Living（传经布道之官），未能理解此处"传道"即"传导"的含义，会使读者曲解大肠的传导作用。

吴本没有译出"传道之官"的官职意义，只是采用意译的方法将其译为 the route for transmitting the drosses，阐释出大肠作为"传道之官"的功能。这种译法虽能实现交际目的，但失去了源语的文化特色。

8. 小肠者，受盛之官，化物出焉。（《素问·灵兰秘典论》）

释义：小肠的功能，是接受脾胃已消化的食物后，进一步起到分化作用。

李本：The small intestine is the organ [similar to] an official in charge of re-ception and is responsible for [further] digestion of foods.

威本：The small intestines are like the officials who are trusted with riches, and they create changes of the physical substance.

文本：The small intestine is the official functioning as recipient of what has been perfected. The transformation of things originates in it.

吴本：The small intestine receives the food from the stomach, it digests the food further, divides them into the essence and the dregs, then absorbs the essence and transmits the dregs to the large intestine.

受盛，即接受、以器盛物的意思。化物，有变化、消化的意思。小肠进一步消化经胃初步消化的饮食物，将水谷化为精微物质，故句中将小肠喻为"受盛之官"。

李本和威本分别使用 similar to 和 be like 两个短语将小肠比作 official，将隐喻显化。其中，李本将"受盛之官"译为 an official in charge of reception，说明这一官职的职能为 reception（接受，接纳），更易于读者理解小肠受盛化物的功能。威本将"受盛之官"译为 the officials who are trusted with riches，对其职能表述不够准确，很容易造成读者的困惑。如将其译为 the officials who are in charge of reception of tributes，则更能体现"受盛之官"的"受盛"职能。

吴本采用意译的方法，用 receive、digest、absorb 和 transmit 等词描述出小肠的功能，易于读者理解小肠泌别清浊、受盛化物的作用，但未能保留"受盛之官"的源语特色。

文本采用直译法，将"受盛之官"译为 the official functioning as recipient of what has been perfected，形象地传达出原文的隐喻含义，较为准确地解释了小肠的功能。

9. 肾者，作强之官，伎巧出焉。（《素问·灵兰秘典论》）

释义：肾是精力的源泉，能产生出智慧和技巧来。

李本：The kidney is the organ [similar to] an official with great power and is responsible for skills.

威本：The kidneys are like the officials who do energetic work, and they excel through their ability and cleverness.

文本：The kidneys are the official functioning as operator with force. Technical skills and expertise originate from them.

吴本：The kidney is an organ with strong functions, when the essence and energy in the kidney are abundant, the body will be strong and the person is skillful and wise in doing things.

肾为人体"先天之本"，主藏精，与人的生长、发育、生殖等密切相关。肾气充盈则人体强壮，故被喻为"作强之官"。

李本、威本和文本都把"肾"比作 official，并分别使用 with 介词短语、who 引导的定语从句和 functioning as 分词短语等修饰手段加以解释，形象地表达出肾的强大功能。吴本则是去掉隐喻形象，直接将"肾者，作强之官"译为 The kidney is an organ with strong functions，用浅显易懂的语言向读者描述肾的功能，易于目的语读者理解，但这种译法未能很好地保留源语的文化特色。

10. 三焦者，<u>决渎之官</u>，水道出焉。（《素问·灵兰秘典论》）

释义：三焦主疏通水液，周身行水的道路，是由它管理。

李本：Sanjiao (triple energizer) is the organ [similar to] official in charge of dredging and is responsible for regulating the water-passage.

威本：The burning spaces are like the officials who plan the construction of ditches and sluices, and they create waterways.

文本：The triple burner is the official functioning as opener of channels. The paths of water originate in it.

吴本：The triple warmer takes the office of dredging water in the watercourse of the whole body, it takes charge of the activity of the vital energy of the body fluid and the regulation and the dredging of the fluid.

三焦居于胃肠道与膀胱之间，引导肠胃中的水液渗入膀胱，是水液下输膀胱的通道。三焦水道通畅，胃肠中的水液就可以顺利渗入膀胱，成为尿液生成之源。将三焦喻为"决渎之官"，形象地说明了三焦疏通人体水道，运行水液的重要生理功能。

李本采用音译加注法将三焦译为 Sanjiao (triple energizer)，音译保留了源语特色，而括号里的注解 triple energizer 解释了三焦主持诸气、总司人体气化的功能特点。在西方，"气"普遍被理解为 energy 或是 vital energy，所以该译法更易于为读者理解[1]。

威本、文本和吴本将"三焦"分别译为 burning spaces、triple burner、

---

[1] 吴海燕，岳峰.中医术语"三焦"英译探析 [J].中国科技术语，2011，13（6）：22.

triple warmer。三个译本中 burn 都具有"燃烧、烧焦"之义，"焦"的含义被局限于较狭小的范围，不及 triple energizer 更能体现三焦的功能特点。

鉴于"决渎之官"在西方语言文化中空缺，四个译本都做了解释性翻译。李本和吴本使用 dredging（挖掘），威本使用 construction（建造、修建），文本使用 opener（开启的工具），较为准确地描述出"三焦"作为"决渎之官"负责挖沟渠和疏通水道的职能。

11. 膀胱者，州都之官，津液藏焉，气化则能出矣。（《素问·灵兰秘典论》）

释义：膀胱是水液聚会的地方，经过气化作用，才能把尿排出体外。

李本：The bladder is the organ [similar to] an official in charge of reservoir and is responsible for accumulation and discharge [of liquids] through Qihua (Qi-trans-formation).

威本：The groins and the bladder are like the magistrates of a region or a district, they store the overflow and the fluid secretions which serve to regulate vaporiza-tion.

文本：The urinary bladder is the official functioning as regional rectifier. The body liquids are stored in it.

吴本：The bladder takes the office of gathering, it stores the water and fluid, after the body fluid is transformed into water by the activating of vital energy, it can be excreted.

膀胱位于下腹部，居肾之下，大肠之前，是一个中空的囊状器官，为人体水液汇聚之所，具有贮存和排泄尿液的生理功能，因此被称为"州都之官"。

对于"膀胱"的翻译，四个译本都用了 bladder 一词，较为准确。但威本在翻译"膀胱"时，多译出 groins（腹股沟），属于误译。

对于"州都之官"的翻译，四个译本既有相同之处，又各有不同。李本和文本都将核心词"官"译为 official，李本使用介词短语 in charge of reser-voir 修饰 official，较好地表达出膀胱作为"州都之官"贮存水液的功能；文本则用分词短语 functioning as regional rectifier（充当地方判决官）来描述州都之官的职能，属于误译。威本将"州都之官"译为 magistrate（地方法官），也曲解了原文语义。吴本采用意译的方法，用动词短语 takes the office of 取代了原文中的隐喻，译出了膀胱的作用，便于读者理解接受。

第四节　战争隐喻及英译

战国时期，群雄争霸，战乱纷争。战争决定各诸侯国的存亡，事关民众生死，成为人们讨论的热门话题。认识到疾病与战争的相似性，《素问》以"治疗疾病就是一场战争[1]"这一结构隐喻为基础，运用与源域"战争"相关的词汇描述目标域"疾病"。这样就将疾病与战争的诸多相似性联系起来，用比较熟悉的战争概念阐释抽象复杂的疾病过程，探讨致病因素的性质和致病特点，说明各种病理变化及病机之间的联系，从而揭示疾病的发生、发展、演变及转归的机理。

《素问》中的战争隐喻反映了一系列的对应关系：战争对应疾病、战场对应人体、敌人对应疾病或病菌等，以及武器对应医药、防御系统对应免疫系统、病愈对应战胜、不愈对应战败等。（图 6-1）

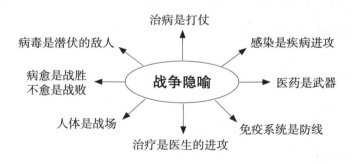

图 6-1　战争隐喻概念系统

本节选取《素问》中有关致病因素的性质、致病因素侵袭方式、正气防御和抵抗方式、正邪对抗方式与结果、预后不良或疾病恶化等方面的战争隐

---

[1]　Ungerer F. & Schmid H. J. *An Introduction to Cognitive Linguistics* [M]. Beijing: Beijing Foreign Language Teaching and Research Press, 2001: 67.

喻，对四个译本的翻译方法和特点进行对比研究及分析。

一、致病因素的性质

（一）贼

"贼"本义指抢劫、偷窃财物的人，也指作乱叛国危害国家的人。《素问》中将引起人体疾病的不正常气候因素隐喻为"贼"，因为外感致病因素与"贼"具有一定的相似性，常在不经意间偷偷侵袭、攻击、伤害人体。以下为与"贼"相关的部分隐喻。

1. 夫上古圣人之教下也，皆谓之虚邪贼风，避之有时。（《素问·上古天真论》）

释义：上古时代的圣人，教导他的下属们说，对于能损伤人体的虚邪贼风，要适时地加以回避。

李本：When the sages in ancient times taught the people, they emphasized [the importance of] avoiding Xuxie (Deficiency–Evil) and Zeifeng (Thief–Wind) in good time.

威本：In the most ancient times the teachings of the sages（圣人）were followed by those beneath them; they said that weakness and noxious influences and injurious winds should be avoided at specific times.

文本：Now, when the sages of high antiquity taught those below, they always spoke to them [about the following]. The depletion evil and the robber wind, there are [specific] times when to avoid them.

吴　本：In ancient times people behaved according to the teaching of preserving health of the sages: All evil energies of various seasons are harmful to people, they attack the body when it is in general debility, and they should be defended anytime and everywhere.

"虚邪"是乘人体之虚伤人的邪气，"贼风"泛指四时不正之气[1]，"虚邪贼风"常乘人体之虚，像盗贼偷窃一样悄无声息地侵袭人体，隐喻在不知不觉中侵袭人体的外恶邪气。

---

[1] 邵学鸿. 对《内经》虚邪贼风的探讨 [J]. 北京中医药大学学报，2007（10）：658.

李本使用音译加注法将"贼风"译为 Zeifeng (Thief-Wind)，音译 Zeifeng 保留了中医术语的汉语语言风格，直译 Thief-Wind 虽然保留了原文的隐喻特色，但是对目的语读者理解 Thief 与 Wind 之间的隐喻关系可能会造成困难。

同样，文本将"贼风"直译为 the robber wind 亦不能帮助读者将 robber（抢劫者）和 wind（风）之间的隐喻意义关联起来，语言交际失败。同时，文本的 the robber wind 暗含"明目张胆地抢劫"之义，这与"贼风"在句中"悄无声息侵袭人体"的特点相去甚远。

威本将"贼风"意译为 injurious winds（有伤害的风），吴本将"虚邪""贼风"合并意译为 all evil energies of various seasons（四时不正之气），两个译文虽然未能有效体现"贼风"悄无声息侵袭人体的特点，但是成功传达了"贼风"是不正之气的内涵意义，实现了语言的转换。

所以，结合李本的音译法和吴本的意译法，采用音译加注法将"贼风"译为 Zeifeng (all evil energies of various seasons)，或许能更好兼顾形与义的表达。

2. 用实为虚，以邪为真，用针无义，反为气贼，夺人正气。（《素问·离合真邪论》）

释义：把实证当作虚证，把邪气当作正气，用针没有法则，邪气就会为害，损伤病人正气。

李本：Taking Shi (Excess) as Xu (Deficiency), regarding Xie (Evil) as Zheng (Genuine-Qi) and failure to abide by the rules for needling will consequently strengthen pathogenic factors and reduce Zhengqi (Healthy-Qi).

威本：Those who use fullness in order to create emptiness, those who use evil in order to bring about normalcy, and those who use the needle without the right way, those physicians will only bring about a contrary (wrong) reaction and hurt the patient's normal health.

文本：If [a practitioner] treats a repletion as if it were a depletion, if he considers evil [qi] as if it were true [qi] and if he applies the needles disregarding what is right to do, contrary [to his intentions] he will be a plunderer of qi in that he removes the proper qi of [that] person.

吴本：When one mistakes the sthenic syndrome as the asthenic syndrome, mistakes the evil–energy as the healthy energy, and applies the needle without any rule, the evil–energy will cause damage and hurt the healthy–energy of the patient.

"气贼"为"正气"之反义，隐喻像盗贼偷窃一样悄无声息侵袭人体的邪气。翻译此句时应注意以下两点：句式结构和"气贼"的译法。

李本使用动名词 taking、regarding 以及名词 failure 将前三个分句"用实为虚，以邪为真，用针无义"译为名词短语充当句子主语，明确指明动词"反为"和"夺"的施动者，准确表达原文的逻辑关系。将"气贼"意译为 pathogenic factors（致病因素），未能保留原文的隐喻特色，但是准确表达了"气贼"的内涵意义，实现内容上忠实于原文。

威本将"气贼"译为 a contrary (wrong) reaction，是把副词"反"误解为形容词"相反的"，修饰名词"贼"，表意不准确；将 those physicians 作为 bring about a contrary (wrong) reaction 的施动者，与原文的逻辑结构不符。

同样，文本将"反为气贼"译为 he will be a plunderer of qi，不仅将动词"为"的施动者"用针无义"误解为 he（a practitioner 行医者），而且将"气贼"直译为 a plunderer of qi（气的盗贼），未能正确理解"气贼"的内涵意义，内容上偏离原文。

吴本将"气贼"意译为 the evil–energy，表意准确，但是 When 引导的从句未能表明"气贼"出现的原因，内容上较为突兀。

3. 浅深不得，反为大贼，内动五脏，后生大病。（《素问·刺要论》）

释义：所以针刺的深浅，如不恰当，反有很大的危害。在内里会伤害五脏，要生大病的。

李本：Hence improper depth [of needling] brings about great disaster that affects the Five Zang–Organs and leads to serious diseases.

文本：When [the proper measure of] shallow or deep [piercing] is not achieved, contrary [to one's intentions] this will cause severe injury and excites the five depots internally. This will generate a serious disease subsequently.

吴本：Therefore, if the depth of the pricking is improper, it can, on the contrary, cause great damage. If the viscus inside is hurt, the patient will contract serious disease.

"贼"用作名词时，本义指做坏事的人，句中隐喻为"祸患、危害"。针刺的"浅深不得"就像做坏事的人，会对人体造成很大的危害。

李本、文本、吴本分别将"大贼"直译为 great disaster、severe injury 和 great damage，分别将动词"为"译为 brings about、will cause 和 can cause 充当句子谓语，体现出"反为大贼"之义。三个译本区别不大，都使用意译法表达"贼"在句中"祸患、危害"之义，同时保留了原文的战争隐喻，成功实现语言和文化的双层转换。

从句式来看，李本将"浅深不得"译为名词短语 improper depth [of needling] 作为主句主语，使用 affects...and leads to 并列句结构表达"内动五脏，后生大病"之间的顺承关系，行文流畅，表意明确，相较于文本和吴本的主从复合句，句式更为简洁清晰。

4. 寒热内贼，其病益甚。（《素问·六元正纪大论》）

释义：这样，寒热之气就会内伤脏腑，它的病就要加重了。

李本：[Then] the interior [will be] damaged by Cold and Heat and the disease will be worsened.

文本：Cold or heat would cause internal injuries. The illness [you try to heal] will become even more severe.

吴本：In this case, the cold and heat evils will injure the viscera internally, and the disease will become worse.

句中将"寒热之气"喻为做坏事的人，会内伤脏腑。"贼"为动词，隐喻义为"造成伤害"。

三个译本都将"贼"当作动词，分别意译为 damage、cause injuries 和 injure，准确表达"贼"在句中"造成伤害"之义，同时保留了原文的战争隐喻。

相比之下，李本将"寒热内贼"译为 [Then] the interior [will be] damaged by Cold and Heat，补译出"内"和"贼"之间的被动关系，利于目的语读者理解原文的内涵意义。吴本将"内贼"意译为 will injure the viscera internally，明确"贼"的对象为脏腑，虽然不如文本的 would cause internal injuries 简洁，但是形和义都更加贴近原文。

（二）客

"客"常用作名词，意为"来宾、宾客"，与"主"相对，引申为外来的盗寇或敌人；作动词时，意为"寄居，旅居"。《素问》中将引起人体病患的外部因素比喻为"客"；有时还将"客"用作动词，用以说明风寒邪气侵犯、寄居人体而致病。下面是与"客"相关的部分隐喻。

1. 厥阴司天，客胜则耳鸣掉眩，甚则咳；主胜则胸胁痛，舌难以言。（《素问·至真要大论》）

释义：厥阴司天，客气胜就患耳鸣眩晕，甚则咳嗽；主气胜就病胸胁疼痛，舌强难以说话。

李本：[When] Jueyin dominates the heavens, the domination of Ke (Guest-Qi) causes tinnitus and dizziness, even cough [if it is] serious; the domination of Zhu (Host-Qi) causes pain in the chest and rib-sides and stiffness of tongue [that makes it] difficult to speak.

文本：When the ceasing yin [qi] controls heaven, in case the visitor [qi] dominates, then [people suffer from] ringing [sounds] in the ears and from swaying and dizziness. When [the domination is] severe, then [the patients] cough. In case the host [qi] dominates, then there is pain in the chest and in the flanks and the tongue has difficulties in speaking.

吴本：When Jueyin is controlling the heaven energy, if the guest energy is overcoming, people will contract tinnitus and dizziness, or even cough; if the host energy is overcoming, people will contract pain in the chest and hypochondrium, and also difficulty in speaking due to stiff tongue.

句中"客"为名词，意为"客气"，隐喻外来的致病因素，与"主"对应。

三个译本都正确理解了"客"在句中"客气"之义，采用直译意译相结合的方法将"客"译为 guest/visitor qi；相应地，将"主"译为 host qi。这样，既忠实于原文内容，又保留了战争隐喻特色。

相较而言，李本采用音译加注法，将"客"译为 Ke (Guest-Qi)，将"主"译为 Zhu (Host-Qi) 为佳译。音译 Ke/Zhu 保留了中医术语的语言风格，直译意译相结合 Guest-Qi/ Host-Qi 解释了"客"和"主"的内涵意义，实现文化与内容的传递。同时李本使用 guest 和 host 这一对反义词表达"客"和"主"的对应关系，使用 Qi 这一约定俗成的译法表达中医术语"气"，用词精准。

2. 风客淫气，精乃亡，邪伤肝也。（《素问·生气通天论》）

释义：风邪侵入人体，渐渐侵害元气，精血就要损耗，这是由于邪气伤害肝脏的缘故。

李本：When wind attacks the body, [it gradually] damages Qi and exhausts Jing (Essence). [This is because of] the impairment of the liver by Xie (Evil).

威本：If the wind enters the body and exhausts man's breath, then his essence will be lost and the evil influences will injure his liver.

文本：When wind settles [in the body] and encroaches upon the [proper] qi, then the essence vanishes, and the evil harms the liver.

吴本：Owning to the wind associates with the liver (liver correspond to the wind and wood), when one is hurt by excessive wind-evil, the essence of life and blood will suffer severe damage. As blood is stored in the liver, the wind-evil will hurt the liver too.

"客"用作动词时，本义为"（人）旅居异国他乡"。句中将风邪喻为人，像做客一样寄居于人体，"风客"指风邪侵入人体。

李本将"客"意译为 (wind) attacks the body，形象地表达出外来风邪对人体的侵害，保留了原文的战争隐喻。

威本和文本分别将"客"译为 (wind) enters the body 和 settles [in the body]，正确理解了"客"的词性和意义，表达出风邪为外来之物并寄居于人体，但是未能传递"风邪对人体的侵害"之内涵意义。

吴本对此句的翻译较为繁冗。将"客"意译为 hurt，强调风邪对人体造成伤害，但是脱离了"客"的本义；同时花费笔墨增译"风"与"肝"之间的关系，解释为何"邪伤肝"会导致"精乃亡"。这一译法有助于目的语读者理解原文，但是行文繁冗，失去原文语言的凝练之美。

3. 此皆卫气所留止，邪气之所客也，针石缘而去之。（《素问·五脏生成》）

释义：这些都是卫气所留止的地方，也是邪气容易留止的处所，如果受了邪气的侵袭，就赶紧用针刺或砭石除掉它。

李本：These are all the places where Weiqi (Defensive-Qi) maintains and Xieqi (Evil-Qi) stays. Needling [at these places] can eliminate [pathogenic factors].

威本：They all protect the life-giving element and prevent evil influences from entering. When acupuncture is applied it causes evil influences to depart.

文本：All these are locations where the guard qi [can] come to a halt and where the evil qi [can] settle as visitor. Needles and [pointed] stones remove the [evil qi] in an encircling manner.

吴本：All of them are the places for the Wei-energy to stay, and they are also the places for the evil-energy to reside, when one is attacked by the evil-energy, it should be removed by acupuncture or by the therapy of stone needle.

句中"客"为动词，与"留止"意义相似，皆有寄居之义，"邪气之所客"意指邪气所留止的地方。

李本和吴本分别将"客"意译为 stay 和 reside，隐喻"邪气"像人一样客居于某处，是对原文的忠实表达。但是李本将"留止"译为 maintain，意义不恰当，因为 maintain 指维持某一水平或状态，不能表示留在某处。相比之下，吴本将"留止"译为 stay，不仅表意准确，而且用词比较灵活。

文本将"客"直译为 settle as visitor，貌似较为形象地表达出邪气是外来之物，但对目的语读者来说，可能很难理解 the evil qi 与 visitor 之间的联系。

威本将"邪气之所客"译为 prevent evil influences from entering（阻止邪气进入），理解原文有偏差，未能正确理解"邪气"与"客"之间的逻辑关系。

4. 风雨之伤人也，先客于皮肤，传入于孙脉。（《素问·调经论》）

释义：风雨伤人是先侵入皮肤，然后传入孙脉。

李本：[When] wind and rain attack human beings, [they] first invade the skin. [Then they are] transmitted to the fine Collaterals.

文本：When wind and rain harm a person, they first settle in the skin, whence they are transmitted into the tertiary vessels.

吴本：When the wind and rain hurt the body, it invades into the skin first, then enters into the minute collateral.

"客"用作动词时，本义为"客居"，句中取其隐喻义"外邪寄居并侵犯人体"。"客于皮肤"指风雨侵入皮肤且对人体造成伤害。

李本和吴本都将"客"意译为invade，区别在于李本将invade用作及物动词，为常用法；吴本将invade用作不及物动词，使用invade into结构，强调风雨侵入皮肤之义。二者既表达出风雨由外向内进入皮肤之义，又体现出风雨对皮肤的侵害这一内涵意义，保留了原文的战争隐喻。

文本将"客"译为settle in，正确表达出"客居"之义，但未能体现出风雨对皮肤侵害的内涵意义。

综上所述，"客"用作动词时，兼具"寄居"和"侵害"两层含义。翻译时应该注意，原文中"客"是单指"寄居"之义，还是强调"由外入侵并造成伤害"之义。

（三）邪

"邪"本义是指品行不正的人，作形容词时，意思为"不正当，不正派"。在《素问》中，"邪"与人体正气相对，隐喻各种致病因素及其病理损害。下面是与"邪"相关的部分隐喻。

1. 故邪不能伤其形体，其病生于内，其治宜毒药。（《素问·异法方宜论》）

释义：这样，虽然外邪不易侵犯他们的躯体，但是，由于饮食、情志等问题，很容易在内脏里发生疾病。在治疗上就需用药物。

李本：[That is why] Xie (Evil) cannot attack their body. Their illness is usually endogenous and can be treated by Duyao (drugs).

威本：Hence evil cannot injure their external bodies, and if they get diseases they strike at the inner body. These diseases are most successfully cured with poison medicines.

文本：Hence, [external] evil cannot harm their physical body; their diseases emerge from within. For their treatment, toxic drugs are appropriate.

吴本：In this case, although their bodies can hardly be hurt by the exogenous evil, but are apt to suffer from visceral illness due to food and emotions. In treating the disease, drug is necessary.

"邪"本义为品行不正的人，句中隐喻能致病的邪气，指外邪。

现代中医学认为，"邪"与人体"正气"构成相对概念，实质为致病因素（pathogenic factor）。WHO 和世中联中医术语标准将"邪、病邪、邪气"意译为 pathogen，将"外邪、客邪"译为 external pathogen。此译法虽然意义上较为准确，但是又过于现代，失去了原文的汉语语言风格 [1]。

一直以来"邪"被理解为 evil，因为古人认为疾病与中邪有关。这一译法虽然意思上不准确，但当前已被很多出版物接受为约定俗成的译法。

四个译本都使用 evil 表达"邪"，其中文本和吴本分别将其译为 external evil 和 exogenous evil，体现出"外邪"之义。李本采用音译加注法将"邪"译为 Xie (Evil)，既表达出"邪"的内涵意义，又保留中医术语的语言风格，顺应中医药对外传播交流的趋势。

2.……外虚内乱，淫邪乃起。（《素问·八正神明论》）

释义：络脉外虚，经脉内乱，所以病邪就乘之而起。

李 本：...cause weakness in the external and disorder in the internal, consequently leading to the onset of diseases.

威本：...there is deficiency at the outside and disorder and confusion in (the body), and excess and evil will arise.

文本：...external depletion [goes along with] internal disorder. As a result, excess evil rises.

吴本：...as a result the syndrome of outer asthenia of the collateral and inner confusion of the channel will occur, and the evil-energy will take advantage to invade.

句中"邪"为名词，隐喻致病之邪气，与"真"为对应概念。

中医病因学中"淫"为"浸淫、过度"之义 [2]，因此"淫邪"常被译为 excessive evil 或者 excess evil，如文本和威本。这种译法将直译与意译相结合，既保留了原文的字面意思，又传达了内涵意义。

李本没有直接翻译"淫邪"，而是采用意译法将"淫邪乃起"译为

---

[1] 李照国.WHO 西太区与世界中医药学会联合会中医名词术语国际标准比较研究：病因部分（一）（英文）[J]. 中西医结合学报，2009，7（3）：285.

[2] 鞠海洋，郑杨，邸鹏举等. 外感病因"淫、邪、疫、毒"基本概念探析 [J]. 亚太传统医药，2015，11（9）：58.

leading to the onset of diseases（导致疾病的发生），表意明确，因为从上下文来看，此处"淫邪"即疾病。

吴本将"淫邪乃起"译为 the evil-energy will take advantage to invade，形象地表达出"乃起"之动作，体现病邪乘之而起的特点；但是将"淫邪"译为 the evil-energy 不合适，一方面未能表达"淫"为"太过"之义，另一方面 evil-energy 常被吴本用来指邪气。

3. 夫<u>邪</u>之入于脉也，寒则血凝泣，暑则气淖泽，<u>虚邪</u>因而入客，亦如经水之得风也。（《素问·离合真邪论》）

释义：凡邪气入于经脉，如为寒邪，则气血凝涩不畅；如为热邪，则气血沸腾而滑利；虚邪贼风入侵于经络，也像经水遇到暴风一样。

李本：[The same is the case] when Xie (Evil) invades the Channels. When it is cold, blood stagnates; when it is hot, Qi flows smoothly and rapidly. The invasion of Xie (Evil) [into the body] is just like the river blown by wind, sometimes leading to something like soaring waves in the Channels.

威本：Now evil influences can enter the pulse. When there is cold the blood congeals; when there is heat the breath comes smoothly and gently. Because of deficiency and evil, alien matter can enter (into the pulse).

文本：Now, when evil enters the vessels, if it is cold, then the blood congeals so that [its flow] is impeded. If it is summerheat, then the qi is saturated with moisture. When subsequently a depletion evil enters [the vessels] and settles [there], then this, too, is similar to when the main waters are affected by wind.

吴本：When the evil-energy invades the channel，if it is a cold-evil，it will cause the blood to become moist. When the wind-evil invades the channel, it is like water being attacked by wind.

"邪"为邪气、病邪，"虚邪"为四时不正之气，当人体正气虚弱之时乘机伤人致病。

李本采用其一贯译法，使用音译加注法将"邪"和"虚邪"都译为 Xie (Evil)，此译法不能体现"邪"和"虚邪"的区别。李本在《素问·上古天真论》中将"虚邪"译为 Xuxie (Deficiency-Evil)[1]，既保留了中医术语的汉语语言风格，又解释了内涵意义，为佳译。

威本和文本分别使用 evil influences 和 evil 表达"邪"，都传递出"邪"在句中的意思。但是，威本把"虚邪"译为 deficiency and evil 不妥，错把"虚"和"邪"当作并列之物。文本将"虚邪"译为 a depletion evil（亏损邪气），误解了"虚"和"邪"的关系。

吴本使用 evil-energy 表达"邪"，同时将"虚邪"译为 the wind-evil，此译法将虚邪与贼风等同，偏离原文意思，是对原文的过度解读。

4. 邪气盛则实，精气夺则虚。（《素问·通评虚实论》）

释义：邪气盛，就是实证，正气被伤，就是虚证。

李 本：Predomination of Xieqi (Evil-Qi) is called Shi (Excess) and insufficiency of Jingqi (Essence-Qi) is called Xu (Deficiency).

威 本：When harmful influences are plentiful then we can speak of fullness; when the essences are decreased we can speak of emptiness.

文 本：When evil qi abounds, then [this is] repletion. When the essence qi is lost, then [this is] depletion.

吴 本：When the evil-energy is overabundant, it is sthenia, when the healthy-energy is injured, it is asthenia.

与"邪"的译法一致，李本使用音译加注法将"邪气"译为 Xieqi (Evil-Qi)，既表达出邪气为不正之气的内涵意义，又保留了中医术语的语言风格。文本将"邪气"译为 evil qi，与李本译法相似，重在传递内容，未保留原文的语言风格。同时，"邪气"为中医学的重要术语，按照专有名词的译法规则，首字母应为大写形式，译作 Evil qi 更佳。

威本将"邪气"意译为 harmful influences（有害的影响），概念过于宽泛，只表达出"邪气"为伤害人体的有害因素，未指明"邪气"的具体内容。

吴本将"邪气"译为 the evil-energy，同"邪"的译法一样，二者无区分度。

---

[1] 李照国.黄帝内经：素问（汉英对照）[M].北京：世界图书出版公司，2005：5.

二、致病因素侵袭方式

《素问》在描述内外致病因素侵袭、损伤人体时，以隐喻的方式大量使用战争进攻类的词汇，如"夺""犯""伤""伐""扰"等。

（一）夺

"夺"的本义为"抢夺"或"丧失"。在《素问》中，"夺"意为"损耗""衰败"或"削弱"等，其主语多为抽象状态的疾病或者邪气。

1. 惊而夺精，汗出于心。（《素问·经脉别论》）

释义：受惊而影响精神的时候，由于心气受伤而汗出于心。

李本：Fright depletes Jing (Essence) and leads to sweating from the heart.

威本：When man is shocked and startled he does violence to his spirit and vitality, and perspiration is produced by the heart.

文本：When one was frightened and has lost essence, the [resulting] sweat originates from the heart.

吴本：When one is frightened, his heart will certainly be hurt.

句中"夺"为动词，源于本义"抢夺"，取其隐喻义"削弱"，"惊而夺精"指受惊会削弱精神。

精是构成和维持人体生命活动的基本物质基础，在现行译法中，essence 已基本上约定俗成地用以翻译"精"和"精气"等概念[1]。李本将"夺"译为 deplete（损耗），使用音译加注法将"精"译为 Jing (Essence)，表意准确，语言简练，是对原文的忠实表达。

威本将"夺精"译为 (man) does violence to his spirit and vitality，不仅把"夺"曲解为 does violence to（破坏），把"夺"的施动者"惊"误解为 man，还混淆了"精"和"神"的概念。同样，文本将"夺精"译为 (one) has lost essence，将"夺"误解为 has lost（丢失），亦曲解了"夺"的施动者。

吴本漏译了原文中的"夺精"。

综上所述，翻译本句时应该明确"夺"的施动者为"惊"。可以采用李本的方法，使用主动语态，将"惊而夺精"译为 Fright depletes Jing (Es-

---

[1]　李照国. 中医文化关键词 [M]. 北京：外语教学与研究出版社，2018：2.

sence），也可以使用被动语态，将"惊而夺精"译为 one is frightened and Jing (Essence) is depleted/hurt。

2. 用针无义，反为气贼，夺人正气，以从为逆。（《素问·离合真邪论》）

释义：用针没有法则，邪气就会为害，损伤病人正气，使顺证变成逆证。

李本：Failure to abide by the rules for needling will consequently strengthen pathogenic factors and reduce Zhengqi (Healthy-Qi). Taking Cong (favorable) as Ni (unfavorable) will cause disorder of Rong (Nutrient-Qi) and (Defensive-Qi).

威本：And those who use the needle without the right way, those physicians will only bring about a contrary (wrong) reaction and hurt the patient's normal health. Instead of bringing about compliance they bring about resistance.

文本：And if he applies the needles disregarding what is right to do, contrary [to his intentions] he will be a plunderer of qi in that he removes the proper qi of [that] person. He considers compliance to be opposition.

吴本：And applies the needle without any rule, the evil-energy will cause damage and hurt the healthy-energy of the patient. In this way, the case of a favourable prognosis will become a case of an unfavourable prognosis.

句中将"用针无义"喻为战争中不恰当的战略，将"正气"喻为我方。"夺"为动词，隐喻义为"消耗、损伤"。

李本将"夺"意译为 reduce，虽然表达出"消耗"之义，但是与宾语"正气"搭配不当。中医学中的"正气"，指机体生命功能和抗病能力 [1]，概念相对抽象，而 reduce 意为"减少"，其受动者多为大小、数量等具体概念。因此，李本如若将"夺"译为 weaken（削弱、减弱程度），与 strengthen 相呼应，可能效果更佳。

同样，威本将"夺"意译为 hurt，虽然表达出"损伤"之义，但是与"正气"搭配不佳，因为 hurt 的受动者多为人，指对身体或情感造成伤害。

文本将"夺"译为 remove 偏离原文意思，因为"夺"意为"削减、损耗"，并非"去除、使消失"之义。

---

[1] 李照国.WHO 西太区与"世界中医药学会联合会"中医名词术语国际标准比较研究：精、神、气、血、津、液部分 [J]. 中西医结合学报，2008（10）：1092.

相较而言，吴本使用中性词 cause damage 表达"夺"，与"正气"搭配，为较佳译法。

3. 邪气盛则实，精气夺则虚。（《素问·通评虚实论》）

释义：如邪气方盛，是为实证，若精气不足，就是虚证。

李本：Predomination of Xieqi (Evil-Qi) is called Shi (Excess) and insufficiency of Jingqi (Essence-Qi) is called Xu (Deficiency).

威本：When harmful influences are plentiful then we can speak of fullness; when the essences are decreased we can speak of emptiness.

文本：When evil qi abounds, then [this is] repletion. When the essence qi is lost, then [this is] depletion.

吴本：When the evil-energy is overabundant, it is sthenia, when the healthy-energy is injured, it is asthenia.

句中"夺"为形容词，与"盛"的概念相对应，隐喻义为"被损伤的，被削弱的"，"精气夺"意即"精气不足"。

李本使用词性转换的方法，将"精气夺"意译为名词短语 insufficiency of Jingqi (Essence-Qi)，充当第二个分句"精气夺则虚"的主语。名词 insufficiency 意为"不足"，准确表达了"夺"在句中"（被损伤而）不足"之义。李本语言简洁清晰，表意准确，体现了译者对中医文化的熟悉和较高的语言技能。

其余三个译本按照原文句式，采用主从复合结构表达"精气夺则虚"。"夺"分别译为 are decreased、is lost 和 is injured，基本能够传达原文意思，但用词不够精准。

4. 脉至如火薪然，是心精之予夺也，草干而死。（《素问·大奇论》）

释义：脉来时像火刚燃起来一样的旺盛，这是心脏的精气已经脱失的脉象，大约到冬初草枯的时候就要死亡。

李本：[If] the pulse beats like, burning fire, it indicates exhaustion of Xinjing (Heart-Essence) [and the patient] will die when grasses become dry [in autumn].

文本：When the [movement in the] vessels arrives like burning fuel, [the patient] will die when the herbs dry.

吴本：When the coming of the pulse is like the beginning of the burning fire,

it shows the refined energy of the heart is exhausting, the patient will die at the be-
ginnibgof winter when the gasses are withered.

"心精之予夺也"意为心精已经脱失，句中"夺"取其隐喻义"被削弱的，衰败的"。

李本和吴本都使用 exhaust 表达"夺"，传递出"脱失"之义。不同的是，李本采用其名词形式 exhaustion 充当动词 indicate 的宾语，符合 exhaustion 的用法。吴本采用其形容词形式 exhausting 作表语，意义不恰当，因为 exhausting 意为"使人筋疲力尽的"，此处应为 exhausted，意为"耗尽的、枯竭的"。

文本漏译了原文中的"是心精之予夺也"。

（二）犯

"犯"的本义为"侵犯，伤害，损害"。在《素问》中，"犯"主要指致病邪气对机体的侵犯。

1. 八正之虚邪，而避之勿犯也。（《素问·八正神明论》）

释义：顺着时序度量八正的病邪，加以避免，就不至于受到它的侵犯。

李本：The Xuxie (Deficiency–Evil) from Bazheng should be avoided.

威本：By means of the regular temperature of the eight principal factors one can avoid the deficiencies and the harmful emanations and one can avoid viola-tions.

文本：{the depletion evils of the eight cardinal [turning points]} one avoids them and thus does not offend them.

吴本：When one measures the evil–energy of the eight main solar terms ac-cording to the time sequence and try to evade it, the invasion of evil–energy can be avoided.

句中"犯"为动词，"避之勿犯"指避免虚邪，不受其侵犯。句中将虚邪喻为敌人，会侵犯机体，具有明显的战争隐喻特色。

李本对本句减译过度，未表达出"勿犯"之义。

威本将"避之勿犯"译为 avoid violations 不恰当，因为 violation 常指对他人隐私的侵犯，不能表示对身体的侵犯。

文本将"避之勿犯"译为 one avoids them and thus does not offend them，动词 offend 较符合原文语境，具有战争隐喻特色，但将"勿犯"的施动者"虚邪"误解为"人"，混淆了施动者和受动者，不能忠实传递原文内容。

相比而言，吴本使用 the invasion of evil-energy can be avoided 表达"避之勿犯"为较好译法。invade 保留了原文的战争隐喻，形象地表达出虚邪对机体的侵犯之义。

2. 故<u>犯</u>贼风虚邪者，阳受之。（《素问·太阴阳明论》）

释义：所以贼风虚邪伤人时，阳分首当其冲。

李本：That is why Zeifeng (Thief-Wind) and Xuxie (Deficiency-Evil) attack Yang.

威本：To rebel and to transgress against the wind will bring about weakness and suffering from bad influences. This will cause suffering to the element of Yang（阳受之）.

文本：Hence, when one is invaded by a robber wind or depletion evil, the yang [conduits] receive it.

吴本：Therefore, when the thief-wind and the debilitating evil invades the body, Yang will be affected first.

句中"犯"为动词，"犯贼风虚邪者"为倒装句，意为贼风虚邪侵犯机体。

李本将"犯"直译为 attack，符合原文语境，但是整句译文过度减译，未能表明贼风虚邪伤害的对象是人体，也未能表达"阳受之"的意思。

威本对原文理解有误，将"贼风"和"虚邪"曲解为因果关系，因而使用 To rebel and to transgress against（反抗、违背）表达"犯"，与原文意思相去甚远。

文本和吴本都使用 invade 表达"犯"，保留原文的战争隐喻，形象地传递出贼风虚邪对机体的侵犯。

3. 当有所<u>犯</u>大寒，内至骨髓，髓者以脑为主。（《素问·奇病论》）

释义：一定有地方遭受了很厉害的寒气，寒气向内侵入骨髓，骨髓是以脑为主。

李本：It is caused by attack of serious cold that penetrates deep into the bone marrow that is mainly stored in the brain.

文本：He must have been invaded by massive cold. Internally, it has reached the bones and the marrow.

吴本：Some part of the body must have been invaded by the cold-evil. When the cold-evil invades the bone marrow, the brain will be invaded as the brain is a main part of the bone marrow.

句中"当有所犯大寒"解释了前句中"人有病头痛以数岁不已"的原因：一定是身体有的地方遭受了很厉害的寒气。此处"犯"为被动义，指机体被大寒侵犯。

李本使用词性转换的方法，将"犯大寒"译为名词短语 attack of serious cold，由此将原文的三个分句译为一个主从复合句。但是译文未能指明大寒侵犯的对象，同时两个 that 定语从句导致整个句子结构较为混乱。

文本和吴本都使用动词 invade 表达"犯"，表意准确，但是文本将 He 当作大寒侵犯的对象，不够准确。相比之下，吴本用名词短语 some part of the body 表达"有所"，明确了大寒侵害的对象是机体某部位，又用 must have been invaded 形象地表达出原文中"当"对已发生事件的肯定推测。

4. 热病生于上，清病生于下，寒热凌犯而争于中。（《素问·六元正纪大论》）

释义：热病生于上部，寒病生于下部，寒热之气互相侵犯而争扰于中部。

李本：Heat disease usually occurs in the upper [part of the body] while cold disease often occurs in the lower [part of the body]. [If] cold and heat attack [each other and] combat [with each other] in the middle...

文本：Heat illness emerges from above; coolness illness emerges below. Cold and heat encroach upon each other and struggle in the center.

吴本：The disease of heat-evil appears in the upper part of the body, the disease of cold-evil appears in the lower part of the body, and the disease of mutual contending of cold and heat appears in the middle part of the body.

句中"凌"和"犯"皆为动词，"凌犯"意为"侵犯、侵扰"，具有战争隐喻特色。

李本使用 attack 和 combat 表达"凌犯"之义，表意准确。文本将"凌犯"译为 encroach 不妥，因为 encroach 多指侵占他人时间、权利或指蚕食土地，与主语 cold and heat 搭配不当。吴本删译"寒热凌犯而争于中"，未能表达出"凌犯"之义。

从句式看，李本使用 while 连接前两个分句，句式工整且意义明确。而吴本追求句式的对称，三个分句都使用 the disease of...appears in 结构，因而对第三个分句进行删译，将"寒热凌犯"译为 mutual contending of cold and heat（寒热相争），未能表达出"凌犯"之义，也就无从保留原文的战争隐喻。

（三）伤

"伤"为"傷"的简化字，篆文为人受箭伤之义，本义为"创伤"。在《素问》中，"伤"主要用作动词，指外来致病因素对机体及五脏六腑的侵犯和伤害。

1. 味伤形，气伤精，精化为气，气伤于味。（《素问·阴阳应象大论》）

释义：味虽能养形，若太过则能伤形，气虽能生精，若太过则能伤精，精虽能化气，若五味之精微太过者，则能伤气。

李本：[Excessive] flavor impairs the body and [excessive] Qi damages the Essence. The Essence can transform into the Qi and the Qi can be damaged by [excessive] flavor.

威本：Through transformation the ethereal spirit becomes air, and air is injurious to the perception of flavors.

文本：Flavor harms physical appearance. Qi harms essence. Essence transforms into qi. Qi is harmed by flavor.

吴本：Although tastes can nourish the physique, but if the five tastes are taken excessively, it will hurt the physique; although the energy can promote the emergence of the essence, but if the energy becomes over-abundant, it will hurt the essence. When the essence of blood is abundant, it can be activated to become energy, but when the five tastes are excessively taken so as to hurt the physique, the energy will also be hurt indirectly, so, the energy can also be hurt by the tastes.

句中"伤"为动词，本义为"伤害"，隐喻义为"致病因素对机体的损伤"。

《黄帝内经素问》隐喻英译对比研究

李本对原文进行直译，字字落实，保留原文句式的工整。同时，结合意译，将"味伤形"补译为 [Excessive] flavor impairs the body，将"气伤精"译为 [excessive] Qi damages the Essence，表达出"味（太过）伤形，气（太过）伤精"之内涵意义，用动词 impair 和 damage 表达"伤"。词汇转换自如，忠实传达了原文的形和义。

威本不仅漏译了原文中的"味伤形，气伤精"，而且将"精"和"气"分别译为 the ethereal spirit（超凡的精神）和 air，误解了二者的概念。

文本对原文进行字对字翻译，将句中三个"伤"皆译为 harm，不仅未能体现"精""气""味"之间的逻辑关系，而且句式、用词稍显单调。

吴本对原文进行大量增译，虽有益于弥补文化缺省，帮助目的语读者理解原文，但是句式过于繁冗复杂，同时译文中反复使用 hurt 表达"伤"，用词单调。

2.……**酸伤筋，辛胜酸。**（《素问·阴阳应象大论》）

……**酸伤筋，辛胜酸。**（《素问·五运行大论》）

释义：……过食酸味能够伤筋，但辛味又能够抑制酸味。

李本 1：...sourness impairs the sinews while pungency dominates over sourness.

李本 2：...sourness impairs the tendons while pungency dominates over sourness.

威本：...The sour flavor is injurious to the muscles, but the pungent flavor counteracts the sour flavor.

文本 1：...[If] sour [flavor causes harm, it] harms the sinews; acrid [flavor] dominates sour [flavor].

文本 2：...Sour [flavor] harms the sinews; acrid [flavor] dominates sour [flavor].

吴本 1：...excessive sour food taken will hurt the tendon, but acridness can overcome the sourness (acrid corresponds to the metal and metal can restrict the wood).

吴本 2：...when the sour taste is excessive, it will injure the tendon, and the acrid taste can restrict the sourness.

"酸伤筋，辛胜酸"在《素问》中出现了两次，对此译者基本保持个人风格的前后一致。对于"伤"的译法，四位译者沿袭自己的一贯用词，李本译为 impairs，威本译为 is injurious to，文本译为 harms，吴本译为 hurt/injure，四个译法皆表意准确，符合原文意思。

不同的是，李本 1 和李本 2 分别将"筋"译为 sinews 和 tendons，这两个名词为同义词，可以相互替换。文本 1 和文本 2 在句式和用词上都基本保持一致，只是文本 1 对原文稍微进行增译。吴本 1 对原文进行了较为复杂的增译，吴本 2 相对简洁，这可能是因为在书中吴本 1 先于吴本 2 出现，因此在理解吴本 1 的基础上无需再对吴本 2 进行赘译。

总体来说，每位译者的风格不会有太大变化，但语言是比较灵活的，只要能够忠实传达原文，译文不必拘泥于固定的用词和句式，适时使用同义词、改变句式，能让行文看起来更加自如。

3. 贼风数至，虚邪朝夕，内至五脏骨髓，外<u>伤</u>空窍肌肤。（《素问·移精变气论》）

释义：贼风虚邪的不断的侵袭，就会内里侵犯到五脏骨髓，外面伤害孔窍肌肤。

李本：Besides, Zeifeng (Thief-Wind) frequently attacks and Xuxie (Deficiency-Evil) repeatedly invades, internally into the Five Zang-Organs and bone marrow, and externally into the orifices, skin and muscles.

威本：Evil influences strike from early morning until late at night; they injure the five viscera, the bones and the marrow within the body, and externally they injure the mind and reduce its intelligence and they also injure the muscles and the flesh.

文本：The robber wind frequently reaches [them]. The depletion evil [is present] in the morning and in the evening; internally it reaches to the five depots, to the bones and to the marrow; externally it harms the orifices, the muscles, and the skin.

吴本：When the thief-evil invades unceasingly, the patient's viscera and bone marrow will be hurt inside, and the orifices and muscle will be hurt outside.

句中"伤"为动词，隐喻义为"贼风虚邪对孔窍肌肤的侵袭伤害"。

李本没有直接翻译"伤"，而是对原文进行意译，使用动词 attacks 和 invades into 表达贼风虚邪进入孔窍肌肤并造成伤害。同时，李本保留原文句式工整的风格，忠实传递原文的形和义。

威本将"伤"直译为 injure，表意准确，将"至"意译为 strike 亦属点睛之笔，体现出"到达并造成伤害"的双层含义。

文本和吴本分别使用动词 harm 和 hurt 表达"伤"，二者皆表意准确。但是，文本将"内至"译为 internally it reaches to，未能体现出贼风虚邪对五藏骨髓造成伤害的内涵意义。相比而言，吴本将"内至"译为 be hurt inside 略胜一筹。

4. 故伤于风者，上先受之；伤于湿者，下先受之。（《素问·太阴阳明论》）

释义：因此外感风邪，多在上部；外中湿气，多在下部。

李本：So when Wind invades [the body], it attacks the upper [part of the body] first; when Dampness invades [the body], it attacks the lower [part of the body] first.

威本：Hence an injury suffered through the wind will first ascend when contracted. An injury suffered through humidity will first descend when contracted.

文本：Hence, if one was harmed by wind, the upper [parts of the body] receive it first. If one was harmed by dampness, the lower [parts of the body] receive it first.

吴本：Thus, when one contracts wind-evil from outside, it is mostly on the upper part, when he contracts wetness-evil, it is mostly on the lower part.

句中"伤"为动词，"伤于"表被动，意为"被……侵犯"。

李本将"伤于风"译为 Wind invades [the body]（风邪侵害机体），使用主动语态表达被动之义，由此使得从句和主句的主语一致，句式简洁工整。

威本将"伤于风者"译为 an injury suffered through the wind 不妥，把语气词"者"误解为名词；将"上""下"分别译为 ascend 和 descend，把名词"上""下"曲解为动词。

文本和吴本都将"伤于风者，上先受之"译为 if/when 从句＋主句，分别将"伤于风"译为 was harmed by wind 和 contracts wind-evil（感染风邪）。两个译法都贴近原文意思，但是两个译文中的 it 都指代不清，容易造成误解。

（四）扰

"扰"本义为"搅扰、扰乱"，引申为侵扰，侵犯。在《素问》中，"扰"主要用作动词，指致病因素对机体的侵扰。

1. 是故暮而收拒，无扰筋骨，无见雾露。（《素问·生气通天论》）

释义：所以到了晚上，阳气收敛于内，行于阴分，这时就应当休息，不要再去劳累筋骨，以耗损阳气于内，也不要到外面接近雾露，以防外邪之侵袭。

李本：When it becomes dark, [Yangqi] stops moving and stays inside the body. Thus the bones and sinews should not be disturbed and [care should be taken] to avoid being exposed to dew.

威本：For this reason (the atmosphere of Yang) should be protected against bad influences, so that they cannot give trouble to the muscles and the flesh, and one should not expose them to the dew and mist of the evening.

文本：Hence, in the evening there is collection and resistance. One must not disturb sinews and bones; one must not encounter fog and dew.

吴本：So in the dusk, one should restrain his Yang energy, should not fatigue his extremities by excessive working so as not to disturb the Yang energy, and not to contact mists and dews by staying outdoor so as to avoid the invasion of cold-wetness evil.

"扰"为动词，本义为"搅扰"，"无扰筋骨"并非指不要搅扰筋骨，句中隐喻为"不要使筋骨劳累"。

李本和文本都将"扰"直译为 disturb，意思贴近原文但并不准确。disturb 的受动者通常为人，多指"干扰正常的秩序，使焦虑不安"，这与原文中"筋骨劳累"的内涵意义相差较大。

威本将"扰"译为 give trouble to（带来麻烦），理解原文有偏差。

吴本将"扰"意译为 fatigue...by excessive working，准确表达出"扰"在句中"使……劳累"之义；但是将"筋骨"译为 extremities 不合适，因为 extremities 意为"身体的四肢"，与"筋骨"的概念不同。

《黄帝内经素问》隐喻英译对比研究

2. 阴争于内，阳扰于外，魄汗未藏，四逆而起。（《素问·阴阳别论》）

释义：阴在内争胜，阳在外干扰，汗出不止，四肢逆冷。

李本：The struggle of Yin inside and the disturbance of Yang outside leads to profuse sweating and coldness of the four limbs.

威本：Yin strives towards the interior; Yang reaches towards the outside, taking the shape of perspiration which cannot be concealed. Disobedience to the four seasons will surely manifest itself.

文本：Yin struggles inside; yang causes trouble outside. [In this case] the po-sweat is not retained, and a four-fold countermovement emerges in the [limbs].

吴本：When Yin is contending inside and Yang is disturbing outside, Yin and Yang will be out of balance. When Yang is not dense outside, the sweat gland will be wide open, and continuous sweating will occur, When Yin is out of order inside, the Yin essence will be out let and cause coldness of the extremities.

句中"争"和"扰"皆为动词，具有明显的战争隐喻特色。"扰"为被动义，意为"被侵扰"，"阳扰于外"指阳在外受到干扰。

李本采用词性转换的方法，将动词短语"阳扰于外"译为名词短语 the disturbance of Yang 担当句子主语，搭配动词短语 leads to 充当句子谓语，说明"阳扰于外"与"魄汗未藏，四逆而起"之间的因果关系，表意准确，语言流畅。

吴本亦使用 disturb 表达"扰"，不同的是吴本将"阳扰于外"译为 Yang is disturbing outside，与"阴争于内"Yin is contending inside 形成排比句。但是，吴本未能正确表达出"阳"与"扰"之间的被动关系，应改为 Yang is disturbed outside。相比之下，李本使用名词 disturbance 表达"扰"，意思为 the fact of being disturbed（被干扰），表意更为准确。

威本和文本分别将"阳扰于外"译为 Yang reaches towards the outside（阳到达体外）和 yang causes trouble outside（阳在体外导致麻烦），未能正确表达"扰"在句中"被干扰"之义。

3. 天气正，地气扰，风乃暴举，木偃沙飞，炎火乃流。（《素问·六元正纪大论》）

释义：天气正常，地气扰动，于是暴风突起，树被吹倒，沙土飞扬，炎火流行。

李本：Tianqi (Heaven–Qi) is in the due [position], Diqi (Earth–Qi) is uneasy, wind blows suddenly, grasses and woods [fall] flat [on the ground], stones and sands fly [with wind], flaming Fire prevails.

文本：The qi of heaven is proper; the qi of the earth is disturbed. Violent winds rise. Trees are bent down and sand flies. Flaming fire prevails.

吴本：The heaven energy is normal, but the earth energy is stirring. The wind will rise all of a sudden, the trees will be blown down, the sand and dust will be flying and the scorching fire energy will be prevailing.

句中"正"与"扰"为对应概念。"扰"意为"不正"，是形容词，描述地气不稳定的状态。

李本将"扰"意译为 is uneasy（不稳定的），与"正"is in the due [position]（在恰当的位置）相照应。uneasy 为形容词，多指人心神不安的，亦指局势动荡不稳定的。李本用 Diqi (Earth–Qi) is uneasy 描述地气被扰动后的不稳定状态，符合原文意思。

文本和吴本分别将"扰"译为 is disturbed 和 is stirring。disturbed 意为"被干扰的"，贴近"扰"的本义，表意准确。stir 常被用作及物动词，意为"搅拌、扰乱……的平静"；用作不及物动词时，stir 指某种情绪产生或者风拂动之义 [1]。因此，如果吴本将 is stirring 改为 is stirred，能更加准确地表达出"扰"在句中"地气被扰动、不稳定的"之义。

原文中"地气扰"描述的是天气正常状态下，地气被扰动、由稳定到不稳定的动态过程。因此，虽然三个译文都成功表达出地气被扰动的状态，但是相较而言，文本使用被动语态 is disturbed 精确表达出地气受到干扰而变得不稳定的过程，更加精准地传递出原文的内涵意义。

4. 木郁之发，太虚埃昏，云物以扰，大风乃至。（《素问·六元正纪大论》）

释义：木郁发作的时候，天空中埃尘昏暗，云气扰动，大风到来。

李本：The burst [due to] stagnation of Wood [is characterized by the state during

---

[1] Merriam–Webster Inc. Merriam–Webster Dictionary [DB/OL]. [2021–10–12]. https://www.merriam–webster.com/dictionary/stir.

which] gloominess of the sky with dusts; clouds and things float; great wind blows; houses and woods are destructed; [grasses and] woods change.

文本：The outbreak of oppressed wood [qi is as follows]: The Great Void is darkened by dust; cloudy things are disturbed. Strong winds arrive. They tear open houses and break trees. The wood undergoes changes.

吴本：In the bursting out of the suppressed wood energy, the sky is gloomy with dust, the clouds are stirring, the gale bale blows, the decorations in the corners of the roots are being blown down by the gale, and the trees are broken and destroyed by the breaking forth of the wood energy.

本句描述了大风即将到来之前天空昏暗，云气扰动的景象。"扰"为动词，隐喻义为"（云物）被扰动"。

对于"扰"的译法，三个译本差别较大。其中，李本将"扰"译为float，与原文的内涵意义不符。句中描述的是大风即将到来之时云物翻腾之景象，float意为"（云彩）在空中飘动"，不能体现出云气被扰动、不稳定的状态。文本将"扰"译为are disturbed（被侵扰的），既贴近"扰"的本义，又体现出隐喻义"云物被扰动"的景象。吴本将"扰"译为are stirring亦很形象，此处stir用作不及物动词，表示"（风）拂动"之义，句中引申为大风即将到来之时云物翻腾的景象。主动语态are stirring表明云物翻腾为自发性动作。

三个译本分别将"云物"译为clouds and things、cloudy things和the clouds，都使用cloud表达"云物"，看似差别细微但是意思不同。句中描述的是大风到来之前云物翻腾的景象，此处"云物"实指云朵，用cloud表达即可，因此吴本的译法最佳，表意准确并且简洁清楚。李本采用直译将"云物"译为clouds and things（云和物），things指代不明，属赘译。文本将"云物"译为cloudy things不当，因为cloudy既意为"多云的"，用于描述天气，又意为"混浊的"，cloudy things易让读者联想到模糊不清的东西，偏离了原文意思。

三、正气防御和抵抗方式

（一）守

"守"本义为"官吏的职责、职守"，引申为保护、防卫之意。在《素问》中，"守"主要指人体正气对致病因素的防御，从而起到保护机体的作用。在战争中，关口和要塞非常重要，因此需要固守；而对疾病治疗来说，经气出入的门户也是非常重要的关口，因此也需要进行特别保护。

1. 恬惔虚无，真气从之，精神内守，病安从来。（《素问·上古天真论》）

释义：思想上要保持冷静，不为贪欲所动，真气就能够顺从人体的功能；精神要守护于内，不要过多地耗散，病邪还能从何处再来侵袭呢！

李本：...and keep the mind free from avarice. [In this way] Zhenqi in the body will be in harmony, Jingshen (Essence–Spirit) will remain inside, and diseases will have no way to occur.

威本：They [the sages] were tranquilly content in nothingness and the true vital force accompanied them always; their vital (original) spirit was preserved within; thus, how could illness come to them?

文本：Quiet peacefulness, absolute emptiness the true qi follows [these states]. When essence and spirit are guarded internally, where could a disease come from?

吴本：When one is completely free from wishes, ambitions and distracting thoughts, indifferent to fame and gain, the true energy will come in the wake of it. When one concentrates his spirit internally and keeps a sound mind, how can any illness occur?

"守"本义为"防守"，常用于战争中对关口和要塞的固守。句中"精神内守"指精神要守护于内，"守"为动词，隐喻义为"守护（机体精神）"。

李本将"内守"译为 remain inside，此译法着重强调"持"而非"守"，偏离了"守"的内涵意义，未保留原文的战争隐喻。与李本一样，威本将"内守"译为 was preserved within，亦偏离了"守"在句中"守护"之义，因为 preserve 同 remain 一样，意为"维持……的原状"。

吴本将"精神内守"意译为 When one concentrates his spirit internally and keeps a sound mind（内聚精神、保持头脑清醒），未能表达出"守"之"守护（机体精神）"之义，与原文意义偏差较大，表意不准确。

文本将"精神内守"译为 essence and spirit are guarded internally，表意准确。一方面动词 guard 形象地表达出"守"的战争隐喻特色，另一方面使用被动语态 are guarded 准确说明"精神"和"内守"之间的逻辑关系，为佳译。

2. 得守者生，失守者死。（《素问·脉要精微论》）

释义：如果五脏能够起到内守的作用，病人的健康就能恢复；否则，病人就濒于死亡了。

李本：Normal functions [of the viscera] ensure life while dysfunctions [of the viscera] cause death.

威本：Those who pay heed to these functions will live and those who neglect to attend to these functions will die.

文本：Those who are able to guard, they live. Those who fail to guard, they die.

吴本：In short, if the five viscera are able to play their roles of guarding inside, the health of the patient can be restored, otherwise, the patient will soon die.

人的五脏在体内各有职守，句中五脏被喻为士兵，守卫人体这个战场。"得守"指五脏能够维护其职守，"守"为名词，意为"职守"。

李本使用词汇转换法，将动词短语"得守"译为名词 Normal functions [of the viscera]，相应地，将动词短语"失守"译为名词 dysfunctions [of the viscera]，表意准确，语言简洁，句式工整，忠实传达原文的形和义。

吴本将第一个分句"得守者生"译为主从复合句，使用 if 从句中补译出"得守"的施动者 the five viscera，搭配谓语动词 are able to play their roles of，逻辑清晰，但是将"内守"译为 guarding inside 不恰当，因为句中"守"意为"五脏的职守"，并非"守护"之义。吴本对第二个分句"失守者死"的译法亦为点睛之笔，使用副词 otherwise，既避免翻译"失守"，又表意准确，句式简洁，一目了然。当然，otherwise 为副词，严谨地说，otherwise 之前的逗号应该改为分号。

威本将"守"意译为 functions，表意准确，但是将"得守"的施动者

"五脏"误解为 Those（病人），混淆了原文的逻辑关系。

文本将"守"译为动词 guard，曲解了"守"在句中"职守"之义。

3. 知其所在者，知诊三部九候之病脉处而治之，故曰守其门户焉。（《素问·八正神明论》）

释义：晓得疾病的所在，就是必须了解三部九候的病脉，知道疾病的变化，才能早期治疗；所以说掌握三部九候，好像看守门户一样重要。

李本：To know the location of a disease means to understand the morbid changes of [the pulse in] the Three Regions and Nine Divisions and to give timely treatment. [To detect the changes of the pulse in the Three Regions and Nine Divisions] is just like to guard the door.

威本：If one knows the location of the disease, one knows through examination that the diseases of the three regions of the body and the nine subdivisions are located within the pulse, and one can thus treat and cure them. Therefore it is said that one should attend to the gates of the pulse.

文本："To know where [the disease] is" is to know how to diagnose, at the nine indicators in the three sections, the locations of the vessels having a disease and to treat them. Hence, this is called "to guard the doors".

吴本：If a physician can discover the location of the disease from the pulse of the three parts and the nine sub-parts and treat in time, it will guard against the invasion of the evil-energy, so it is called the "guarding of entrance".

"三部九候"是病脉由行出入之所[1]，句中被喻为建筑物的门户。因此"守其门户"指看守门户，"守"为动词，意为"看守、守卫"。

李本、文本和吴本分别将"守其门户"直译为 to guard the door、to guard the doors 和 guarding of entrance，译法基本一致，都使用 guard 表达出"守"在句中"守卫"之义，使用 door 或 entrance 表达出"门户"的字面意思，保留了原文的隐喻特色。相比而言，李本在 to guard the door 前面补译出 is just like，将原文的隐喻显化，明确表达出"守其门户"的内涵意义。

威本将"守其门户"译为 attend to the gates of the pulse 不妥，因为 attend

[1] 张介宾.景岳全书 [M]. 太原：山西科学技术出版社，2006：43.

to 意为"照料、致力于",偏离"守护"之义,而且 the gates of the pulse 表意模糊。二者未能有效传递原文信息。

4. 静以待时,谨守其气,无使倾移。(《素问·五常政大论》)

释义:要耐心地观察,谨慎地守护着正气,不要使它耗损。

李本:...quietly observe natural changes, protect [the genuine] Qi and avoid any violation.

文本:Carefully guard the [patient's] qi, lest it moves towards imbalance.

吴本:When invigorating or adjusting the energy, one must observe carefully and guard the healthy energy prudently against waste and consumption.

四时的气序,是不可违反的,因此只能"静以待时,谨守其气"。句中"气"被喻为战争中的我方,需要谨慎守护。"守"为动词,意为"守护、守卫"。

李本将"守"译为 protect(保护⋯⋯不受伤害),文本和吴本都将"守"译为 guard(守卫)。三个译本都保留了原文的战争隐喻,但相较而言,文本和吴本使用 guard 强调"在正气耗损之前,警惕守护"之义,更加贴近原文"谨守其气"的意思。

(二)攻

"攻"的本义为"进攻",施动者是己方军队,受动者是敌方军队。在《素问》中,"攻"主要指治疗疾病,施动者是医生,受动者是疾病,多在动词之前指出所使用的工具。

1. 粗工凶凶,以为可攻,故病未已,新病复起。(《素问·移精变气论》)

释义:大吹大擂,自以为能够治愈。结果呢,原来的疾病没有治愈,又添上新的病证了。

李本:Unskillful doctors think that attack therapy can be used. As a result, they, instead of curing the old diseases, make the patients suffer from new ones.

威本:Poor medical workmanship is neglectful and careless and must therefore be combatted, because a disease that is not completely cured can easily breed new disease or there can be a relapse of the old disease.

文本:Uneducated practitioners behave very aggressively, believing they can launch an attack. Before the old disease has ended, a new disease emerges in addition.

吴本：He boasts of his curative effect about his treating, supposing that the disease can surely be cured, but finally, the former disease is still remaining, and some new diseases are added.

技术不高明的医生，不根据四时的变化治疗疾病，等到疾病已经形成了，还大吹大擂，自以为能够治愈。句中将医生喻为战争中的我方，将疾病喻为战争中的敌方，"攻"为动词，隐喻义为"治疗疾病"。

李本将"以为可攻"意译为 attack therapy can be used（可用攻法），将"攻"看作名词，译为 attack therapy（进攻之法），既保留了原文的战争隐喻，又表明"攻"在句中"治疗方法"的内涵意义。

同李本一样，文本也将"攻"理解为"攻法"，将"可攻"译为 launch an attack（发动进攻）。此译法具有明显的战争隐喻特色，但是未能表明"攻"在句中"治疗方法"的内涵意义，致使读者很难理解 launch an attack 与 disease 之间的关系。

吴本将"可攻"译为 the disease can surely be cured，补译出"可攻"的对象 the disease，使用动词 can be cured 表达"攻"，体现出"攻"在句中"治疗疾病"之义，但是未能保留原文的战争隐喻，失去了"攻"的文化意义。

威本将"攻"译为 be combatted，虽然保留了原文的战争隐喻，但是将"攻"的对象"疾病"误解为 Poor medical workmanship（粗糙的医疗工艺），表意不准确。

2. 必齐毒药攻其中，镵石针艾治其外也。（《素问·汤液醪醴论》）

释义：必定要内服药物，外用镵石针艾，然后病才能治好。

李本：Nowadays [people] have to use Duyao (drugs) to treat internal [diseases] and Chanshi (ploughshare-shaped stone), Acupuncture and moxibustion to treat external diseases.

威本：The present generation must respect（齐）the poisonous medicines, which assault the diseases within their bodies and they should hold in awe acupuncture and treatment with moxa, which cure the diseases of the external body.

文本：The people of today, they must administer toxic drugs to attack in their

《黄帝内经素问》隐喻英译对比研究

center, as well as chisel stones, needles, and moxa to treat their exterior.

吴本：In nowadays, when people contract disease, it is neccessary to treat them with medicine internally or with acupuncture stone pricking or moxibustion externally to cure the disease.

句中"其中"和"其外"分别指机体的内部和外部疾病，被喻为战争中的敌方。"攻"与"治"为并列概念，"攻"即"治"，意为"治疗疾病"，对象为疾病。

李本和吴本都使用动词 treat 表达"攻"，将"攻其中"分别意译为 treat internal [diseases] 和 treat them with medicine internally（注：them 代指前句中的 disease），此译法虽然失去原文的战争隐喻特色，但是准确表达了"攻"在句中"治疗疾病"之内涵意义。

威本将"攻其中"译为 assault the diseases within their bodies，准确理解"攻"在句中"治疗疾病"之义。assault 用作动词时多指"暴力袭击"，也指"发动军事进攻"。此译法保留了原文的战争隐喻，基本实现信息传递与文化交际的双重目标。

文本将"攻其中"译为 attack in their center 不妥，将"攻"直译为 attack 虽然保留了原文的战争隐喻，但是未指明 attack 的对象，不能体现"攻"在句中"治疗疾病"的内涵意义。同时，将"其中"译为 in their center，说明未能正确理解"其中"在句中"机体内部疾病"之义。

3. 毒药攻邪，五谷为食，五果为助……（《素问·脏气法时论》）

释义：毒药是用来攻邪的，五谷是用来营养的，五果是用来作为辅助的……

李本：Duyao (drugs) [can be used] to attack Xie (Evil), the five kinds of grain [can be used] to nourish [the body], the five kinds of fruit [can be used] to assist [the five kinds of grain to nourish the body]...

威本：The poisons and medicines attack the evil influences. The five grains act as nourishment; the five fruits from the trees serve to augment...

文本：Toxic drugs attack the evil. The five grains provide nourishment. The five fruits provide support...

吴本：Poisonous drugs are to expel evils. The five kinds of cereals are to nourish the body, the five kinds of fruits are for supplementing...

句中"毒药攻邪"指使用药物祛除邪气，"邪"被喻为敌方，"毒药"是克敌的工具。"攻"为动词，隐喻义为"祛除（邪气）"。

李本、威本和文本都将"攻"直译为attack，保留了原文的战争隐喻，表达出"毒药"对"邪"的侵袭之义，基本忠实传达原文意思。

吴本采用直译意译结合法将"攻邪"译为expel evils。动词expel常指"将……除名或驱逐出境"，也可指"排出气体或毒素等"。expel evils准确表达出"攻邪"在句中"祛除邪气"之义，同时也保留了原文的战争隐喻，为佳译。

从句式结构来看，虽然四个译本都按照原文句式译为三个分句，但是李本连续使用三个 [can be used] 结构对原文进行补译，句式更为工整，一目了然。同时，李本补译出"食""助""益""充"的对象，更为具体地传递出原文意思，较之其他三个译本略胜一筹。

4. 发表不远热，攻里不远寒。(《素问·六元正纪大论》)

释义：发表不必忌热，攻里不必忌寒。

李本：[When] relieving [pathogenic factors from] the exterior, [the use of drugs] Heat [in nature] should not be avoided; [when] attacking the interior, [the use of drugs] Cold [in nature] should not be avoided.

文本：If [you wish to] open the [body's] exterior, you do not [need to] stay away from heat; if [you wish to] attack the interior, you do not [need to] stay away from cold.

吴本：When dispelling the superficial evils, the medicine of hot nature should not be omitted, when dispelling the evils in the interior, the medicine of cold nature should not be omitted.

句中"发表"与"攻里"为对应概念，"发表"指发散表邪，"攻里"指祛除内邪。"攻"为动词，隐喻义为"祛除（内邪）"。

李本和文本都将"攻里"直译为attack the interior，动词attack保留了原文的战争隐喻，表达出"攻"在句中"祛除内邪"之义。但是将 the interior 当作"攻"的宾语不恰当，未明确指明"攻"的对象为"内邪"。

吴本将"发表"和"攻里"分别译为 dispelling the superficial evils 和

dispelling the evils in the interior，使用同一个动词 dispel 表达"发"和"攻"。dispel 意为"驱散、消除"，虽然与"发"和"攻"的字面意思相差较远，但是准确表达出二者在句中"祛除邪气"之内涵意义。同时，吴本明确指明"发"和"攻"的对象分别为 the superficial evils（外邪）和 the evils in the interior（内邪），表意准确，一目了然。

（三）卫

"卫"，从行，从韦。"韦"意为"层叠"，"行"指"出行""道路"。故"卫"的本义为安全部队沿道路两侧警戒。在《素问》中，"卫"字出现频率极高。"卫"可以用作名词，是卫气的简称，常出现卫气、营卫、荣卫等说法。"卫"也可以用作动词，指卫气卫外的功能。

1. 卫者，水谷之悍气也。（《素问·痹论》）

释义：卫是水谷所化成的悍气。

李本：Wei (Defensive-Qi) is the Hanqi (Swift-Qi) of water and food.

文本：The guard qi, that is the violent qi of water and grain.

吴本：The Wei-energy is the rough energy which is transformed from water and cereals.

"卫"从战争中的"戍卫"引申而来，指正气对人体的保卫，具有战争隐喻色彩。句中"卫"用作名词，指通过吸收水谷的营养而形成的保护人体的正气。

李本使用音译加注法将"卫"译为 Wei (Defensive-Qi)，音译 Wei 保留了中医特有的文化内涵，注解中 defensive（防御的，保护的）既对气的特性进行界定，又传达出战争隐喻色彩。同时，目的语读者在熟悉中医文化之后，反倒更喜欢使用源语言，例如 Qi（气），能理解这是中华文化的独特概念[1]。因此，李本有助于目的语读者理解原句的中医概念，从而更好地理解中医文化。

文本采用直译、音译相结合的方法，将"卫"译为 guard qi，直译 guard 具有明显的战争隐喻色彩，音译 qi 传递出"卫"在句中的具体所指——卫

---

[1] 黄婉怡，张佛明，宋兴华等.从"文化引领"谈中医英译策略 [J].中医药导报，2019，25（21）：136.

气，有利于目的语读者对"卫气"的理解和接受。

吴本采用音译和意译相结合的方法，将"卫"译为 Wei-energy。音译 Wei 保留了中医文化特色，但未明确说明"卫"在句中的准确意义，给目的语读者带来理解上的困难。"气"为中医学特有术语，含义丰富，将"气"意译为 energy（能量，精力），有利于目的语读者的接受。但此译法不能准确表达"气"的含义，易造成对中医术语的误解。

2.故天运当以日光明，是故阳因而上，<u>卫</u>外者也。（《素问·生气通天论》）

释义：所以说天的运行不息，是借太阳的光明，人体的健康无病，是赖轻清上浮的阳气保卫。

李本：Thus the normal movement of the heavens depends on the normal shining of the sun. Similarly, Yangqi [in the body] must flow upwards to protect the exterior [of the body].

威本：The movements of Heaven are illuminated by the sun. Yang rises up to protect man's body externally.

文本：The fact is, the movements [of the celestial bodies] in heaven require the sun to be lustrous and brilliant. Hence the yang [qi] follows [the sun] and rises; it is that which protects the outside.

吴本：So the unceasing operation of heaven depends on the brightness of the sun, and the bodily health of a man depends on the clear and floating of Yang energy which guards against outside.

句中"卫"为动词，表示阳气对人体的保卫、保护，蕴含战争隐喻色彩。

李本、威本和文本均采用直译法，将"卫"译为动词 protect（保护），较忠实且简洁地传达出阳气对人体的保护作用。此外，protect 在英语中也来自战争语域，有利于帮助目的语读者从熟悉的认知域出发去理解原句的战争隐喻。但是文本误解了 protect 的对象，将"卫"的对象"人体"误解为 outside（外）。

吴本将"卫"译为 guard against（守卫），不仅明确指明"卫"和"外"之间的逻辑关系，同时保留源语的战争隐喻特色。

3. 阳者，<u>卫</u>外而为固也。（《素问·生气通天论》）

释义：阳是保卫人体外部而坚固腠理的。

李本：While Yang protects the exterior to keep it firm.

威本：Yang serves as protector against external danger and must therefore be strong.

文本：As for the yang, it protects the exterior and is firm.

吴本：...and Yang is to defend the periphery of the body and is guarding outside.

句中"卫"为动词，意为"保护"。

李本和文本相同，均将"卫"直译为 protect，以"阳"作主语，行文简洁，忠实原文，表现了阳气守卫人体这一战争隐喻。威本采用词性转化的方式，将动词"卫"意译为名词 protector，把阳气比作人体的守护者。英国翻译理论家纽马克曾总结了隐喻的七种翻译方法，其中之一是将隐喻翻译成明喻[1]。该译法既准确阐述了医理，又把战争隐喻转化为明喻，形象生动、易于理解。

吴本选用 defend（保护、保卫）翻译"卫"，意义与原文贴合；同时 defend 直接来源于英文战争语域，目的语读者可从自己熟悉的语境出发来理解原句中的战争隐喻。

四、正邪对抗方式

（一）搏

"搏"，从手，从専，本义为"用武术套路对打"。后来引申为"搏斗"，指徒手或用刀、棒等激烈地对打。在《素问》中，"搏"用来表达人体内部的正气与致病因素相互较量。

1. 阴虚阳搏谓之崩。（《素问·阴阳别论》）

释义：阴脉虚而阳脉搏击的，是阴虚而阳盛，火热迫血妄行，在妇人而为血崩症。

---

[1] Newmark, P. *Approaches to Translation* [M]. Shanghai: Shanghai Foreign Language Education Press, 2001: 84–96.

李本：[If] the Yin [pulse] is Xu (deficiency or asthenia) and Yang [pulse] is vigorous, it will cause Beng (sudden and profuse uterine bleeding) in women.

威本：When Yin is empty and hollow and Yang is full and abundant, the result is called a "collapse" (menorrhagia).

文本：When the yin is depleted and the yang beats, this is called "collapse".

吴本：When Yang is contending, it is the over-abundant of Yang, when Yin is in debility and Yang is over-abundant, the blood will be forced to run rashly and cause metrorrhagia.

句中"搏"为动词，意为"搏动、搏击"，由源域战争引申而来，暗指阴脉和阳脉处于一种相互斗争、此消彼长的关系中。

李本准确理解了原文中的隐喻关系，在 Yin 和 Yang 后增译 pulse，准确地向目的语读者指出具有斗争关系的两类本体——阴脉和阳脉。同时，使用词性转化的方法，将"搏"意译为形容词 vigorous（充满活力的），形象生动地传达出阳脉搏动之旺盛。

威本将"搏"意译为形容词 full and abundant（大量的、充足的），但这两个词侧重事物的数量之多，偏离了"搏"的隐喻义。

吴本与威本类似，将"搏"意译为形容词 over-abundant（过剩的），在一定程度上偏离了原文。

文本将"搏"直译为 beat（搏动），译文简洁明了，表达出阳脉旺盛搏动之义。

2. 三阴俱搏，二十日夜半死。（《素问·阴阳别论》）

释义：三阴（肺脾）之脉，都搏击于指下，经过二十天就会在夜半死亡。

李本：[If the pulses related to] three Yin (the spleen and the lung Channels) all beat vigorously [under the pressure of the fingers], [the patient] will die in the midnight after twenty days.

威本：When the three Yin attack and rush toward each other death will ensue at midnight after twenty days.

文本：When all third yin beat, [the patient] dies within 20 days at midnight.

吴本：When the pulses of the third Yin (lung and spleen) all pulsate under the fingers, the patient will die at midnight of the twentieth day.

"搏"原指战争双方的搏击交战，在本句中指人体内部的正气与致病因素相互较量。

李本把"搏"意译为 beat vigorously（旺盛地搏动），形象地表达出原文的隐喻，即脉搏的激烈跳动仿佛战争的一方在主动迎敌而上。

威本也再现了原文中的战争隐喻，其选用的两个动词 attack（进攻）和 rush（猛冲）在英语中常用于与战争相关的语域。经脉如同在战场上一样相互攻击冲撞，让读者体会到脉搏之紊乱，实现源语和目的语在词汇意义与文化内涵上的对等。

文本将"搏"翻译为 beat（搏动），忠实地传达了词义。

吴本将"搏"直译为 pulsate（跳动）。"搏"在原文中指脉搏激烈搏动，犹如迎战的应激状态，而 pulsate 指在正常状态下脉搏有规律地跳动、搏动，没有准确地表达"搏"的含义，也无法很好地传达出原文所包含的战争隐喻。

3. 搏阳则为巅疾，搏阴则为喑。（《素问·宣明五气》）

释义：病邪入于阳，阳过盛则为巅顶疾患；病邪入于阴，阴过盛则不能言。

李本：Combat [of Xie] with Yang causes head diseases; combat [of Xie] with Yin causes hoarseness.

威本：When the evils strike at Yang, they cause insanity（巅）; when they strike at Yin, they cause loss of speech（喑）.

文本：When it strikes at the yang, then this causes peak illness. When it strikes at the yin, then this causes muteness.

吴本：When the evils enter into Yang to cause adverseness of the vital energy, then disease will occur; when the evils enter into Yin to cause the damage of Yin-fluid, dumbness of the patient will occur.

在原文的战争隐喻中，人体被隐喻为战争发生的场所。"搏阳"意为邪气与人体的阳气互相对抗，"搏阴"指邪气与阴气的较量。

李本将"搏"译为 combat（与……搏斗）。combat 经常用于战争这一概念域，保留了原文的战争隐喻色彩；同时，李本加注增译出和 Yang 较量的对象"邪"[Xie]，战争中敌我双方搏斗的概念被移植到人体内阴阳与邪气搏斗这一领域中，使读者可以根据熟悉的战争概念更好地理解疾病的发展过程。

威本和文本将"搏"译为 strike（攻击）。strike 在英语中常用于战争语境，方便目的语读者理解。威本中 when 引导的时间状语从句采用主谓宾结构，strike 的主语为 the evils，宾语为 Yang，目标域中的"邪"和"阳"通过来自源域战争的 strike 产生联系，使读者清晰地理解邪气对阴阳的攻击。可见，威本对战争隐喻的翻译是成功的。

吴本将"搏阳"意译为 when the evils enter into Yang，侧重解释邪气侵入阳和阴这一医理现象，但未能译出"搏阳"和"搏阴"中所包含的战争隐喻。

（二）争

"争"，其金文字形上为"爪"（手），下为"又"（手），中间表示某一物体，像两人争一样东西。本义为"争夺"，后引申为"较量，抗衡"。在《素问》中，"争"用来表达人体内部的正气与致病因素之间的抗衡较量。

1. 阴争于内，阳扰于外。（《素问·阴阳别论》）

释义：阴在内争胜，阳在外干扰。

李本：The struggle of Yin inside and the disturbance of Yang outside...

威本：Yin strives towards the interior; Yang reaches towards the outside.

文本：Yin struggles inside; yang causes trouble outside.

吴本：When Yin is contending inside and Yang is disturbing outside.

"阴争于内"意为阴气在体内互相较量、抗衡。

李本将"争"译为名词 struggle。struggle 表示艰难的斗争，表达出体内五脏之阴气互相抗衡较量之意；但这种将原文动词"争"转译为名词的处理方法在一定程度上丢失了原文阴气之间的激烈较量之感。

和李本类似，文本也将"争"直译为 struggle（斗争），不同之处在于文本保留了原文"争"的动词词性，从而表现出体内阴气失去平衡，仿佛战争中的各方力量互相斗争牵制。这种处理方法很好地实现了从源域战争到目标域疾病的映射，利于读者理解。

吴本将"争"译为动词 contend（斗争、竞争），该词的选用符合原文意思；值得注意的是，在时态上，吴本选用了现在进行时 when yin is contending，更加形象地表达出体内阴气互相争锋之意。

威本将"争"意译为 strive（奋斗、力求），侧重努力奋斗以达成目标；

而原文中的"争"来自战争域，意为"较量，抗衡"，故与来自战争语域的 struggle 和 contend 相比，威本在一定程度上曲解了原文之意，没有正确表达出原文的隐喻。

2. 一阳独啸，少阳厥也，阳并于上，四脉<u>争</u>张。（《素问·经脉别论》）

释义：如果二阴经脉独盛，这是少阴热厥，虚阳并越于上，心脾肝肺的脉气争张的缘故。

李本：When double Yin [Channels] are vigorous, it is due to reverse flow of Shaoyang together with Yangqi and dilatation of the four Channels.

威本：When one element of Yang alone (influences the viscera), there is a whistling and hissing tone like the hiccoughs, produced by the lesser Yang. Yang also strives with the upper (parts of the body) and the four pulses and seeks to dominate.

文本：When the first yang [qi] hisses alone, [this is a situation of] minor yang recession. The yang collects above and the four vessels compete.

吴本：If the second Yin channel is solely over-abundant, it is caused by the cold extremities due to heat-evil of Shaoyin and asthenic Yang above, and the energies of heart, spleen, liver and lung are contending.

"争"从源域战争通过认知隐喻投射到目标域疾病之中，指四种脉气相斗相争。

文本将"争"译为动词 compete（竞争、对抗），该词常用于与斗争、冲突相关的语域，符合目的语读者的认知模式，能使其从熟悉的概念出发，更好地理解中医经脉运行的状况。

同样地，吴本也选用一个经常出现在战争语境的词 contend（斗争、争夺）来翻译"争"，实现了目的语和源语在战争隐喻表达上的对应。

李本将"四脉争张"译为 dilatation of the four Channels（四种经脉的扩张），但实际上原文指来自心脾肝肺的脉气互相较量争胜。由此看来，李本过度简化，未将"争"所包含的战争隐喻较贴切地翻译出来。

句中"争张"的主语为四脉，威本将主语误译为 Yang；且"争张"被译为 dominate（支配、占优势），未表达出"争张"的本义和战争隐喻。

3. 今邪气交<u>争</u>于骨肉而得汗者，是邪却而精胜也。（《素问·评热病论》）

释义：现在邪正在骨肉之间交争而能够出汗，这是由于邪气退而精气胜的原因。

李本：Sweating during the combat between Xieqi (Evil–Qi) [and Zhengqi (Healthy–Qi)] indicates recession of Xie (Evil) and domination of Jing (Essence).

威本：Now, when the evil influences are interlocked in battle with the bones and the flesh, then perspiration should come forth so that the evil (airs) remove themselves and the pure essence excels.

文本：Now, when evil [qi] and [proper] qi interact in a struggle in the bones and in the flesh and when this leads to sweating, [this indicates that] the evil retreats and the essence dominates.

吴本：In the combat of evil–energy against the healthy–energy between the bone and muscle, if the refined–energy wins, the evil–energy will be excreted along with the sweat, and the patient will be recovered.

句中"争"用作动词，指正气与邪气交缠相争。

李本将"争"译为名词 combat（斗争），并借用 between...and... 补译出未在原文出现的正气 [Zhengqi (Healthy–Qi)]，明确指出战争隐喻中的两个本体——正气与邪气。这两个本体通过介词短语 between...and... 与 combat 连用，使读者联想到敌我双方，从而理解原文中正气与邪气交缠斗争的中医医理。值得注意的是，李本省译原文中的"骨肉"，该词指身体，是正气与邪气交锋的场所，对应的源域是战场。但由于 combat 所引出的战争隐喻模型的铺垫，读者会自然地从战场对应到人体，"骨肉"的省译不会带来困惑，因此李本较好地实现了翻译的跨文化交流功能。

吴本和李本相同，选用 combat 翻译"争"，也是可取的。

文本将"争"译为 in a struggle（在斗争中），忠实且通顺地翻译了原文。

威本采用直译，将原文动词"争"转换词性直接翻译为 battle（战斗），符合原文的战争隐喻。但威本将与邪气抗衡的对象错译为骨肉，而非正气，对战争隐喻本体的理解出现了偏差。

4. 下气上争不能复，精气溢下，邪气因从之而上也。（《素问·厥论》）

释义：在下的阴气，向上浮越，与阳相争，而阳气不能内藏，精气漏泄，阴寒之气得以从而上逆。

李本：[However, the struggle of Qi in the lower is impossible] to avoid being exhausted. [As a result,] Jingqi (Essence-Qi) leaks from the lower and Xieqi (Evil-Qi) runs up-wards accordingly.

文本：The qi from below moves upwards to fight [with the proper qi for its space], [Hence, the proper qi above] cannot restore [its loss]. The essence qi over-flows and moves down; evil qi, then, follows it and moves upwards.

吴本：...it causes the Yin energy below to float up and contend with the Yang energy, As the Yang energy can not be stored inside, the Yin energy which is cold will be reversed up to become the cold-type jue-syndrome.

句中"下气"指阴气，其向上运行与阳气相争。"争"为动词，隐喻义为"阴气和阳气较量抗衡"。

文本将"争"译为动词 fight（打架）。该词来源于英文中的战争语境，选词准确。同时，文本在 fight 后用括号加注的方式指明下气抗争的对象为正气，该隐喻翻译是成功的。

吴本选用动词 contend（竞争），其也常用于战争概念域中，且 contend 的施动者为阴气（the Yin energy），受动者为阳气（the Yang energy）。译文句子结构一目了然地指出阴气与阳气犹如敌我双方互为对抗，翻译到位。

李本采用直译法，把"下气上争"翻译为 the struggle of Qi in the lower，基本忠实于原文；但如果补译出"下气上争"的对象是阳气，则能更准确地翻译出原文的战争隐喻。

五、正邪对抗结果

（一）失

"失"，本义为"失掉、丢失"，表示从手中丢失。在《素问》中，"失"用来表达人体内部的正气与致病因素之间的抗衡和较量的结果。

1. 得神者昌，失神者亡。（《素问·移精变气论》）

释义：如果病人面色光华，脉息和平，这叫"得神"，预后良好；如果病人面色无华，脉不应时，这叫"失神"，预后不佳。

李本：[If] the Shen is not lost, the illness is curable; [if] the Shen is lost, the illness is incurable.

威本：and then it becomes apparent that those who have attained spirit and energy are flourishing and prosperous, while those perish who lose their spirit and energy.

文本：If one gets a hold of the spirit, the [patient] will prosper; if the spirit is lost, [the patient] perishes.

吴本：If the complexion of the patient is lustrous, and the pulse beat is calm, it is called the "spiritedness", the disease can be healed. When the complexion of the patient has no lustre, and his pulse fails to correspond with seasonal variations, it is called the "depletion of spirit", the disease can by no means be cured.

句中"失神"指精神的丧失。

威本采用直译法将"失"译为 lose，这与战争域相对应。lose 常用于战争语境，指战争的失败，例如，lose a war 意为"输掉一场战争"。

李本、文本与威本类似，采用 lose 的形容词 lost 来翻译"失"，表达精神丧失的状态。根据 lose 所代表的战争语义，目的语读者很容易体会到正气被致病因素打败的结果是精神的丧失。这三个译本较好地译出了原文的战争隐喻。

值得改进的是，威本可以调整语序，把 while those perish who lose their spirit and energy 改为 while those who lose their spirit and energy perish，这样更符合英文的表达习惯以及原文的内容与形式。

吴本将"失"译为 depletion（损耗，锐减），在表达神志丧失之意上略有偏差。

2. 三部九候皆相失者死。（《素问·三部九候论》）

释义：如果三部九候都失其常度的主死。

李本：[If] the pulse states in the Three Regions and Nine Divisions are all in disharmony, [it indicates impending] death.

威本：When the three regions and the nine subdivisions mutually err against each other death will result.

文本：When all the [movements in the vessels at the] nine indicators in the three sections do not conform with each other, [this indicates] death.

吴本：If the three parts and the nine sub-parts of the pulse are all irregular, it shows the patient will die.

"失"在原文中的隐喻义为位于三部的脉搏在致病因素的作用下不相协调、运行反常、失去规律。

李本采用意译法，将"失"译为 be in disharmony（不和谐）。harmony 指事物处于和谐共生的关系之中，在中文语境中有"合则两利，斗则俱伤"的说法，在英文中也有 in an era of peace and harmony 的表达，因此 harmony 的否定词 disharmony 既清晰地解释了人体上中下三个部位脉搏的失常，又贴切地传达出原文中的战争隐喻。

文本选用动词 conform（相符）的否定形式，指脉搏不相符合，互为冲突，进而和战争域产生联系，实现了目的语和源语在词汇意义和文体风格上的对等。

威本将"失"翻译为 err against。err 意为"犯错误、出差错"，虽然表达出脉搏失常的医理现象，但缺少对战争隐喻的再现。

吴本选用形容词 irregular（不规律的）来翻译"失"，仅表达出字面意思，未译出战争隐喻。

3. 以从为逆，荣卫散乱，真气已失。（《素问·离合真邪论》）

释义：使顺证变成逆证，以致病人荣卫散乱，正气消耗，邪气旺盛。

李本：Taking Cong (favorable) as Ni (unfavorable) will cause disorder of Rong (Nutrient-Qi) and (Defensive-Qi), loss of Zhenqi and retention of Xie (Evil) in the body.

威本：Instead of bringing about compliance they bring about resistance. Blood and vital substances become scattered and spoiled, the normal constitution becomes completely lost.

文本：He considers compliance to be opposition, causing camp and guard [qi] to disperse in disorder. The true qi has been lost already.

吴本：In this way, the case of a favourable prognosis will become a case of an unfavourable prognosis, the Rong-energy and the Wei-energy of the patient will be confusing, his healthy-energy will be exhausting.

句中"失"指真气的消耗、丧失。

李本、威本、文本对"失"的译法相似，均采用了直译。李本选用动词 lose 的名词 loss，威本和文本则选用其形容词 lost。lose 常与 game、war、 argument、election 等词搭配，是直接表达战争结果的词汇。因此，直译不仅保留了原文的信息，准确地表达出真气丧失的医理现象，而且也再现了原文的隐喻。

李本、威本和文本的不同之处在于对句式结构的处理上。汉语多意合，三个并列的四字短语"以从为逆，荣卫散乱，真气已失"之间含有因果关系，即"以从为逆"所导致的结果是"荣卫散乱，真气已失"。李本准确理解句子的逻辑关系，将三个短语处理为动名词或名词短语结构，并在第一个名词短语"以从为逆"后添加谓语动词 will cause，以主谓宾结构的长句体现原文的因果关系，也符合英语句法结构。

文本通过非谓语动词 causing 做状语将前两个并列短语处理成因果关系，也是可取的。

威本未能理解三个并列短语之间的逻辑关系，将其分别翻译成独立的句子，且第二个句子和第三个句子之间没有连词，建议改为 Instead of bringing about compliance they bring about resistance. Therefore, blood and vital substances become scattered and spoiled, and the normal constitution becomes completely lost.

吴本采用意译，选用 exhaust（耗尽、耗竭）翻译"失"，暗含着在与邪气的斗争中，正气逐渐损耗之意，表达出原文中的战争隐喻。但吴本受汉语意合思维的影响，用逗号连接三个分句，不符合英文形合的句子结构，可以改为 In this way, the case of a favourable prognosis will become a case of an unfavourable prognosis, thus the Rong-energy and the Wei-energy of the patient will be confusing, and his healthy-energy will be exhausted.

4.不当其位者病，迭移其位者病，失守其位者危。（《素问·五运行大论》）

释义：不当其位的会生病，左右相反的会生病，见到相克之脉病就危险。

李本：[If the pulse] does not appear in the right region, [it leads to] disease; [if the pulse has] changed the locations, [it leads to] disease; [if the pulse has] lost its position, [it indicates that the disease is] severe.

文本：When they oppose the qi [that controls heaven], then there is disease. When they do not occupy their proper position, [this indicates] disease.

吴本：When the energy is on the left and the pulse is on the right, it is the diseased pulse in the wrong position, when the corresponding pulse often shifts its position, it is also the diseased pulse.

"失守其位"指脉搏因致病因素的侵袭偏离其在体内的正常位置。

李本采用直译法，通过括号加注的方式补译出主语 the pulse，将"失守其位"译为 [if the pulse has] lost its position，表达脉搏因致病因素侵袭而丢失其守位，仿佛交战的一方因敌人进攻而丢失其领地，不仅忠于原文，也暗含战争隐喻。

文本将"失"译为 do not occupy，occupy 有"通过武力军事占领"之意，因此文本既译出原文脉搏位置变化，也将战争隐喻表现出来。

吴本将"失守其位"译为 shifts its position，虽将脉搏位置的变化表达出来，但 shift 未能表达出脉搏因致病因素侵袭而被动转换位置这一含义。

（二）衰

衰，与"盛"相对，指力量的减退，衰落，没落。在《素问》中，"衰"用来表达人体内部的正气与致病因素之间的抗衡和较量的结果，有"衰老、虚弱"或"减退、减少"之义。

1. 今五脏皆衰，筋骨解堕，天癸尽矣。（《素问·上古天真论》）

释义：现在年岁大了，五脏皆衰，筋骨无力，天癸竭尽。

李本：Now the Five Zang-Organs have declined, the bones become weak and the Tiangui is exhausted.

威本：But when, at this stage, the five viscera are dry, the muscles and bones decay, the generative secretions are exhausted.

文本：[At this age] now the five depots are all weak and the sinews and the bones have become sluggish. The heaven*gui* is used up entirely.

吴本：As one's five viscera are then all declining, the tendons and bones are all becoming weak, and the Taingui is also exhausted.

句中"衰"指五脏的衰弱。

李本和吴本将"衰"直译为动词 decline（在质量、数量或重要性上减少、下降），体现出正气与致病因素互相抗衡导致五脏功能衰弱这一结果，也暗含战争隐喻中敌方胜出而我方衰败的含义。尤金·奈达在《翻译科学探索》中指出，原文读者对原文的反应须和译文读者对译文的反应基本一致[1]。李本和吴本成功地把原文的信息和内涵传达出来，实现了读者反映的对等。

文本将"衰"译为形容词 weak（虚弱的），在一定程度上表达了脏腑功能减弱的事实。

在威本中，"衰"被翻译成 dry（干燥的），曲解了原文意思，属于误译。

2. 七日巨阳病衰，头痛少愈；八日阳明病衰，身热少愈。（《素问·热论》）

释义：到第七天，太阳病就会减轻，头痛也就会稍好一些；到第八天，阳明病会减轻，身热也会稍微消退。

李本：In the seventh day Taiyang disease alleviates and headache is mild; in the eighth day, Yangming disease alleviates and fever is mild.

威本：The sickness of the great Yang improves somewhat on the seventh day and the head aches less. On the eighth day the "sunlight" improves, and the body becomes less hot [feverish].

文本：On the seventh day, the disease in the great yang [conduits] weakens. The headache has somewhat abated. On the eighth day, the disease in the yang brilliance [conduits] weakens. The body heat has somewhat abated.

吴本：On the seventh day, the disease of Taiyang will turn to the better and the headache will be somewhat alleviated; on the eighth day, the disease of Yangming will turn to the better and the fever of the body will come down slightly.

句中"衰"指疾病的减轻、减弱。

四个译本均将"衰"处理为动词，但在选词上有较大差异。李本和文本选用表疾病减轻的动词，而威本和吴本选用了表疾病改善的动词。

李本将"衰"译为 alleviate（减轻痛苦或症状），传达出"疾病减轻"之义。但是 alleviate 常用作及物动词，因此李本将 Taiyang disease alleviates 改为 Taiyang disease is alleviated 更为合适。

文本将"衰"译为 weaken（减弱），表达出疾病威力减弱的战争隐喻。

威本和吴本没有正面翻译"衰"，而是分别将"病衰"意译为 The sick-

[1]　Eugene A. Nida. *Towards a Science of Translating* [M]. Leiden: E. J. Brill, 1964: 159.

《黄帝内经素问》隐喻英译对比研究

ness...improves 和 the disease...will turn to the better，表示疾病向着好的方向发展，贴近原文意义。美中不足的是，语言搭配不太规范，因为动词 improve 和 turn to the better 在表示"好转"之义时，主语应为 patients，而非 sickness 或 diseases。

3. 极则阴阳俱衰，卫气相离，故病得休。（《素问·疟论》）

释义：发病达到极点，则阴阳之气都已衰退，卫气和邪气相离，病就休止。

李本：[When the disease becomes] extremely serious, Yin and Yang begin to decline and Weiqi (Defensive–Qi) is separated from [Xieqi], and therefore preventing the occurrence of the disease.

文本：When it has reached its peak, then yin and yang are both weak and the guard [qi] and the [evil] qi have disassociated themselves from each other. Hence, the disease can rest.

吴本：When the attack of the disease is in the extreme condition, both the Yin and Yang energies will be declining, when the Wei–energy is devorced from the evil–energy, the disease will cease.

句中"衰"表阴阳之气的衰退减弱。

李本和吴本均将"衰"直译为不及物动词 decline（减弱、减少）。该词经常和 the military power、the war deaths 等与战争有关的主语搭配，这使 decline 具有战争中的一方偃旗息鼓、气势逐渐减弱的内涵，可以帮助目的语读者从较为熟悉的战争语域出发，投射到抽象的中医话语体系中，从而更好地理解阴阳之气衰弱的医理现象。因此，该译法是可取的。

但李本和吴本在时态上存在差异。李本选用一般现在时，借助 begin to do 短语表示阴气和阳气开始衰弱；吴本选用将来进行时 will be declining，表示将来某一时间疾病的状态。相比之下，将来进行时更能表达出阴阳之气逐渐衰弱的病理状态，因此，吴本的译法效果更佳。但是，吴本受到汉语意合结构的影响，用逗号连接所有的分句，这不符合英语形合的结构特征。应将其改为 When the attack of the disease..., ...will be declining; when the Wei–energy..., the disease will cease.

文本选用形容词 weak 翻译"衰"，表现出当疾病来临时阴气和阳气虚弱的状态。

4.各安其气，必清必静，则病气<u>衰</u>去，归其所宗。(《素问·至真要大论》)

释义：使五脏之气各安其所，清静无所扰乱，病气自然就会消退，那么其余气也就各归其类属。

李本：[Once] Qi (Healthy–Qi) is calmed and stabilized, Bingqi (Morbid–Qi) will decline and all [kinds of Qi] will return to the due positions.

文本：Always pacify the respective qi. It must be cleared and it must be calmed. As a result, the disease qi will weaken and leave and return to its origin.

吴本：In this way, the five viscera will each get to its due position without disturbing each other, the evil energy will be diminishing in due course, and the other energies will be each to its category without partial overabundance and resume its own normal state.

"衰"为动词，"病气衰去"指病气消退，句中将"病气"喻为敌人，当五脏之气各安其所时，病气就会不战而败自然消退，体现了战争隐喻。

李本沿袭其一贯用法，将"衰"译为 decline，表示病气的逐渐减弱之势，符合读者的认知，实现由源语到目的语的转化。

文本选用 weaken（虚弱、衰弱），也表现出病气渐渐减弱的过程。

吴本选用将来进行时 will be diminishing 解释"衰"的含义，diminish 意为"减弱、减少"，其与将来进行时的连用更能生动地描绘出疾病的变化趋势，巧妙传达出原文的内涵和战争隐喻。

（三）胜

"胜"，本义为"胜任、禁得起"。在《素问》中，"胜"用来表达人体内部的正气与致病因素之间的抗衡和较量的结果，有"充盛、过盛"或"得胜"之义，还可以指五行生克中的相胜。

1.阴<u>胜</u>则阳病，阳<u>胜</u>则阴病。阳<u>胜</u>则热，阴<u>胜</u>则寒。(《素问·阴阳应象大论》)

释义：如果阴气偏胜了，那么阳气必然受到损害。同样，阳气偏胜了，那么阴气也一定受到损害。阳气偏胜就会生热，阴气偏胜就会生寒。

李本：Predominance of Yin results in the disease of Yang while predominance of Yang leads to the disease of Yin.

威本：If Yin is healthy then Yang is apt to be defective, if Yang is healthy then Yin is apt to be sick.

文本：When yin dominates, then the yang is ill; when yang dominates, then the yin is ill.

吴本：The Yin and Yang within a human body must always be kept in balance. The over-abundance of Yin will cause Yang diseases, and the over-abundance of Yang will cause Yin diseases.

句中阴气和阳气是互相较量的双方，一方的获胜、占据上风被称为"胜"，具有强烈的战争隐喻色彩。

李本在意译的同时进行了词性转换，把动词"胜"翻译为名词 predominance（优势）。该词的英文释义为 the state of having more power or influence than others。由英文释义可以看出，该词可以准确地诠释出阴气或阳气的偏胜，能够表达出一方胜过另一方的战争隐喻，有利于传播源语中的隐喻文化。

文本和李本在"胜"的翻译上有相似之处，选用 predominance 的同根词 dominate。该词的英文释义为 to control or have a lot of influence over sb./sth.，也具有一方胜过另一方的含义，与汉语里的战争隐喻是对等的，因此有助于目的语读者深入理解原文中阴盛或阳盛的内涵。

李本和文本的不同之处在于，李本选用名词 predominance，文本选用动词 dominate。从词性的作用来看，dominate 更生动地体现出一方控制另一方的战争隐喻内涵；从句子结构来看，李本选用名词使句子更简明、更具逻辑性。

威本将动词"胜"意译为形容词 healthy，表明阴或阳的特性。这种译法曲解了"胜"的含义，也未将其蕴含的战争隐喻表达出来。

吴本将"胜"意译为名词 over-abundance，传达出阳气或阴气的过盛，但在表达战争隐喻上有所欠缺。

2. 五脏有病，则各传其所胜。(《素问·玉机真脏论》)

释义：五脏如果有病，就会传给各自所克之脏。

李本：[For example,] the diseases of the Five Zang-Organs are transmitted to the organs to be restricted respectively.

威本：When the five viscera are sick then each passes it on to that which is inferior.

文本：When [one of] the five depots has a disease, it is always transmitted to the [depot] which [the transmitting] can dominate.

吴本：If one of the five viscera is ill, its evil-energy will be transmitted to the viscera it restricts.

句中"胜"为动词，指五行生克中的相胜，"其所胜"意为所克之脏。

中医五行中的"相克"常被译为 restriction，"所胜"常被译为 element being restricted。李本、吴本分别将"其所胜"意译为 the organs to be restricted 和 the viscera it restricts，正确理解"胜"在句中"内脏之间互相制约"的内涵意义，准确传达原文内容，表现了敌我制衡的态势，较好地保留战争隐喻色彩。

威本将"其所胜"译为 which is inferior（地位、级别较低的内脏）是将"胜"误解为"战胜"，与"相克"之义相去甚远，未能正确理解并传递原文。

文本将"其所胜"译为 the [depot] which [the transmitting] can dominate，首先是将"胜"误解为"掌控"，虽然具有战争隐喻色彩，但是未能正确传达原文内涵意义；同时，也将"胜"的施动者"五脏"误解为"传"（the transmitting），未能正确理解原文。

3. 今水不胜火，则骨枯而髓虚。（《素问·痿论》）

释义：现在水不能胜火热，就会骨枯髓空。

李本：Failure of water to control fire will lead to dryness of bones and deficiency of marrow.

文本：Here now, the water does not dominate the fire. As a result the bones dry and the marrow is depleted.

吴本：And presently, the water is unable to overcome the heat of fire, the marrow will be emptied.

句中"胜"用作动词，指水火中的一方处于优势，能控制另一方。

李本未拘泥于字对字的翻译，而是从整个句子的逻辑出发，将"今水不胜火"译为名词词组 Failure of water to control fire，充当"则骨枯而髓虚"的主语，表达出水火互相较量的战争隐喻。

文本将"胜"翻译为 dominate，该词体现出"胜"表控制的意思。

吴本将"胜"直译为 overcome，指一方能战胜、解决另一方，也表达出水和火之间争胜的关系。

综上所述，李本、文本和吴本均选用一些经常出现在战争语境的词汇，如 control、dominate、overcome，表示水争胜于火。

（四）耗

耗，假借为"消"，本义为"亏损、消耗"。在《素问》中，"耗"用来表达致病因素对人体正气侵犯导致的结果，有"消耗、匮乏"之义，也可以指"轻用、不加珍惜地随便使用"。

1. 以欲竭其精，以耗散其真。（《素问·上古天真论》）

释义：以致精气竭尽，真气耗散。

李本：[As a result,] their Jingqi (Essence–Qi) is exhausted and Zhenqi (Genuine–Qi) is wasted.

威本：Their passions exhaust their vital forces; their cravings dissipate their true (essence).

文本：Through their lust they exhaust their essence, through their wastefulness they dissipate their true [qi].

吴本：They are addicted to drink without temperance, keep idling as an ordinary, indulge in sexual pleasures and use up their vital energy and ruin their health.

句中"耗"为动词，表示人体受到侵犯导致的结果是真气消耗，隐喻战败的一方精疲力竭。

李本以"真气"作主语，将原文的主动语态改为被动语态，将"耗散其真"译为 Zhenqi (Genuine–Qi) is wasted。waste 意为"浪费、滥用"，语意契合原文，忠实传达出当今不注意养生、随意浪费真气的事实；但 waste 在表达"耗"所蕴含的战争隐喻上张力不够，有所欠缺。

威本和文本使用动词 dissipate（消散、挥霍）表达"耗"，传递出"真气耗散"之义；同时，英语中 dissipate 常用于战争隐喻，例如 dissipate the anger、dissipate the fog of war 等，因此这一译法较好传达了原文的内容与文化特色。

吴本对原文进行意译，将"耗"译为 use up，该短语简明清楚地表达出"真气耗尽"之义，但未能保留战争隐喻特色。

2. 孤精于内，气耗于外。（《素问·汤液醪醴论》）

释义：内里精血虚损，外面卫气耗散。

李本：...internal stagnation of Jing (Essence–Qi), external exhaustion of Qi...

威本：The spirit is confined to the interior of the body, while wasteful and destructive airs attack from the outside.

文本：The po–soul resides alone. The essence is weakened in the interior.

吴本：Their symptoms appear to be the emptiness of the body fluid, the withering of the spiritual activities, consumption of the essence and blood inside, and the dispersion of the Wei–energy outside.

句中"耗"指真气在体外消耗的结果。

李本将"气耗于外"译为名词短语 external exhaustion of qi（气的外在枯竭）。exhaustion（耗竭）准确地传递出"耗"在句中的内涵意义，同时也保留了战争隐喻特色。

文本使用被动语态将"气耗于外"译为 The essence is weakened in the interior。此译法省略施动者，用 weakened 偏重表达气损耗的状态。weaken 暗含一方被另一方减弱、削弱，具有战争隐喻色彩。

威本将"气耗于外"译为 wasteful and destructive airs attack from the outside（邪气从体外进攻），是对原文的误解。首先，原文中的"气"并非指邪气，而是指守卫人体的正气；其次，对"气"的误译导致威本将"耗"译为 attack，这与"耗"在句中"正气消耗"之意相差甚远。

与李本一样，吴本也将"气耗于外"译为名词短语 the dispersion of the Wei–energy outside。dispersion 意为"分散、散布"，而原文"耗"指"消耗、匮乏"，因此意思与原文不太贴切。

3. 惊则气乱，劳则气耗，思则气结。（《素问·举痛论》）

释义：过惊则气混乱，过劳则气耗损，思虑则气郁结。

李本：...[excessive] fright disorders Qi; overstrain consumes Qi; [excessive] contemplation binds Qi.

文本：When one is frightened, then the qi is in disorder. When one is exhausted, then the qi is wasted. When one is pensive, then the qi lumps together.

吴本：When one is in excessive melancholy，the energy will be confusing；when one is over fatigue, the energy will be consumed; when one is anxious and worrying, the energy will be stagnated.

句中"耗"为动词，"气耗"表被动义，意为"气被消耗"。

李本、吴本都使用 consume（消耗、耗费）表达"耗"，符合句意。不同的是，李本采用主动句结构，将"劳则气耗"直译为 overstrain consumes Qi，传递出"操劳过度耗费真气"之义，明确指明"劳"和"气"之间的逻辑关系。而吴本采用被动句结构，将"劳则气耗"意译为 when one is over fatigue, the energy will be consumed。在"疾病是战争"这一隐喻模式下，二者都选用 consume 表达"耗"，表达了正气犹如战争中的士气一样被渐渐地消耗的含义，保留战争隐喻特色。相比而言，李本语言更为鲜明。

文本将"气耗"译为 qi is wasted（气被浪费）。动词 waste 意为"浪费、未充分利用"，偏离了"耗"在句中的内涵意义，有失妥当。

4. 病深者，以其外耗于卫，内夺于荣。（《素问·疏五过论》）

释义：这种病所以会日渐加深，就是因为情志抑郁，在外耗损了卫气，在内劫夺了荣血的关系。

李本：Aggravation of the disease is due to external consumption of Wei (Defensive-Qi) and internal loss of Rong (Nutrient-Qi).

文本：When the disease is in the depth, this is because the guard [qi] is diminished in the outer [regions of the body] and the camp [qi] has been removed from its inner [region].

吴本：As the disease is caused by the depression of the spirit, the Wei energy will be wasted outside, and the Rong energy which nourished the blood will be depleted inside, and the condition will become worse day after day.

句中"耗"为动词，"外耗于卫"指卫气在外被损耗。

李本简译原文，将"外耗于卫"译为名词短语 external consumption of Wei (Defensive-Qi)（卫气的外在损耗），忠实传达原文内容。

文本选用被动语态 be diminished 表示卫气被损耗。diminish 意为"减弱、减少"，该词有利于读者理解体内卫气不断被减弱的过程，也暗含两者相争，一方势力逐渐减弱的战争隐喻。

吴本采用被动语态，将"外耗于卫"译为 the Wei energy will be wasted outside。wasted 意为"浪费、白费"，与原文"卫气被消耗"的意思不符，属于误译。

六、预后不良或疾病恶化

（一）亡

"亡"，本义为"逃跑、逃亡"，引申为"失去"。在《素问》中，"亡"用来表达致病因素对人体正气侵犯，导致疾病进一步恶化，预后不良。

1. 风客淫气，精乃亡，邪伤肝也。（《素问·生气通天论》）

释义：风邪侵入人体，渐渐侵害元气，精血就要损耗，这是由于邪气伤害肝脏的缘故。

李本：When wind attacks the body, [it gradually] damages Qi and exhausts Jing (Essence). [This is because of] the impairment of the liver by Xie (Evil).

威本：If the wind enters the body and exhausts man's breath, then his essence will be lost and the evil influences will injure his liver.

文本：When wind settles [in the body] and encroaches upon the [proper] qi, then the essence vanishes, and the evil harms the liver.

吴本：Owning to the wind associates with the liver (liver correspond to the wind and wood), when one is hurt by excessive wind-evil, the essence of life and blood will suffer severe damage. As blood is stored in the liver, the wind-evil will hurt the liver too.

由于对句中"亡"的理解不同，四个译本出现了直译和意译两种译法。李本和吴本采用意译法，将"亡"理解为精血的损耗、遭受损失；威本和文本采用直译法，将"亡"理解为精血的彻底消亡、消失。

李本增译主语"风"，使用主动语态将"精乃亡"译为 (wind) exhausts Jing (Essence)（风亡精），体现出"精被损耗"之义。

吴本将"亡"译为 suffer severe damage（遭受严重的损失）。这两种译法均能表现出风邪入侵导致精损耗，同时亦保留了战争隐喻特色。

《黄帝内经素问》隐喻英译对比研究

威本和文本采用直译法，分别将"亡"译为 be lost（丢失）和 vanish（消失）。此译法过度加深"亡"的程度，未表达出精血在致病因素侵袭下损耗的医理。可见，译者主体性过强会导致过度加工，在一定程度上影响目的语读者对中医文化的正确理解。

2. 逆从倒行，标本不得，亡神失国。（《素问·移精变气论》）

释义：假如认识病情时把顺逆搞颠倒了；处理疾病时又不能取得病人的配合。这样的话，就会使病人的神气消亡，身体受到损害。

李本：Errors in distinguishing the favorable from the unfavorable [changes of the countenance and pulse will result in] disagreement between the Biao (the diagnosis and treatment) and Ben (the pathological changes of the patients), inevitably leading to depletion of Shen (spirit or vitality) [in treating diseases] and national subjugation [in governing a country].

威本：When those who rebelled against the laws of nature obtained power, the medicines prepared from the topmost branches and roots were no longer given, the divine spirit perished and the country deteriorated.

文本：If [acting] contrary to and [acting] in compliance with [the norms] are reversed, and if tip and root do not match, [in the course of the treatment the healer] loses his spirit, [just as in government the ruler] loses his country.

吴本：If the source of the disease in comprehended in a wrong sequence, or fail to obtain the cooperation of the patient, the treatment will not succeed. When one assists a king to rule the country like this, the country will be subjugated.

句中"亡"为动词，"亡神"指神气消亡。

李本采用词性转化的方法，将"亡神"意译为名词短语 depletion of Shen，充当动词 lead to 的宾语。depletion 意为"损耗、锐减"，侧重数量上的大量减少，因此虽然在一定程度上可以表示神的损耗，但并不十分贴切。

威本和文本都采用直译法，保持译文与原文的结构一致。威本将"失神"译为 the divine spirit perished。perish 为不及物动词，意为"丧失、毁灭"，传达出"神"受到侵犯而丧失的过程，符合目的语读者认知中的战争隐喻模式。文本补译出"失神"的施动者 the healer，将其译为（the healer）loses his spirit，虽不如威本形象生动，但也简明准确，利于读者理解。

吴本漏译"亡神"。

3. 真气得安，邪气乃<u>亡</u>。(《素问·疟论》)

释义：那正气不伤，邪气也就完了。

李本：Treatment [at this stage] can calm Zhenqi (Genuine-Qi) and eliminate Xieqi.

文本：The true qi will find peace and the evil qi will perish.

吴本：A treating in time will not injure the healthy energy and the evil-energy can be removed.

句中"亡"为动词，"乃亡"与"得安"相对，隐喻疾病发作时及时调治能够使邪气消亡。

李本增译主语 treatment，将"亡"译为 eliminate，其宾语为"邪气"。eliminate 意为"清除、消除"，同时还具有消灭、杀死敌人或对手之义。由此可见，在英文语境中 eliminate 已隐含战争隐喻，因此李本对"亡"的翻译实现了从源语到目的语的正确映射。

文本选用 perish 来翻译"亡"。该词为不及物动词，意为"丧失、毁灭"，既正确解读了原文，又形象地传达出邪气消亡所蕴含的战争隐喻。

吴本选用及物动词 remove，使用被动语态，将"邪气乃亡"译为 the evil-energy can be removed。removed 意为"移除、移去"，体现出邪气被祛除的医理，但缺少战争隐喻色彩。

4. 阴气者，静则神藏，躁则消<u>亡</u>。(《素问·痹论》)

释义：五脏的阴气，安静时就精神内藏，躁动时就易于耗散。

李 本：When Yinqi [of the Five Zang-Organs] is calm, Shen (Spirit) maintains inside; when Yinqi [of the Five Zang-Organs] is restless, [Qi] is exhausted.

文本：As for the yin qi, if it is kept calm, then the spirit is stored; if it is agitated, then it wastes away and perishes.

吴本：When the Yin energy of the five solid organs is calm, the spirit will be kept inside, when it is irritating, it will apt to be dispersed outside.

句中"静"与"躁"，"藏"与"亡"对仗工整，语句优美。在字义上，"亡"与"藏"相对，表示五脏阴气的耗散。

在句式上，李本采用主从复合句结构，构成两个排比句；在选词上，以形容词作表语，保持与原文形式的统一，体现出对仗之美。李本用形容词 exhausted 表达气的耗散。exhausted 指过度操劳带来的精神、精力的耗竭，既传达出因为躁动导致阴气耗散的医理，也保留了原文的隐喻特色。

文本采用直译法，将"消亡"译为 waste away and perish，将阴气耗散的信息传达给目的语读者；但字对字的直译也造成意义的重复和语言繁琐。perish 本身就具有 waste away 所表达的"逐渐消失"的含义，因此若只保留 perish，删去 waste away，译文会更简明。

吴本将"亡"译为 be dispersed。disperse 意为"分散、散开"，仅表达出阴气的分散，未将阴气耗尽的意思表达出来，因此译不达意。

（二）败

"败"，本义为"毁坏、搞坏"，后引申为战争的"失败、战败"。在《素问》中，"败"也用来指疾病进一步恶化，预后不良。

1. 所谓阴者，真脏也，见则为<u>败</u>，<u>败</u>必死也。（《素问·阴阳别论》）

释义：所谓阴脉就是五脏真气呈败露之象的真脏脉，如果这种败象显现了出来，那就一定要死了。

李本：The so-called Yin pulse refers to Zhenzang (Genuine-Zang) [pulse] [marked by loss of Weiqi (Stomach-Qi)]. The appearance of such pulse is [the sign of] the deterioration [of the Five Zang-Organs] and the deterioration [of the Five Zang-Organs] inevitably leads to death.

威本：Of the intestines some belong entirely to the Yin element, and when these become visible they become impaired; and when these intestines are impaired death follows.

文本：As for the so-called yin [qi], these are the true [qi of the] depots. When they appear, this indicates destruction. Destruction entails death.

吴本：Yin indicates the pulse condition of indicating the exhaustion of visceral energy which is of entirely no stomach-energy. It may occur in all the pulses of the five solid organs. In clinic, most of them represent the syndrome of corruption. As the viscera-energy is corrupted and the stomach-energy is severed, the patient will surely die.

句中"败"为名词，从"战败"引申而来，指疾病的恶化。

李本使用名词 deterioration（恶化、退化）表达"败"，该词准确无误、贴合原文。同时，deterioration 在英文中也常指两国关系的恶化，如 a serious deterioration in relations between the two countries，其本身也包含战争隐喻的内涵，有利于读者从熟悉的战争概念出发去理解中医语言的战争隐喻。

吴本选用名词 corruption（堕落、腐化）和形容词 corrupted（腐化的、腐败的）对"败"进行意译。这两个词侧重指权力、政府的腐败，也指身体的腐化。将"败"转换为 corruption 和 corrupted，贴近原文战争隐喻的深层内涵，表达出疾病的恶化之意。

威本将"败"译为 impaired（被损害），表现出疾病在五脏的恶化，该词的选用是成功的。但威本将"脏"译为 intestine，原文中"脏"指"五脏"，而 intestine 指"肠"，属于误译。

文本选用名词 destruction 来翻译"败"。destruction 意为"摧毁、毁灭"，总体上能够传达出疾病恶化的态势，但严重程度过高，不如 deterioration 贴合原文。

2. 下工救其已成，救其已<u>败</u>。（《素问·八正神明论》）

释义：而不高明的医生，却等病已形成或疾病已经败坏时才治疗。

李本：Poor doctors give treatment only after the onset or aggravation of a disease.

威本：The inferior physician begins to help when (the disease) has already developed; he helps when destruction has already set in.

文本："The inferior practitioner stops what has already fully developed" [is to say:] he [attempts to] rescue what is already ruined.

吴本：A poor physician can not discover the disease at the beginning, he can only treat the disease when it has already taken shape.

句中"败"隐喻病情的恶化。

李本采用词性转化法，将"败"译为名词 aggravation（恶化）。该词既指病情的恶化，也可用于战争语境中，表示冲突加剧、关系恶化。因此，李本准确实现目的语和源语的对应，译文准确。

威本将"败"译为名词 destruction，该词虽能表现出病情恶化之义，但表示的恶化程度过重、范围过大，不如李本的 aggravation 精妙。

文本将"败"译为名词性从句 what is already ruined。意译使译文流畅自然，中心词 ruined 也常用于战争语境，传达出战争隐喻。

吴本不拘泥于原文的句式结构，将"救其已败"意译为 ...treat the disease when it has already taken shape。此译法以目的语读者为中心，便于理解，但过度意译使译文失去了原文中的战争隐喻和中医文化特色。

3. 邪溢气壅，脉热肉<u>败</u>，荣卫不行，必将为脓。（《素问·气穴论》）

释义：如果外邪亢进，正气壅塞，脉热肉坏，荣卫不能通行，肌肉必定要肿脓。

李本：Exuberance of Xie (Evil) and stagnation of Qi, feverishness of Channels and decay of muscles as well as stoppage of Rong (Nutrient–Qi) and Wei (Defensive–Qi) lead to suppuration.

文本：When evil overflows [from the tertiary network vessels], the [paths of the] qi are congested. The vessels turn hot and the flesh rots. The camp and the guard [qi] do not move. This will cause pus [to develop].

吴本：When the evil–energy invades and resides in the valley and groove, the healthy–energy will become stagnated to cause the blood–heat and the deterioration of the muscle, the Rong and Wei energies will be unable to pass through and the muscle will become swelling.

句中"败"指人体肌肉因外邪过盛而溃烂、败坏。

李本将"肉败"译为名词短语 decay of muscles。decay 意为"腐烂、腐朽"，准确地表达出原文"败"的含义。

文本将"败"译为动词 rot。rot 和 decay 为同义词，意为"腐烂、腐朽"，忠实地传达出人体肌肉溃烂的情形。

吴本将"肉败"译为名词词组 the deterioration of the muscle。deterioration 意为"恶化"，其常与病情、关系等搭配，因此与 muscle 搭配有失妥当。

4. 故贵脱势，虽不中邪，精神内伤，身必<u>败</u>亡。（《素问·疏五过论》）

释义：譬如原来的封君公侯，一旦降职罢官，虽然不中外邪，而精神上先已受伤，身体一定要败坏，甚至死亡。

李本：[If a noble person has] lost the position, [he will certainly suffer from] internal damage [due to depression], though there is no invasion of Xie (Evil) [from the outside].

文本：The fact is, when a [man of] noble rank is stripped of his power, even though he was not struck by an evil [qi from outside], his essence and spirit have been harmed inside and [hence] his body must face destruction and death.

吴本：Such as, when a former prince or duke who has been dismissed from office and demoted, although he is not attacked by the outer evil, yet his spirit is injured already. His body will be harmed and he can even die.

句中"败"为动词，隐喻身体状况恶化。

李本仅翻译了前三个分句，漏译了"身必败亡"。

文本采用直译，将"身必败亡"译为 his body must face destruction and death，保留了原文的意思，是可取的。

吴本和文本类似，采用直译法将"身必败亡"译为 His body will be harmed and he can even die，忠实地翻译出原文。与文本相比，吴本语言更加地道，更符合英语的行文习惯。

综上，吴本和文本均采用战争语境中表败亡的词，如 destruction、death、die，来翻译原文中的战争隐喻，将战争结果投射到表示疾病变化结果的概念域中，成功实现了隐喻的翻译。

《黄帝内经素问》隐喻英译对比研究

小 结

本章介绍了《素问》中有关阴阳学说、精气学说、脏腑学说和战争隐喻等结构隐喻的用法，并对四个译本进行了对比分析。由于译者的文化背景、汉语底蕴、职业特点、受众读者等各不相同，对源语的诠释和翻译方法也不尽相同，各译本既有相似之处，又各具特色。

本章共列举十余个有关"阴阳""阴""阳"隐喻的例句，它们在不同语境中的含义不尽相同。李本以直译为主，能够根据语境较灵活地变通"阴阳"的翻译或适当增补，如将"把握阴阳"译为 the law of nature，将"所谓阴阳者，去者为阴，至者为阳"译为 "The Yin and Yang [pulses can be defined in this way], the receding [pulse] is Yin and the coming [pulse] is Yang"。威本多采用直译加注，注重保留中医文化，常将"阴阳"译为 Yin and Yang，并根据语境适当进行注释，如"法于阴阳"译为 the Yin and the Yang [the two principles in nature]。此外，威本增补内容较多，虽利于读者的理解，但语言略显拖沓。文本与吴本采用音译法较多，有时未能准确理解"阴阳"在语境中的具体含义，故不能很好地传递原文信息。

"精""气"相关隐喻主要体现在水精、精微、肾精、天气、地气、精气以及各脏腑之气等术语中。李本注重源语文化的外传与外译，惯用汉语拼音 Jing 和 Qi 对译"精"和"气"。在翻译"脏腑"之气时，借用西医解剖学中对诸脏的表述进行注释。文本主要采用意译法和音译法对"精"和"气"进行英译，多用 essence 和 qi 来对译"精"和"气"。吴本主要采用意译法，将"精"译为 substance，将"气"译为 energy。由于其中医师的职业特点，而且读者群体多为患者，吴本更加通俗化，不注重术语表达规范和中医文化的外传，专注信息传递。威本主要采用意译法，将"精"以多种译法呈现，如 spirit、essence、vitality、energy 等；将"气"译为 force、influence、vapor 等。遣词较为随意，不注重术语表达规范，也弱化了文化传递。

脏腑器官通常被喻为相傅、将军、中正、臣使、仓廪、传导、受盛、作强、决渎、州都等，生动形象地解释了人体五脏六腑复杂的生理功能、病理变化规律及相互关系。李本多采用音译法，例如将"三焦"和"气化"分别译为 Sanjiao (triple energizer) 和 Qihua (Qi-transformation)；同时多借助 similar to 将原文中的隐喻做显化处理，便于读者理解隐喻的内涵意义，达到跨文化交际的目的。而威本由于受其自身文化背景和语言环境的限制，对多处隐喻的翻译出现理解偏差。例如，将"气化"译为 vaporization（蒸发、汽化），误将"气"理解为"汽"；将"传道之官"译为 the officials who propagate the Right Way of Living（传经布道之官），未能正确理解汉语文化中这些官职的真正含义，这在很大程度上限制了中医文化的对外传播。文本多紧扣原文进行释义，简明译出脏腑部位对人体的作用。例如，将"肝"译为 the official functioning as general，直接将"肝"比作"具有将军职能的官员"，较为忠实地体现了源文化的内涵，但未指出"肝"与"将军"的共通之处，不利于读者理解原文隐喻，影响对中医文化的接受度。吴本多采用增译法对脏腑部位对应的官职职能进行解释。例如，将"仓廪之官"译为 an officer who is in charge of the granary，同时增译了 digesting, absorbing, spreading, storing 四个动词说明脾胃的职能，从而帮助读者较好地理解各脏腑部位在人体内的职能。

战争隐喻用以解释疾病的产生、发展、防治以及结果等，疾病与战争之间的隐喻映射主要体现在动词（夺、犯、伤、扰、守、攻、卫、博、争、胜、失、衰、耗、亡、败）和少数名词（贼、客、邪）。对于名词的翻译，李本多采取音译加注法，例如将"贼风"译为 Zeifeng (Thief–Wind)，将"客气"译为 Ke (Guest–Qi) 等。威本倾向于采用意译法，但有时会出现误译或者词不达意，例如将"气贼"译为 a contrary (wrong) reaction，将"邪气"译为 harmful influences 等。文本多采用直译法，但是有时曲解了原文的意思，例如将"气贼"译为 a plunderer of qi（气的盗贼），这与"气贼"在句中"致病因素"之义相去甚远。吴本多采用意译法，几乎没有误译和歧义，但是也容易出现用同一译法表达不同术语的现象，例如将"气贼""淫邪""邪""邪气"皆译为 the evil–energy，表意不够精确。同时，由于表示战争隐喻的动词常常随着语境变化而意义多变，因此四个译本多使用意译法翻译动词。例如，"客"兼具"寄居"和"侵入"两层隐喻义，因此常被译成 settle、reside、stay、enter 或者 attack、invade into。当"客"强调"侵入"之义时，李本译为 attack 或 invade，吴本译为 hurt 或 invade into，这与"犯"的译法是类似的。李本将"犯"译为 attack，文本和吴本将"犯"译为 invade，虽然"客"和"犯"的字面意思差别较大，但是二者的内涵意义相近，译法也就类似。

综上所述，李本采用拼音加注法，既保留了中医术语的汉语语言风格，又传递了原文的战争隐喻特色；忠实于原文，书面语程度高，句式简洁，尽显凝练之美。因此李本在信息传递、遣词造句、句式结构、文化保留、术语翻译规范等方面都略胜于其余三个译本。

第七章　社会关系隐喻及英译

社会关系隐喻是指参照社会生活中用来表达人际关系的各种具体或抽象概念所形成的中医隐喻概念，如君臣、父母、母子、夫妻、主客等。这类隐喻以人类的社会关系作为喻体，通过人们对社会关系的认识来理解人体脏腑器官的关系和功能。母、子、孙等本来都是人的亲属关系，但在《素问》中用来隐喻人体不同部分之间的关系。在说明不同器官的功能时，《素问》用政府机构的功能进行隐喻，不但形象，而且解释力强。《素问》中，社会关系隐喻主要包括官职隐喻、父母隐喻、母子隐喻等。

第一节　官职隐喻及英译

所谓官职，是指在国家各级机构中担任一定职务的官吏，涉及职官的名称、职权范围和品级地位等。一直以来，中医界就流传着"医道通治道"的说法，即中医医理与治国之术相通。这是一种逻辑类比，更是一种隐喻的思维方式。在这种思想的指导下，古人通过各种隐喻努力寻找中医医理与治国之术的相通之处。在这种文化背景下，很多中医学词语便与治理国家和社会结构的词语产生了千丝万缕的联系，并以隐喻的方式实现从源域（社会学）到目标域（中医学）的映射。

在《素问》中，为了更好地说明五脏六腑的功能，出现了很多官职隐喻，形象地把五脏六腑隐喻成各种官职。

1. 心者，君主之官也，神明出焉。（《素问·灵兰秘典论》）

释义：在人体内，心的重要性就好比君主，人们的聪明智慧都是从心生出来的。

李本：The heart is the organ [similar to] a monarch and is responsible for Shen-ming (mental activity or thinking).

威本：The heart is like the minister of the monarch who excels through insight and understanding.

文本：The heart is the official functioning as ruler. Spirit brilliance originates in it.

吴本：The heart is the supreme commander or the monarch of the human body, it dominates the spirit, ideology and thought of man.

句中将"心"喻为"君主"，通过官职隐喻说明心的功能。

文本采用 A is B 的结构，将"君主之官"译成 the official functioning as ruler，将原文隐喻的内容显化，较为准确地译出与心对应的官职的职能，从而帮助读者理解心的功能。

李本使用短语 be similar to，将隐喻转换为明喻，以明喻的形式呈现隐喻的内容。将"君主之官"译成 the organ [similar to] a monarch，但读者仍然不好理解 the organ 与 a monarch 之间的相似之处，因此在达意上有一定不足。

吴本同样采用 A is B 的结构，将"君主之官"译成 the supreme commander or the monarch of the human body，读者理解起来仍有一定困难，未能很好地实现交际目的。

威本采用 be like 结构将原文中的隐喻转换为明喻，译文用词比较丰富，体现了译者以英语为母语的语言优势。但是，译者受自身文化背景的局限，将"君主之官"译成 the minister of the monarch（君主的大臣），出现误译。

2. 愿闻十二脏之相使，贵贱何如？（《素问·灵兰秘典论》）

释义：我希望听你讲一下十二脏器在人体内的相互作用，有无主从的区别？

李本：I'd like to know the functions of the twelve Zang-Organs and their positions. Could you explain it for me?

威本：I desire to hear how it is possible that the twelve viscera send each other that which is precious and that which is worthless.

文本：I should like to hear [the following]: How do the twelve depots engage each other, and what is their hierarchy?

吴本：I would like you to tell me the mutual relations between the twelve viscera in human body and their principal and subordinate status in functions.

"相使"泛指官职，"贵贱"指职位的高低。句中将十二脏喻为帝王体制中分工不同的官职。

吴本将"相使"意译为 the mutual relations between the twelve viscera，较为准确地表达出十二脏之间的相互关系；另外，吴本将"贵贱"译成 principal（主要的）和 subordinate（从属的），较好地说明"贵贱"的含义，即十二脏之间的主从关系。

李本采用直译和音译相结合的方法，将"十二脏"译为 twelve Zang-Organs，保留了源语的文化特色。但译文中的 functions（功能）和 positions（职位）未能准确地表达出"相使"和"贵贱"的含义。

文本将"相使"意译为 engage each other，强调十二脏之间的相互联系和相互作用。但 engage 表示"相通、相互联系"时，应与介词 with 搭配。此处可改为 engage with each other。另外，文本将"贵贱"译为 hierarchy（等级制度），也不准确。

威本未能正确理解"相使"作为官职的意义，误译成 send each other（相互派遣）[1]。另外，威本将"贵""贱"直译为 precious（宝贵的）和 worthless（没有价值的），仅停留在表面意义，没有真正理解句中"贵贱"的内涵，导致完全没有传达出原文的意思。

3. 凡此<u>十二官</u>者，不得相失也。故<u>主</u>明则下安……<u>主</u>不明则<u>十二官</u>危……（《素问·灵兰秘典论》）

释义：以上十二脏器的作用，不能失去协调。当然，君是最主要的。它如果得力，下边就能相安……反之，如果君不得力，那么十二官就成问题了……

李本：These twelve organs should not lose balance. If the monarch (the heart)

---

[1] 罗茜. 模因论视角下《黄帝内经·素问》隐喻翻译研究 [J]. 景德镇学院学报，2016，31（5）：65.

is wise (normal in functions), the subordinates (the other organs) will be peaceful (normal in function)... [If] the monarch (the heart) is not wise (abnormal in function), all the twelve organs will be in danger...

威本：These twelve officials should not fail to assist one another. When the monarch is intelligent and enlightened, there is peace and contentment among his subjects...But when the monarch is not intelligent and enlightened, the twelve officials become dangerous and perilous...

文本：All these twelve officials must not lose [contact with] each other. Hence, if the ruler is enlightened, his subjects are in peace... If the ruler is not enlightened, then the twelve officials are in danger...

吴本：The above twelve viscera must be coordinating and supplementing to each other. As the heart is the monarch in the organs, it dominates the functions of the various viscera, so when the function of heart is strong and healthy, under its unified leadership, all the functions of the various viscera will be normal... but when the monarch is thick-headed, that is, when the function of the heart is incapable, the mutual relations between the viscera in the body will be damaged...

"故主明则下安""主不明则十二官危"包含两层意思，一是指字面上的君臣关系，二是隐喻含义，指心（君主）和其他脏腑（臣子）的关系。

李本将"主""明""下""安"分别译为 monarch (the heart)、wise (normal in functions)、the subordinates (the other organs) 和 peaceful (normal in function)，用加注的方式将喻指对象补充出来，既有助于读者对译文的理解，又有利于信息的准确传递和源语文化的对外传播。

吴本不囿于原文的叙述顺序，采用增译法分别论述心（heart）与其他脏腑（various viscera）的关系。由此可见，吴本不受原文语言形式的限制，更注重语义的传达，增译后的详细译文更利于读者的理解。

威本和文本对十二脏与官职的隐喻关系进行直译，译文较为简洁，基本能够说明十二脏之间相互协调的重要性。两个译本分别将"主"译为 monarch（君主）和 ruler（统治者）。结合原文语境可知，句中"君"喻指作为"君主之官"的"心"，因此译为 monarch 更为恰当。

4. 君位臣则顺，臣位君则逆。（《素问·六微旨大论》）

释义：君居臣位是顺的，臣居君位是逆的。

李本：[If] the Monarch is in the position of the Courtier, [it is] the favorable [condition]; [if] the Courtier is in the position of the Monarch, [it is] the adverse [condition].

文本：When the ruler takes the position of the official, then this is compliance. When the official takes the position of the ruler, then this is opposition.

吴本：When the monarch situates in the position of the courtier, it is the agreeable condition, when the courtier situates in the position of the monarch, it is the adverse condition.

句中"君"和"臣"分别指君火和相火，这两个名称本身就是一种官职隐喻。君火，指心火，因为心为君主之官，故而得名。君火居于上焦，能够主宰全身。相火居于下焦，可以温养脏腑。二者各安其位，促使机体发挥正常功能。

三个译本均采用直译法，说明君火和相火之间的相互关系。

就"君""臣"两词的翻译，李本和吴本都译为 monarch（君主）和 courtier（朝臣），较为准确地表达出君与臣的意思，帮助读者理解二者的关系。

文本将这"君""臣"译为 ruler（统治者）和 official（官员），仅表达出广义的上下级关系，无法准确表达出君与臣的对应关系。

5. 君一臣二，奇之制也；君二臣四，偶之制也。（《素问·至真要大论》）

释义：君药一味，臣药二味，是奇方之法；君药二味，臣药四味，是偶方之法。

李本：Odd [prescription is] composed of one Monarch [drug] and two Minister [drugs]; even [prescription is] composed of two Monarch [drugs] and four Minister [drugs].

文本：One ruler, two ministers, that is an uneven composition. Two rulers, four ministers, that is an even composition.

吴本：When applying one monarch medical herb and two courtier medical herbs, it is the method of making an odd prescription; when applying two monarch med–

ical herbs and four courtier medical herbs, it is the method of making an even pre-scription.

句中将主药、辅药分别喻为君、臣，从而阐述方剂中的君臣佐使理论。

李本补译出隐喻的具体内容 prescription，用"君"和"臣"喻指"君药"和"臣药"，有助于读者的理解；补译出 prescription，将隐喻显化，使语义更加清楚明了，从而较好地达到跨文化交际的目的。

文本在句式上与原文对应，用 one ruler、two ministers 对应"君一臣二"，但是仅使用 ruler 和 ministers 两个词来翻译"君臣"，却未对这一隐喻做出详细解释，读者仍然难以理解。

吴本采用意译法，将"君""臣"译为 monarch medical herb 和 courtier medical herb，增译出 herb 一词，使译文清楚地表明君药与臣药之间的关系，有效地传递了信息，便于读者理解。

6. 主病之谓君，佐君之谓臣，应臣之谓使，非上下三品之谓也。（《素问·至真要大论》）

释义：主治疾病的药味就是君，辅佐君药的就是臣，供应臣药的就是使，不是上中下三品的意思。

李本：[The drugs for] treating disease are called the Monarch [drugs]; [the drugs for] assisting the Monarch [drugs] are called the Minister [drugs]; [and the drugs for] corresponding to the Minister [drugs] are called the Envoy [drugs]. [These three categories of drugs in a prescription] are not the so-called the upper, medium and lower grades [of drugs].

文本：[The drug] which rules the disease is called "ruler". [The drug] which assists the ruler is called "minister". [The drugs] which respond to the minister are called "messengers". This has nothing to do with the three ranks [of drugs as cate-gorized] in the upper, [middle], and lower [ranks].

吴本：The main medical herb for treating the disease is the monarch herb, the assistant medicine for helping the monarch medicine is the courtier herb, and the medicine for supporting the courtier medicine is the envoy herb. They do not mean the three grades of upper, medium and lower ones.

君、臣、佐、使原指君主、臣僚、僚佐、使者四种人，分别起着不同的作用。句中使用官职隐喻，根据药物在中药处方中所起的不同作用，分别隐喻君药、臣药、佐药、使药，称之为君、臣、佐、使。

李本和文本均补译出该隐喻的具体内容 drug，都使用被动语态，将"谓"译为 be called，与原文句式相对应。这样既体现源语的文化特色，又确切地传达原文隐喻的含义。

文本将"君药"和"主治"译为 ruler（统治者）和 rule（统治），这两个词在表达治疗上，明显不及李本、吴本的 monarch 和 treat 准确规范。

与文本和李本采用的句式不同，吴本用 for 引导的介词短语来修饰 herb 和 medicine，准确地表达了君药、臣药、佐药、使药的作用，实现信息的有效传递。

第二节　父母隐喻及英译

父母是人类生命的创造者，承担着抚养和培育后代的重大责任。在子女幼年时期，父母为他们提供各种生活必需品以及心理和情感关怀，是人类成长过程中最为重要的社会关系角色之一。正是基于对父母的这些感知和体验，古人将天地自然视为父母，同时也就将人类视为天地自然的孩子。与父母一样，天地自然通过交合可以孕育世间万物。如果天地之气无法上下交通，则万物不得滋养而枯槁，生命也将无法绵延而死亡。通过运用父母隐喻，人类在心理上对天地自然产生了非常强烈的亲切感和敬畏感，也能更加形象地反映出天地自然对人类的作用和影响。

1. 阴阳者，天地之道也，万物之纲纪，变化之<u>父母</u>……《素问·阴阳应象大论》）

释义：阴阳的道理，是宇宙间的普遍规律，是一切事物的纲领，是万物发展变化的起源……

李本：Yin and Yang serve as the Dao (law) of the heavens and the earth, the fundamental principle of all things, the parents of change...

威本：The principle of Yin and Yang [the male and female elements in nature] is the basic principle of the entire universe. It is the principle of everything in creation. It brings about the transformation to parenthood...

文本：As for yin and yang, they are the Way of heaven and earth, the fundamental principles [governing] the myriad beings, father and mother to all changes and transformations...

吴本：...Yin and Yang are the ways of heaven and earth... Yin and Yang are the guiding principles of all things... Yin and Yang are the parents of variations...

阴阳的对立统一是自然界的根本规律；宇宙万物的发生、发展、运动、变化、消亡，其根源皆在阴阳。句中将"阴阳"喻为人们熟悉的"父母"，更易于说明阴阳是万物变化产生的根源。

对于"父母"的翻译，李本、吴本将其译为 parents（父母），文本译为 father and mother（父亲和母亲），解释了阴阳为万物变化之源，较忠实于原文。威本则将其译为 parenthood（父母身份、亲子关系），不如 parents、father、mother 等词准确贴切。从译文长度上来看，吴本最长，原因在于，吴本不仅翻译了原文，还解释原文中论述的道理，帮助读者不仅知其然，更知其所以然。

对于"道"这一文化词语的翻译，因为在英语文化中并未找到相应的映射，李本使用音译加注法，译为 the Dao (law)，帮助读者不仅理解其内涵意思，还能接触到汉语"道"所蕴含的文化信息 [1]。

2. 天有八纪，地有五里，故能为万物之父母。（《素问·阴阳应象大论》）

释义：天有八节的气序，地有五方的布局。因此，天地能成为万物生长的根本。

李本：The heavens demonstrates the eight solar terms and the earth displays the rules of Wuxing (Five-Elements). That is why [the heavens and the earth are regarded as] the parents (source) of all things.

威本：In Heaven there are eight regulators; upon earth there are five principles; and by means of these all living creatures can be transformed into parents.

文本：Heaven has the eight arrangements; the earth has the five structures. Hence,

---

[1] 李莫南. 概念整合理论映照下的《黄帝内经》隐喻翻译 [D]. 南京中医药大学，2013：29.

[heaven and earth] can be father and mother of the myriad beings.

吴本：The reason of the heaven and earth can be the parents of all things is that the heaven has its invisible refined energy and the earth has its visible substance.

句中将"天地"喻为"万物之父母"，形象地说明了天地自然创造并培育世间万物。

李本将"父母"直译成 parents，然后用括号内 source 对隐喻含义进行解释 [1]，既帮助读者更好地理解隐喻，又可以保留源语特色。同时，借用方括号将省略的 the heavens and the earth are regarded as 补译出来，使行文更为连贯。

文本和吴本均采用直译法，将"父母"分别译成 father and mother 和 parents，仅翻译出"父母"的字面意思，未能揭示出背后蕴含的隐喻内涵，不利于读者的深入理解。

威本并未理解本处隐喻，误将"万物"理解为"父母"，将其译为 all living creatures can be transformed into parents，曲解了原文意思。

3. 人能应四时者，天地为之父母。（《素问·宝命全形论》）

释义：人如果能适应四时的变化，那么自然界的一切都会成为他生命的泉源。

李本：[For those who can] abide by [the changes of] the four seasons, the heavens and the earth are their parents.

威本：Man has the ability to conform to the four seasons. Heaven and Earth act as his father and mother.

文本：If someone is able to correspond to the four seasons, heaven and earth are [his] father and mother.

吴本：If a man can adapt to the change of the four seasons, then, all things in nature will become the source of his life.

句中将"天地"喻为"父母"，将人喻为天地之子，因为天地合气造就人的生命，天之阳气地之阴精养育了人。

四个译本都译出天地之气对人的孕育，使读者理解"天地"为"父母"

[1] 翟书娟，刘艾娟. 概念隐喻视角下《黄帝内经》的英译研究 [J]. 海外英语，2016（6）：113.

这一隐喻。

李本、威本和文本都将"父母"译为 parents 或 father and mother，能较为直观地使读者理解"天地"如"父母"一样，造就孕育人的生命。

而吴本则将其译为 the source of his life，与其他三个译本相比，这种表述过于抽象，未能较好地实现与源语意义的对应。

4. 鬲肓之上，中有父母。（《素问·刺禁论》）

释义：膈肓上面是供给气血维持生命的心、肺两脏。

李本：Over the diaphragm there are parents.

文本：Above the ge-huang, in the middle there are father and mother.

吴本：Above the diaphram, there is the sea of energy which maintains the life.

句中"父母"用以隐喻心、肺二脏。肺主气，心主血，共营卫于身，故为父母。

李本、文本将"父母"分别直译为 parents 和 father and mother。此译法虽然在形式上忠实于原文，但皆未译出喻指对象的具体内容，不能实现有效交际的目的。

吴本舍弃"父母"的字面意思，将其意译为 the sea of energy which maintains the life，明确表明"父母"在句中指的是维持机体生命的气海，即心肺二脏。

5. 三阳为父……三阴为母……（《素问·阴阳类论》）

释义：三阳相当于高尊的父亲……三阴相当于善养育的母亲……

李本：Triple-Yang [is equivalent to the position of] father... Triple-Yin [is equivalent to the position of] mother...

文本：The third yang is father... The third yin is mother...

吴本：The third Yang is equivalent to the honorable father... the third Yin is equivalent to the mother who is good at breeding...

句中将三阳经喻为"父"，因为三阳经总领诸经，高尊如父；将三阴经喻为"母"，因为三阴经能够滋养诸经，像母亲养育子女一样。

对于"父""母"的翻译，李本、文本和吴本都将其译为 father 和 mother，但细节上有所不同。

李本采用括号加注的形式，借助短语 is equivalent to the position of，表明三阳、三阴如父如母一样，对人体起着外围屏障的作用，准确译出三阳和三

《黄帝内经素问》隐喻英译对比研究

278

阴对于人体的作用。

文本采用 A is B 的结构，将"三阳为父"译作 The third yang is father，将"三阴为母"译作 The third yin is mother，直接将三阳和三阴分别说成是父与母，简洁明了地描述出三阳和三阴在人体内的重要作用。

吴本采用增译的方法，使用 honorable 和 who 引导的定语从句分别修饰 father 和 mother，形象地说明三阳犹如高贵的父亲，三阴犹如母亲那样具有濡养诸经的作用，准确表述出"三阳"和"三阴"在人体内的作用，使译文表达更加清楚，有效地传递信息。

第三节　母子隐喻及英译

中医学认为，五行是相生相克的。同样，五脏之间也存在相互资生的关系，即一脏对另一脏具有滋养、助长、促进的作用。如木生火，即肝为心之母；水生木，则肾为肝之母；土生金，则脾为肺之母等。在病理状况下，一脏患病会传变到其所生的另一脏。如脾土为母，肺金为子，肺气虚弱，可发展为脾失健运，是谓"子盗母气"；又如肝木为母，心火为子，肝阳上亢，可发展为心火亢盛；又如脾土为母，肺金为子，脾胃虚弱，也可累及肺气不足，是谓"母病及子"。

在人类社会中，母亲扮演着生养和培育子女的角色，失去母亲就意味着失去生活和情感的依靠。母亲和子女的这种关系与五藏之间的相生关系十分类似。因此，中医理论将五脏之间的相生关系隐喻为母子关系。中医学在表达脏腑在疾病过程中的传变规律和治疗原则时，大量使用"母病及子""子病犯母""子盗母气""虚则补其母""实则泻其子"等与母子隐喻相关的术语。通过隐喻的方式以母子关系来表达五脏之间的相互关系，更易于理解和解释。

1. 东方生风，风生木，木生酸，酸生肝，肝生筋，筋生心，肝主目。
(《素问·阴阳应象大论》)

释义：东方属春，阳气上升而生风，风能滋养木气，木气能生酸，酸味能养肝，肝血又能养筋，筋又能养心，肝气上通于目。

李本：The east produces wind, the wind promotes [the growth] of trees, the trees produces sour [taste], the sour [taste] nourishes the liver, [the blood stored in] the liver nourishes the sinews, the sinews nourishes the heart and the liver controls the eyes.

威本：The East creates the wind; wind creates wood; wood creates the sour flavor; the sour flavor strengthens the liver; the liver nourishes the muscles; the muscles strengthen the heart; and the liver governs the eyes.

文本：The East generates wind; wind generates wood; wood generates sour [flavor]; sour [flavor] generates the liver; the liver generates the sinews; the sinews generate the heart; <The liver rules the eyes>.

吴本：The east corresponds to spring..., so the east produces the wind... so, the wind produces the wood. Wood... produces sour... so, the sour produces the liv-er... so, liver produces the tendons... so the tendon produces the heart... so, the liver determines the condition of the eyes.

此句是古人对自然界四时万物以及人体生理、病理各种过程之间相互联系和制约的认识，是五行学说在医学上的具体运用。文中连续使用了多个"生"字，将"生"和"所生"之间看成母子关系，运用一系列的母子隐喻，把自然界的东方、春、风、酸等，通过五行的木与人体的肝、筋、目联系起来，表达了天人相应的整体观念，让读者感觉好像一幅自然界各种联系和制约过程的总图解。

四个译本均译出了该母子隐喻。对于"生"的翻译，四个译本各不相同。李本将"东方生风""木生酸"中的"生"译为 produce（生产），"风生木"中的"生"译为 promote（提升），"酸生肝，肝生筋，筋生心"中的"生"都译为 nourish（滋养）。结合该句释义，"东方生风"和"木生酸"中的"生"指"生成"，译为 generate（生成）较为准确。"风生木""酸生肝，肝生筋，筋生心"中的"生"指"滋养"，所以李本用 nourish 一词较为恰当。

威本将"生"都译为 create（创造），吴本都译为 produce，不能准确地传达源语的文化内涵。而文本将"生"都译为 generate，也是不合适的。

2. 欲知其始，先建其母。（《素问·五脏生成》）

释义：打算知道某病是从哪脏里发生的，先要考察那一脏脉的胃气怎样。

李本：To know the onset of a disease, [one must] decide its Mu (pathogenic factors) first.

威本：In order to know (the proper time) for this beginning one must first establish which of the ten stems is to be the first month of the year.

文本：If one wishes to know its starting point, one first establishes its mother.

吴本：When treating the disease, one must know which viscera the disease comes from, and investigates the condition of the stomach-energy of the said viscera. If the stomach-energy of a certain viscera is deficient, one should set up its stomach-energy which is the mother of all other viscera energies first (earth is the mother of all things, and stomach associates with earth).

句中把疾病的原因喻为"母"，疾病也就相当于"子"。根据生活经验可知，先有母，后有子，以母子进行隐喻，更容易理解病因和疾病之间的关系。

李本将"母"音译为 Mu (pathogenic factors)，并通过括号加注的形式，译出了该隐喻所指的具体内容，指出"母"喻指病因，便于读者理解该隐喻的内涵，从而更好地理解病因和疾病之间的关系。

威本将"母"译为 one which of the ten stems is to be the first month of the year，会使读者产生困惑，无法使读者真正理解该隐喻所表达的母子关系。

文本将"母"直译为 mother，对"母"所喻指的意义没能进行解释，使读者很难理解"母"的真正内涵，从而不能实现交际目标和有效的文化传播。

吴本将"母"意译为 which viscera the disease comes from，而且增译 If the stomach-energy... energies first (earth is the mother of all things, and stomach associates with earth)，详细阐述五行当中"母"与"子"之间的相生关系，易于读者理解该隐喻。

3. 此六者，地气之所生也……此五者，天气之所生也……（《素问·五脏别论》）

释义：这六者，是感受地气而生的……这五者，是感受天气而生的……

李本：The brain, marrow, bones, vessels, gallbladder and uterus are all produced [under the influence of] Diqi (Earth-Qi)... The stomach, the large intestine, the small intestine, the Sanjiao (triple energizer) and the bladder are all produced [under the influence of] Tianqi (Heaven–Qi)...

威本：...these six organs, have been produced by the atmosphere of the earth... these five viscera, have an evil odor...

文本：...these six are generated by the qi of the earth... these five are generated by the qi of heaven...

吴本：The six organs... are generated in accordance with the earth–energy... The five organs of stomach... are generated in accordance with the heaven–energy...

奇恒之腑禀承地气而生，能储藏阴质，就像大地包藏万物一样，藏而不泄；传化之腑禀承天气而生，其作用像天一样的健运周转，泻而不藏。句中运用母子隐喻，将天和地隐喻成奇恒之腑和传化之腑的母亲。

对于动词"生"的翻译，李本和威本都将其译为 produce（批量生产），文本和吴本则译为 generate（生成、产生），但是根据此处的具体语境"奇恒之腑禀承地气而生"和"传化之腑禀承天气而生"，"生"意为"生成"，根据 produce 和 generate 两个词的语义侧重点，译为 generate 较为妥当，故文本和吴本的翻译较为准确。

4. 五脏受气于其所生，传之于其所胜，气舍于（其）所生，死于其所不胜。（《素问·玉机真脏论》）

释义：五脏所受的病气来源于它所生之脏，传给它所克之脏，留止在生己之脏，死于克己之脏。

李本：[Among] the Five Zang–Organs, [one organ] gets affected by Qi from the organ that it promotes and transmits to the organ that it restricts. Qi maintains in the organ that it promotes and [causes] death when transmitted to the organ that restricts it.

威本：The five viscera receive the impact of the life–giving force from those who generate them, and they pass it on to those whom they subjugate. Their force of life is bestowed upon those whom they beget, but they bring death upon those who cannot overcome their diseases.

文本：[Each of] the five depots receives qi from the [depot] which it generates; it transmits it to the one which it dominates. The qi rests in [that depot] by which [the transmitting depot] is generated. Death results [when it is] in that [depot] which [the transmitting depot] cannot dominate.

吴本：The evil-energy of a certain viscera originates from the viscera that it produces... transmits to the viscera which it restricts... retains in the viscera that produces it... and the patient will die when the transmission reaches the viscera that restricts it...

句中运用母子隐喻论述病传的问题，即病气由本脏及于他脏的传行和演变情况。每脏有病，皆可及于其余四脏，而且病气的传行，以胜相传，即由母传子。

四个译本对"生"和"胜"的理解不尽相同。这两个词是指五脏之间的相生相克关系，"生"指事物的发生和生长，"胜"即克，表示约束，制约。对于"生"，威本和文本都译为 generate，表达出生长的含义，比李本的 promote（提升）和吴本的 produce（生产）更为准确。

对于"胜"，李本和吴本都译为 restrict（限制、约束），威本译为 subjugate（征服、使臣服），文本则译为 dominate（支配、统治）。根据此处具体语境，李本和吴本译为 restrict，更能准确地描述出"胜"的含义。

小　结

本章介绍了《素问》中的社会关系隐喻，包括官职隐喻、父母隐喻、母子隐喻等，并对四个译本进行对比分析。各译本既有相似之处，又各具特色。

对于官职隐喻的翻译，李本借助 similar to 这一类的喻词将隐喻转换为明喻，且在必要的时候进行增译和补译，使译文更加完整连贯，更加符合英语句式的表达习惯，更易于目的语读者理解源语言文化特色，更好地领悟中医文化。威本对中国古代的官职没能形成一个准确的认识，无法正确理解官职的意义，因此译文出现一些不够准确规范的情况，有时甚至会漏译、误译。文本在行文方面比较忠实于原文，在对原文隐喻进行诠释的同时，试图原汁原味地呈现中医面貌，让西方读者真正领略中医内涵，但有时会过于追求贴近原文的表达，反而不能完整准确地表达源语的真正含义。吴本多以意译和增译为主，打破原文的语言形式，对官职隐喻进行解释，使读者较为容易地理解隐喻的真正内涵。但意译有时不能很好地保留源语的文化特色，无法使读者真正领略中医文化特色。

对于父母隐喻，李本通过括号加注的形式，忠实准确地传达原文语义，同时括号内的注释又对父母做进一步解释，完整表达文中隐喻的真正内涵。威本由于缺乏系统的中医理论知识，在译文的准确性方面有所欠缺，可能导致读者难以理解文中的隐喻现象。文本采用直译法比较忠实地译释原文，但有时会因囿于原文的表达形式，致使译文过于简洁，无法完整地译出原文隐喻的含义。吴本则是不吝篇幅地进行增译，帮助读者更加详细地了解中医文化。但译文经常打破原文的句式限制，使译文在一定程度上丢失源语的文化特色。

母子隐喻部分涉及的中医术语较多，四位译者都在必要的时候采用括号加注的形式进行补充翻译。对于中医术语的翻译，四位译者选词不尽相同。李本多采用音译加注法，而威本则多是进行意译，但是对一些术语的翻译不够准确，甚至出现误译。文本基于忠实于原文，对母子隐喻紧扣原文进行译释，虽然简明扼要地译出原文的内容，但有时语言过于简洁，致使译文不够完整准确。吴本多采取增译和补加注释的方法，能够较为完整地译出原文隐喻的真正内涵，便于西方读者了解博大精深的中医文化。

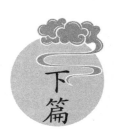

下篇

《素问》隐喻英译研究

第八章 《素问》译者的翻译风格

第一节 李照国的翻译风格

李照国是著名的中医药翻译家，曾任世界中医药学会联合会翻译专业委员会会长、中国中西医结合学会中医外语专业委员会副主任委员、世界中医药学会联合会中医名词术语国际标准化审定委员会委员等职，一直致力于中医药文化的翻译与国际传播。李照国的学习经历很丰富，知识背景也很宽广。他具有西安外国语大学英语学士学位、西安医科大学专门用途英语硕士学位和上海中医药大学中医学博士学位，为上海外国语大学翻译学博士后。多年来，他一直从事翻译教学和中医药翻译工作，笔耕不辍，出版专著二十余部，译著三十余部，发表各类论文数百篇。自 1985 年起，李照国着手《黄帝内经》的英译工作。经过近二十年的不懈努力，于 2005 年完成。同年，《黄帝内经》英译本出版，并于 2007 年入选国家《大中华文库》工程。

李本充分遵循《大中华文库》工程的宗旨，全面系统地介绍中国传统文化、向世界展示中华民族的光彩和魅力。李本翻译的基本原则是"译古如古，文不加饰"，目标是"最大限度地保持原作的写作风格、思维方式和主旨思想"[1]。

一、风格分析

（一）语言风格

李本在语言运用上重视对原文的还原，力图保留原文的写作风格，翻译

---

[1] 黄光惠.《黄帝内经·素问》概念隐喻英译研究 [D]. 福建师范大学，2013：53.

时遵循"去冗就简"的原则，即在翻译中尽可能不添加不必要的词汇，弱化原文中复杂深奥的文学修辞，删除原文中的重复内容，确保行文流畅、语句精练。李本在语言上注重语句对仗工整，遵循原文的结构形式和表达方式，符合学术文本正式、严谨的文体特征，适合具有一定中医学术背景的读者阅读。李本常直接采用与原文一致的平行结构，保证每个分句主干部分的信息统一，而从属部分的信息则用以体现不同的病症或表征等内容。对于读者而言，这种处理方式不仅可以降低理解难度、突出重点信息，而且可以保持语言结构的工整划一，彰显译文的韵律之美和文学色彩，从而兼顾阐释医理和传递中医文化特色的需要。

在对隐喻的处理上，李本力求用简练准确的词汇、语法结构和表达方式传递隐喻的内涵。例如：

原文：以天地为之阴阳，阳之汗，以天地之雨名之；阳之气，以天地之疾风名之。暴气象雷，逆气象阳。（《素问·阴阳应象大论》）

译文：To compare the heavens and the earth to Yin and Yang [in the human body], sweating [induced by the movement of] Yang is just like rain in nature, the movement of Yangqi is just like strong wind in nature.

李本将"天地"译为"the heavens and the earth"，将"疾风"译为"strong wind"。两处隐喻均进行直译。前者使用连词 and 构成并列结构，保留原文的结构形式，使用 heaven 的复数形式表示"天空"，与其单数形式所表达的"天堂"之意区分开来，且具有一定的文学性；后者使用形容词 strong 表达"疾"，较为贴切，在形式上也还原了原文的偏正结构。

由于古汉语表达简洁凝练，而且具有较高的文学性，经常出现省略、通假等语言现象，因此，在很多情况下，若不增词很难保证译文结构的完整和语法的正确。李本通常会根据具体语境增补相关的词汇和内容。例如：

原文：寒热内贼，其病益甚。（《素问·六元正纪大论》）

译文：[Then] the interior [will be] damaged by Cold and Heat and the disease will be worsened.

该句将"寒热之气"隐喻为做坏事的人，"贼"为动词，隐喻义为"伤害"，语言非常精练。为充分说明"内"与"贼"的关系，李本将"寒热内贼"译为 the interior [will be] damaged by Cold and Heat，方括号内补译助动词 will 表达将来时态，补译 be 与其后的 damaged 表达主语 the interior 和宾语 Cold and Heat 之间的被动关系。补译不仅保证句子结构的完整和语法的准确，而且利于读者准确把握原文内容。

尽管有英语语言文学专业学习经历，李照国毕竟是一位以汉语为母语的译者。相对于以英语为母语的译者而言，他在英语语言的运用上仍然存在少量不甚到位的情况，有时甚至影响到译文的衔接与连贯。例如：

原文： 脉至如喘，名曰暴厥。暴厥者，不知与人言。（《素问·大奇论》）

译文： [The disease with] the pulse that is surfing is called Baojue (sudden syncope) and [the patient] is unconscious and unable to speak.

喘，《说文·口部》云："疾息也。"喘，有"疾"义。"脉至如喘"，乃谓"脉至而疾"也。"喘"指水之湍急，此处以湍急的水流隐喻发生暴厥时出现的急脉之脉象特征。李本将"喘"译为 surfing（冲浪），补译主语中心词 the disease，并且使用定语从句对其进行修饰，努力实现译文语句的完整。但是，surf 的选用不甚妥当，在意思上无法与 disease 形成符合逻辑的主谓关系，因此造成译文与原文在意思上有所出入，未能准确传递原文所描述的急脉之脉象特征，可能会令读者费解。

（二）翻译策略

李本在翻译隐喻时大量采用音译、音译加注、直译和直译加注等译法。李照国认为，中医基本理论中的核心概念，如阴阳、五行、精、神等，均含有国情，无论直译还是意译都无法完全清楚地表达内涵[1]。对于此类概念，李本多采用"音译为主，释义为辅"的翻译策略。因此，对于《素问》中蕴涵丰富文化内涵的隐喻内容，李本在翻译时通常先进行音译，然后以括号的方式补充注释，用以说明现行通用译法或者原文衍文、补充原文缺失的内容，便于读者准确理解和接受。例如：

原文： 饮入于胃，游溢精气，上输于脾。脾气散精，上归于肺，通调水道，下输膀胱。水精四布，五经并行。（《素问·经脉别论》）

译文： When water is taken into the stomach, the Jingqi (Essence-Qi) is distributed around and is transported to the spleen. The spleen distributes Jing (Essence)

[1]　李照国. 译海心语 [M]. 上海：上海中医药大学出版社，2006：99–100.

and transports it upwards to the lung. [The lung] regulates water passage and transports [water] to the bladder. [In this way,] the Jing (Essence) of water is distributed all through the body and into the five Channels.

本句中的三处"精"均含有不同的隐喻意义,"游溢精气"中的"精气"是对"水汽"的隐喻;"脾气散精"中的"精"是对"水谷精微"的隐喻;"水精"则是对"水液"或者"津液"的隐喻。李本采用音译加注的方法将"精气"译为 Jingqi (Essence-Qi),将"脾气散精"中的"精"译为 Jing (Essence),将"水精"译为 Jing (Essence) of water。音译保留了中医特有概念,有利于传播中医文化,括号内的注解则可以帮助读者更好地理解三处隐喻所喻指的不同内容。

对于自然隐喻、动物隐喻、战争隐喻等,中西方读者均较容易理解,能够在译文中找到对应的词汇和译语,因此李本一般采用直译或者直译加注的方法,简洁明了地传递其隐喻内涵。例如:

原文:**如鸟之喙者,此谓不及,病在中**。(《素问·玉机真脏论》)

译文:[if] the pulse appears like the beak of a bird, it is called Buji (insufficiency), indicating diseases in the interior.

"喙",即鸟嘴。"如鸟之喙者"是用以隐喻脾脉来时锐而短的状态。李本将"如鸟之喙"直译为 like the beak of a bird,并且补译出主语 the pulse,语言简洁准确,忠实于原文,较好地实现语言、交际、文化的转换目标。

不过,对于古汉语中特有的、带有显著中医学特色且在英语中很难找到对应语的隐喻,翻译时只能进行意译。例如"内-外"空间隐喻表示色诊、脉诊两种诊断方法及表示房事时,译者主要采用意译的方法,以实现原文内涵的准确传递。例如:

原文:**名曰肺痹,寒热,得之醉而使内也**。(《素问·五脏生成》)

译文:...known as Feibi (Lung-Bi Syndrome). It is caused by cold-heat and sexual intercourse after drinking of alcohol.

句中的"内"并非字面意思,而是特指房事。这一含义为古汉语中特有,在英语中无法找到对应的词汇,不宜使用直译的方法。因此,李本采用了意译,将其译为 sexual intercourse,清晰准确地解释"内"的特殊含义,便于读者理解。

（三）翻译目标的实现

李照国在《黄帝内经》英译本前言中指出，该译本的意义在于向对中医感兴趣但不懂中文的读者介绍《黄帝内经》。遗憾的是，该译本在海外的接受度尚未达到预期。殷丽对海外图书馆的馆藏量、发表在国外权威期刊上的海外同行专家撰写的书评以及对亚马逊网站的读者评论等方面进行调查。结果显示，李本的海外接受度不高，具体表现在李本在海外图书馆馆藏量较少、国外权威学术期刊上没有查找到任何书评或评价、亚马逊网站的读者评论寥寥无几。这说明无论是在海外普通阅读市场还是在学术领域的接受状况，《素问》国内译本都与海外英译本的接受状况有着不小的差距[1]。因此，作为国家文化输出工程的内容之一，李照国译本的海外接受度是不够理想的，既未在学术型读者中实现预期的好评，也未能获得一般读者的青睐。背后的原因是多方面的，包括书籍的定价、出版社和译者的影响力、学界推介等，值得进一步深入思考和探究。

二、原因分析

（一）原文解读

李照国先后获得文学学士（英语专业）、文学硕士（专门用途英语专业）和医学博士学位（中医学专业），在英语语言文学和中医学领域均有很高的造诣。作为中医学博士且长期致力于中医翻译教学、实践及相关研究，李照国具有丰富的经验和较好的研究基础，对于《素问》的理解较为准确和深入，对文中各类隐喻的阐释也十分到位，因而译文整体准确度较高。在四个译本中，李本的误译、漏译等现象出现最少，较好地传递了原文的形与意。

（二）文化意识

李照国注重中医文化的对外传播，在翻译中更加关注如何实现语言和文化的转换，因而对于文化缺省的相关隐喻内容大量使用音译加注和直译加注的译法。对于中医基本概念、专有名词等则以音译为主，意译为辅。同时，

---

[1] 殷丽. 中医药典籍国内英译本海外接受状况调查及启示——以大中华文库《黄帝内经》英译本为例 [J]. 外国语（上海外国语大学学报），2017，40（5）：33–43.

为保持原文风格，李本在对篇章翻译的处理上尽可能遵循原文的结构形式和表达方式，因而同样选择直译为主的译法。这些翻译方法均强调保留原文蕴含的文化内涵，符合弘扬中华民族文化的最终目标。

李本的翻译工作完成于 21 世纪初，当时的中医发展已进入新时期，中西方文化交流日渐频繁。尽管译者常居国内，但已有较多的渠道和方式查阅和获取各类中英文参考资料。因此，该译本参照历代医家的多种注释，译文中也出现大量脚注和注释，这反映出译者严谨的治学态度。

第二节　威斯的翻译风格

爱尔萨·威斯（IlzaVeith）是美国医学史博士。在约翰·霍普金斯大学（Johns Hopkins University）医史研究所攻读博士期间，威斯于 1945—1946 年完成《素问》第 1 章至第 34 章的翻译和评注。面对工具书缺乏、古文晦涩难懂等困难，威斯确定的翻译原则为："只翻译《黄帝内经》的内容大意，而不去深究字义。"她在前言中写道："这部典籍的翻译，仅代表自己作为医史学家的方法，并非汉文字学家的方法。希望自己的初步研究能成为对该书进行进一步研究的起点，尤其特别关注众多语言学问题。"[1]1949 年，威连姆斯和威尔金斯出版社（Williams & Wilkins）首次出版该部译著。

尽管威本仅完成对《素问》第 1 章至第 34 章的翻译，但这是《黄帝内经》第一个较为完整的英译本，其目标读者为对中医了解甚少的英语国家读者。该译本行文流畅，语言生动优美，可读性强，易于为广大西方读者理解和接受。威本自出版以来已再版数次，在国外学术界和对中国传统文化感兴趣的读者中均具有较大的影响力。

---

[1]　黄光惠.《黄帝内经》西传推动西方医学发展 [N]. 中国社会科学报，2019–08–30（5）.

一、风格分析

（一）语言风格

威斯的母语为英语，对英语的驾驭能力相比其他语言背景的译者自然更胜一筹，尤其是在处理隐喻等文学性较强的内容时，表现出较强的语言优势。由于熟知英语国家读者的用词和语法习惯，威本往往不拘泥于原文的词汇，而是尽可能进行巧妙转换。这样做不仅保留原文的语言美感，而且增强译文的可读性。例如：

原文：惊而夺<u>精</u>，汗出于心。（《素问·经脉别论》）

译文：When man is shocked and startled he does violence to his spirit and vitality, and perspiration is produced by the heart.

句中的"精"指精神、神气。受惊会影响精神，因心气受伤会引起汗出于心。威斯根据对"精"的隐喻内涵的理解，使用并列短语 spirit and vitality 进行意译，并且运用 when 引导时间状语从句，表明前后两个分句之间的逻辑关系。该译法虽然在语言上未能保留中医学"精"的概念，却较为准确地实现了其内涵的表达，因此，更易于读者理解和接受，有利于交际目标的实现。

对原文的理解和解读是威斯翻译过程中的难点和弱点，尤其是对中医特有概念及其相关隐喻的理解出现较多偏差。因此，威本译文虽然语言流畅，文字优美，深受西方读者欢迎，但是误译、漏译等现象较为常见。例如：

原文：味归形，形归气，气归<u>精</u>，<u>精</u>归化；<u>精</u>食气，形食味，化生<u>精</u>，气生形。（《素问·阴阳应象大论》）

译文：The flavors belong to the physical body. When the body dies the ethereal spirit is restored to the air, having thus undergone a complete metamorphosis (having thus become naturalized 归化). The ethereal spirit receives its nourishment from the air and the body receives its nourishment from the flavors. The ethereal spirit is created through metamorphosis, the physical shape assumes life through breath.

该句以"气""味""精"和"形"为例解释阴阳互根，句中的四处

"精"均指阴精，即人体的津液之一，是对"构成人体精微物质"的隐喻。威本将"气"与"味"，"精"与"形"之间的转化译为 metamorphosis（形变、质变），并在括号内进行补译和注释，在一定程度上便于西方读者理解"归""化生"和"生"等词语的内涵。但是，将"精"译为 the ethereal spirit（超凡的精神），显然是因错误解读而造成的误译。此类情况在威本中较为常见，也从侧面反映出译者只求翻译大意、不追究深意的原则。

（二）翻译策略

与内容相比，威本更重视对原文语言的还原，最大限度地忠实于原文，以实现语言的转换。因此，在对隐喻的处理上，威本多采用直译法。例如：

原文：邪入于阳则狂，邪入于阴则痹，搏阳则为巅疾，搏阴则为喑。（《素问·宣明五气》）

译文：When the eight evils reside within the elements of Yang in man, then the result is wildness（狂）; when the eight evils reside within the elements of Yin in man, then the result is numbness. When the evils strike at Yang, they cause insanity（巅）; when they strike at Yin, they cause loss of speech（喑）.

本句中，人体被隐喻为战场，"搏阳"喻指邪气与人体阳气的对抗，而"搏阴"则隐喻邪气与人体阴气的较量。此处，威本将"搏"直译为 strike（突击，攻击）。在英语中，strike 常用于战争语境，而威本正是借助 strike 说明"邪"与"阴"和"阳"之间的联系，使西方读者很容易理解该处隐喻的内涵，即邪气对阴阳的攻击。

威本非常注重译文的可接受性和可读性，努力帮助读者消除理解障碍，因此翻译中会采用意译的方法阐释原文中一些较为复杂的抽象概念和现象。对于文化内涵丰富的隐喻，威本也经常运用归化策略，对相关概念和内容进行语言转换，根据具体情况选择直译或意译。如果隐喻内容在英语中有对应的词汇或表达，则进行直译，实现语言的转换和内容的传递。例如：

原文：二七而天癸至，任脉通，太冲脉盛，月事以时下，故有子。（《素问·上古天真论》）

译文：When she reaches her fourteenth year she begins to menstruate and is able to become pregnant and the movement in the great thoroughfare pulse（太冲脉）

is strong. Menstruation comes at regular times, thus the girl is able to give birth to a child.

本句用"天癸"隐喻能够促进生殖机能的物质，即女子的月经。威本将"天癸至"译为动词 menstruate（行经，月经来潮），同时将下文的"月事"译为名词 menstruation。两词前后呼应，实现语言的衔接和连贯。

对于在英语中较难或者无法找到对应词的概念，威本常采用意译的方法进行解释说明。例如：

原文：此四支八溪之朝夕也。（《素问·五脏生成》）

译文：The four limbs and their eight flexible joints are in use from early morning until late at night.

句中的"溪"是对人体"关节"的隐喻。八溪，即八虚，指上肢部的肘关节、肩关节，下肢部的膝关节、髋关节，左右侧共八处。威本将"八溪"意译为 their eight flexible joints（八个灵活的四肢关节），比较准确地传递"溪"所隐喻的内容，成功实现交际目标。但是，此译法未能还原"溪"这一中医学的特有概念，因而在文化层面的转换上存在一定欠缺。

（三）翻译目标的实现

威斯重视译文的可接受性和可读性，因此，威本在实现语言和交际目标上较为成功，能够尽最大可能实现语言转换，还原隐喻对象的特征，而且语言简练，文字优美，易于读者理解和接受。

但是，威本的文化传递效果相对较弱。尤其在面对众多较难理解的与隐喻相关的中医术语、概念和关系时，该译本的文化目标更是无法成功实现。翻译目标的实现情况也有所不同。在处理战争隐喻等中英文化差异较小的隐喻时，译文整合适应程度相对较高，文化目标实现较好，而对于文化差异较大的空间、阴阳、官职等隐喻的处理则不甚理想，多处出现释义不明、译不达意等现象，甚至存在误译和漏译。尽管如此，作为《素问》真正意义上的首部较为完整的译本，威本基本实现了预期目标，受到西方读者的认可和欢迎，并为后来其他译者的翻译工作提供了有益的参考和借鉴。

二、原因分析

（一）原文解读

威斯于 1945 年开始进行《素问》英译工作。当时中国正处于抗战时期，中外文化交流相对较少，因此，她能够获取的资料十分有限。由于没有渠道获得现代汉语版本，威斯只能选用文言文体的宋本《黄帝内经》作为源本。由于中医学专业知识不足，再加上缺乏中医、哲学等方面的专业词典，她在理解古汉语上费时费力，而且无法深入，对中医医理和术语的理解不太到位，甚至出现误读，对中医隐喻思维的掌握也存在一定欠缺，翻译过程可谓困难重重。但是，在中医文字的翻译策略和对术语的阐释方法等方面，威斯仍然有自己的独到见解，因而能够最终顺利完成翻译工作，并获得较大成功。

（二）文化意识

威本完成时间较早，首次出版于二十世纪中期。当时在世界医学领域，西方医学占据主导地位，而中医学处于边缘化的境地。作为医史学博士，威斯翻译的主要目标是从医史学的角度初步介绍和探讨《素问》，因此更注重向读者传递原文的基本意义，而非语言背后的深刻文化内涵。另外，作为一名外国译者，威斯不可能承担中华文化对外传播的使命和责任，因而在翻译过程中文化意识相对较弱，以至于很少关注语言背后的文化内涵及文化传递目标的实现。

第三节　文树德的翻译风格

文树德（Paul U. Unschuld）是德国著名医史学家和汉学家，曾任德国慕尼黑大学医史研究所所长，长期从事中国医学史研究，在中医文献和古籍英译方面颇有建树。他曾翻译过《黄帝内经》《难经》《本草纲目》等中医药典籍，在翻译过程中形成了独具风格的中医翻译观。

文树德是西方"考据派"的代表人物 [1]。在中医翻译过程中，他因从独特视角解读中医文献以及与众不同的翻译方法而独树一帜。他专注《黄帝内经》翻译研究二十余年，发表和出版了一系列与《黄帝内经》研究相关的学术论文和专著。2011 年，文树德与美国学者田和曼、中国学者郑金生合作完成译著《黄帝内经素问译注》（*Huang Di Nei Jing Su Wen: An Annotated Translation of Huang Di's Inner Classic — Basic Questions*），由加州大学出版社出版。该译著秉承文树德对中医文献翻译一以贯之的翻译理念和方法，注重语言和内容的考据，在语言形式、内容、风格方面最大限度地保留《素问》之原貌。

一、风格分析

（一）语言风格

文树德认为，译文应充分考虑中医思维模式，探究古代医学中比象、隐喻的原意，从中医形成的时代背景中寻找中医语言的含义。他反对按照西方人的思维方式解读和阐释结构精美、语意深刻的中医概念和术语，主张从文史、文献和文化等方面入手加深对中医语言的理解，以中文的习惯和传统进行表达，在语言形式和内容上保留原文的风格。

在语言形式上，文树德参照《素问》成书时代的古汉语语法和句式等，严格遵循原著的章节顺序，力求在语序和句式上与原文保持一致。隐喻的翻译多采用原文的结构形式，行文简洁紧凑，能够较好地呈现原文语言的凝练之美。需要指出的是，遵循原文语序和句式结构并不等于简单的逐字翻译。宏观上，文树德注重遵循原文的语言形式，但在翻译词组和短语时，倾向于选择符合英语习惯的表达。例如：

原文：寒热内贼，其病益甚。（《素问·六元正纪大论》）

译文：Cold or heat would cause internal injuries. The illness [you try to heal] will become even more severe.

本句将"寒热之气"隐喻为做坏事的人。"贼"在句中名词动用，意为"伤害"。文本准确解读原文中的战争隐喻，将"寒热"译为 cold or heat，充当句子主语，将动词"贼"译为符合英文表达习惯的动词短语 cause injuries，

---

[1]　李照国 . 中医翻译研究教程 [M]. 上海：三联书店，2019：138.

表意准确而简洁。译文遵循原文的语序、句式结构和词性，在语言形式上和原文保持一致，较好地保留原文风格。

原文：脉至如涌泉，浮鼓肌中，太阳气予不足也。（《素问·大奇论》）

译文：When the [movement in the] vessels arrives like [water] gushing from a fountain, at the surface, and drumming in the muscles, qi and flavor are diminished.

本句将浮而有力的脉象隐喻为涌动的泉水，生动形象而又直观易懂。译文从整体上遵循原文句式，将喻词"如"译为 like，用以连接本体和喻体。对"涌泉"一词，文树德并未按汉语词序逐字翻译，而是使用符合英文习惯的表达，用后置定语 gushing from a fountain 对中心词 water 进行补译。这种译法重视保持原文结构，但又不拘泥于个别词语，既能保留原文风格，贴合原文内容，传递文化意象，又符合英文表达，方便目的语读者理解。

在语言内容上，文树德注重探究成书时代的社会文化语境，考察中医语言与社会和生活的关联性，力求原汁原味地呈现原文。他反对以西代中、用西医术语硬套中医术语的做法，认为这会混淆中西医差异，无法准确传递中医理念，引起西方对中医学的误解[1]。他认为，只有用古人自己的术语来阐明他们的理念、理论和行为作法才能明断中医英译中出现的分歧[2]。在对隐喻的翻译中，这一理念贯穿其中，他注重探究隐喻的原意，追本溯源，谨慎选择能够传递中国文化的词汇，做到内容上的忠实，重现原文的隐喻表达。例如：

原文：余闻上古之人，春秋皆度百岁，而动作不衰。（《素问·上古天真论》）

译文：I have heard that the people of high antiquity, in [the sequence of] spring and autumn, all exceeded one hundred years. But in their movements and activities there was no weakening.

句中"上"来隐喻时间的久远，"上古"指远古时期。文树德深究其源，巧妙地将"上古"译为 high antiquity。high 一般指空间位置的高，亦指在数量、质量等方面超出常规，用在此处能够凸显时间的久远。译文中"上"对

---

[1] 郑金生. 文树德教授的中国医学研究之路 [J]. 中国科技史杂志，2013，34（1）：8.

[2] 张晓枚，陈锋，陈宁等. 文树德英译本《黄帝内经》文化负载词英译探究 [J]. 环球中医药，2018，11（7）：1087.

应 high，"古"对应 antiquity，既在形式上遵循原文，又在内容上形象地传达"上"的隐喻意义。

原文：内<u>舍</u>五脏六腑，何气使然？（《素问·痹论》）

译文：When [the disease] proceeds into the interior and lodges in the five depots and six palaces, which qi causes that?

句中"舍"本意指"居住的房子"，此处用作动词，有"贮藏，容纳"之意。本句将人体内部的五脏六腑隐喻为能够藏匿邪气的容器。lodge 在英文中既可作名词也可作动词，名词意为"房舍"，动词有"居住"之意。文树德将"舍"译为 lodge，该词在词性和意思上均和原文对等，在形式和内容上均忠实于原文。

（二）翻译策略

文树德重视对原文的还原。为最大限度重现原文的语言形式和内容，他主要运用"经文直译"加"全面、严谨、学术型的大量注释"的翻译策略[1]。

在翻译隐喻时，他善于使用直译的方法，尽可能避免使用西医术语，力求重现原文中隐喻对象的特征。例如：

原文：夏者火始治，心气始长，脉瘦气弱，阳气留溢，热熏分腠，<u>内</u>至于经。（《素问·水热穴论》）

译文：In summer, the fire begins to govern. The qi of the heart begins to stimulate growth. The vessels are lean and the qi is weak. The yang qi remains [at its place] and overflows. The heat steams the interstice [structures]; internally it reaches the conduits.

句中"内"是空间隐喻的代表，意为"向内"，表示热气在体内的运行方向。文本采用直译的方法，将"内"直译为 internally，词性和意义均与原文相应，准确再现热气运行的路径。

除直译外，文树德另一特色是"文献式"翻译，即大量使用注释提供相关历史文献资料，从词源或不同中医流派的理解等方面对直译内容进行补充。注释最多的主要有两类：①对因直译而显得行文不通的经文进行意译。②对某些含义复杂或深奥的字词提供相关词源信息或文化背景资料，让目的语读

---

[1]　徐冰.《黄帝内经·素问》英译研究 [D]. 上海外国语大学，2017：20.

者更准确地理解《素问》中概念的含义和渊源。

（三）翻译目标的实现

文树德本着严谨的翻译态度和自创的翻译理念，展示了西方学者解读《素问》的独特视角，在欧美和国内颇受肯定和欢迎[1]。整体来说，文树德的翻译目的是让英语读者了解真正的中医，而不是近代以来被西方观念扭曲的"中医"[2]。文树德对于隐喻的翻译，字斟句酌，总体上来说较为客观，一定程度上保留了隐喻的文化内涵。直译从语言形式上重现隐喻，但有时过于追求形式的统一，会使目的语读者曲解原文，不利于隐喻和文化的传递。因此，文树德补充大量注释，将相关背景知识介绍给读者，力求实现中医内涵的准确传达，一定程度上弥补了直译的不足。文树德虽为汉学家，但其母语并非汉语，再加上中医语言模糊深奥，很多隐喻的喻指对象比较抽象，其相似性不易推测，导致他对一些中医专有术语与其喻指对象的关系理解不够透彻，对中医文化及隐喻思维的解读和把握存在一定欠缺，有时出现释义不明、行文晦涩、译不达意的遗憾。例如：

原文：得守者生，失守者死。（《素问·脉要精微论》）

译文：Those who are able to guard, they live. Those who fail to guard, they die.

"守"是战争隐喻的体现。在战争中，士兵固守关口和要塞，而在治疗疾病时，五脏如同士兵一样守卫人体经气出入的门户。句中"得守"指五脏能够维护其职守，"守"为名词，意为"职守"。

译文采用直译的方法，句式简洁工整，在语言形式上基本忠实于原文。"守"在句中的意思为"职守"，但文树德将其译为动词 guard（保卫），有曲解原文之嫌。而且，他将"得守"的施动者"五脏"误解为 Those（病人），混淆原句的逻辑关系，未能将句中的战争隐喻如实地呈现给读者。

[1] 张晓枚，陈锋，陈宁等.文树德英译本《黄帝内经》文化负载词英译探究 [J]. 环球中医药，2018，11（7）：1085.

[2] 徐冰，张莹.《黄帝内经·素问》四个英译本的翻译策略和接受 [J]. 外国语言与文化，2019，3（3）：104.

二、原因分析

（一）原文解读

文树德不仅是一位译者，同时还是一位医史学家，尤其擅长医学思想史领域的研究[1]。在 2003 年出版的《黄帝内经素问——古代中国医经中的自然、知识与意象》一书中，"他全面系统介绍《素问》的历史、命名、版本及注家等内容，深入评价了《素问》的自然观、人体观、疾病观、养生思想以及各种治疗法则"[2]。通过二十余年的研究，文树德逐步加深对《素问》的理解，上至深层的中医医理，下至外在的语言形式，都较为熟悉，为《黄帝内经素问译注》中的隐喻翻译打下坚实的基础，总体上取得了较为理想的翻译效果，得到译界和中医界的认可。但是，中医理论博大精深，中医语言模糊深奥，《素问》中亦有很多在中医界尚存争议的内容，再加上一些隐喻晦涩难解，译者不容易把握喻指对象和喻体之间的相似性，对于非母语译者来说尤为如此。这些因素综合起来，增大了翻译的难度，译文难免出现不足。

（二）文化意识

文树德在翻译过程中尤其注重文化意识的体现。他认为，翻译中医典籍必须了解成书的历史背景，并结合中国传统文化和中医思维模式来解读中医学。这种文化意识恰恰决定了他的翻译策略。对于隐喻的翻译，他坚持探究古代医学中比象、隐喻的原意，遵循成书时代的语法、句法和古汉语知识，选择恰当的词汇，并配合大量注释，为读者提供更多的文化背景知识，让读者全面了解原著内容，原汁原味地反映成书时代的人们对中医的认知。反过来，这种忠实于原著、忠实于历史的翻译策略对中医翻译和中国文化传播起到了积极的推动作用，便于目的语读者领略中医文化内涵。

[1]　徐冰，张莹.《黄帝内经·素问》四个英译本的翻译策略和接受 [J]. 外国语言与文化，2019，3（3）：103.

[2]　张晓枚，陈锋，陈宁等 . 文树德英译本《黄帝内经》文化负载词英译探究 [J]. 环球中医药，2018，11（7）：1087.

第四节　吴连胜、吴奇的翻译风格

吴连胜、吴奇父子是美籍中医师，他们在多年行医经验的基础上，选用唐代王冰原注的《黄帝内经》，于1995年完成了《黄帝内经》（*Yellow Emperor's Canon Internal Medicine*）的英译，并荣获第三届世界传统医学大会"最高荣誉金奖"。该译本风格独特，前无序言，后无附录，引用内容未标注文献来源，衍文略去不译，属于应用型版本[1]。该译本的目标读者为对中医感兴趣的西方读者，因此译者根据自己的实践经验，将晦涩深奥的古文阐释为简单直白的具体操作步骤或用药方法，以期将基本的中医医理和医术传递给读者，用于治病和保健。该译本注重展现中医的临床实践价值，操作性和指导性较强。

一、风格分析

（一）语言风格

译者身份和目标读者决定译本的语言风格。由于吴氏父子是从业医师而非语言学家，译本的目标读者是期望了解中医并学习中医保健之术的西方普通读者，因此他们翻译的着眼点与其他译者颇为不同。他们重内容，轻形式，追求流畅具体、通俗易懂的译文，而非字斟句酌、语法准确的学术型语言。对于隐喻的翻译，特别是当喻指对象较为抽象或者不甚明显时，吴氏父子往往根据他们的行医经验进行阐释翻译。

从语言形式看，吴氏父子并不追求对等，在翻译过程中，经常进行意译，不断变换词汇、句式、语序，以达到阐释医理、指导实践的目的。例如：

原文：开鬼门，洁净府，精以时服。（《素问·汤液醪醴论》）

译文：Then, try to make the patient to perspire thoroughly, and keep his urination

---

[1]　杨渝，陈晓.《黄帝内经》英译文本分类述评（1925–2019）[J]. 中医药文化，2020，15（3）：43.

unobstructed, besides, give the patient, according to the condition, some medicine on due time.

句中"开鬼门"和"洁净府"是典型的容器隐喻，吴本没有采用直译的方法，而是通过释义的方式将两个隐喻分别意译为 make the patient to perspire thoroughly（使病人充分出汗）和 keep his urination unobstructed（保持排尿通畅）。译文回避了"鬼门"和"净府"两个富含中国文化的隐喻词汇，未受限于原文的语言形式，但是准确地解释原文意思，便于读者理解。

原文：**东方青色，<u>入通于肝</u>，<u>开窍于目</u>**。（《素问·金匮真言论》）

译文：Yang emerges in the east and the colour of east is green, the human liver is also green and corresponds to wood, as the energy of universe is connected with the human energy, so the east energy communicates with the liver. The liver channel gets access to the brain and connecting the eyes, so eyes are the orifices of the liver.

吴本对此句同样采用阐释性翻译，变换了"开窍于目"的句式，化被动为主动，译为 eyes are the orifices of the liver（眼为肝之窍），并增译出东方、青色、肝、木、目之间的联系，同时使用因果连词 so 凸显句中的逻辑关系。译文在语言形式上并未忠于原文，导致译文较为繁琐，未能重现原文简洁凝练之美，但是对"东方""青色"和"肝"之间的关系进行了阐释说明，合理解释中医医理，帮助读者理解句中提到的事物之间的抽象关联，更易于目的语读者接受。

从语言内容看，吴氏的阐释译法不求解释概念来源及可能出现的歧义解读，只求将深奥的古文阐发为简练的养生口诀 [1]。译文不标注任何参考文献或脚注，而是将所有解释融入文中，对隐喻的翻译以传递信息为主，不拘泥于语言形式，以实现内容的可读性为目的，选择西方普通读者更易于理解的表达方式进行阐释，因此译文中不乏使用西医术语解释中医概念的情况。例如：

原文：**寒则腠理闭，气不行，故气收矣。炅则腠理<u>开</u>，荣卫<u>通</u>，汗大<u>泄</u>，故气泄**。（《素问·举痛论》）

译文：The cold-evil causes the channel and collaterals to become rough, and the circulation of the Ying and Wei energies to become obstructed. So, it is called

---

[1] 徐冰，张莹.《黄帝内经·素问》四个英译本的翻译策略和接受 [J]. 外国语言与文化，2019，3（3）：107.

the "collecting of energy". The heat causes the opening of the striae and the excessive excretion of the Ying and Wei energies along with the sweat. So, it is called the "excretion of the energy".

此句采用意译的方法对医理进行解释说明，将"行"译为西医术语 circulation（循环），将体现容器隐喻的"腠理开"译为 opening of the striae，将"泄"译为西医术语 excretion（排泄）。译文通过借助西医术语进行解释，使读者更易于理解和接受中医文化。但是，该译法在一定程度上将中医西化，在隐喻翻译和文化传递上的效果略显不足。

原文：……其气九州（九窍）、五脏、十二节……（《素问·生气通天论》）

译文：...In the universe, there are nine states (namely Ji, Yan, Qing, Xu, Yang, Jing, Yu, Liang and Yong), and man has nine orifices (seven orifices: two ears, two eyes, two nostrils, and one mouth; two Yin orifices: external urethral orifice and the anus); there are five musical tones in the universe, man has five solid organs responsible for storing the mental activities (liver stores soul, heart stores spirit, spleen stores consciousness, lung stores inferior spirit, kidney stores will); there are twelve solar terms in the universe, and man has twelve channels...

吴本对句中具有隐喻特征的"九窍"采用直译加释义的方法，首先将其译为 nine orifices，然后在括号内补充说明"九窍"的具体所指：七阳窍（眼二、耳二、鼻孔二，口一）与二阴窍（前阴一，后阴一）。对于"九州""五脏"也采用同样的译法。从形式上看，译文复杂繁琐，但从内容上看，译文准确清楚，可读性大大提升，更易于读者理解和接受中医文化。

（二）翻译策略

为实现译文的应用功能，传播中医的医理和诊治方法，吴本的归化特征非常明显。在对隐喻的翻译中，吴氏倾向于选择符合读者语言习惯的表达，用西医术语解释中医内涵，借助阐释来翻译富含中国文化的隐喻。译文不追求忠实于原文，不强求语言形式的对等和工整，灵活使用增译、补译、减译、创译等翻译方法，借助简单、近乎直白的语言解释隐喻，将个人行医经验融入其中传授给读者。例如：

原文：肾汗出逢于风，内不得入于脏腑，外不得越于皮肤。（《素问·水

热穴论》）

译文：When the wind-evil invades the body during the sweating, his sweat pores will close all of a sudden, as the perspiration has not completed, the sweat can not return to its viscus inside, neither can it be discharged to the skin outside.

句中"内"和"外"是典型的方位隐喻，表示肾汗在体内的运行路径，具有"向内"或"向外"的意思。吴本采用增译的方法，补充原文中隐而未明的内容 his sweat pores will close all of a sudden, as the perspiration has not completed（汗孔骤闭，余汗未尽），详细解释中医医理，使句意更加清晰。同时，译文中选择了 perspiration、viscus、discharge 等西医术语解释中医内容，便于读者的理解和接受。

原文：**春有惨凄残贼之胜，则夏有<u>炎暑燔烁</u>之复**。（《素问·气交变大论》）

译文：...if the metal energy is subjugating the insufficient wood, there will be cold and destitude metal energy in spring and the son energy of the wood (fire energy) will retaliate to cause hot weather like burning fire in summer.

句中"炎暑燔烁"意为气候炎热，如同烈火燃烧一般。炎暑和燔烁之间的相似性在于灼热感，但是原文没有出现喻词，二者之间的关联需要读者自行体会。对于读者来说，直译出来的译文不易理解，因此吴氏采用意译的方法将其译为 hot weather like burning fire in summer，增译喻词 like 连接"炎暑"与"燔烁"。这种阐释使二者之间的相似性一目了然，更易于读者理解和接受。

（三）翻译目标的实现

吴氏父子将深奥晦涩、意蕴丰富的《素问》通过阐释译法进行解读翻译，行文简洁朴实。对于隐喻的翻译，吴氏主要采用意译的方法，在一定程度上以牺牲语言形式为代价提高译文的可读性。语言形式虽然未完全遵循原文，略显繁琐，但总体上可以满足读者了解和学习中医的需求，使他们能够更顺畅地理解原文，把握中医医理和隐喻特征，接受中医方法和文化，展现中医临床价值，在很大程度上促进《素问》的推广和中医文化的传播。值得指出的是，吴氏并非语言专家，在翻译过程中出现对同一术语进行音译、直译、意译的混乱情况，还有一些语言错误。因此，译文在严谨性上存在一定的不足。例如：

原文：故风无常府，卫气之所发，必开其腠理，邪气之所合，则其府也。(《素问·疟论》)

译文：Therefore, although the invading location of the evil-energy is not certain, yet, whenever the Wei-energy corresponds to it, the striae will open, the evil-energy will retains and causes disease.

句中将腠理隐喻为人体体液渗泄、气血流通的门户，具有"开""合"功能。吴本对该容器隐喻做了阐释，说明风邪入侵的地方并不固定，只要卫气与之相应，腠理打开，邪气就会停留并引起疾病。译者并未直译出体现容器隐喻的"府"字，但是形象准确地解释了中医医理。译文中的 will retains and causes 出现语法错误，情态动词后应使用动词原形。类似的语言错误在吴本中多次出现，说明吴氏父子在语言运用上不甚严谨，影响译文的准确性。

原文：开阖不得，寒气从之，乃生大偻。(《素问·生气通天论》)

译文：It is normal when the skin striae of a man opens in spring and close in winter. If it does not open when it should open and does not close when it should close, it will leave the opportunity for the cold-evil to invade. When the cold-evil penetrates deep and damages the Yang energy, he may contract hunchback. This is because of the damaged Yang energy can no more soften the tendons.

吴本增译主语 skin striae。striae 为 stria 的复数形式，意为"条纹，细沟"。在意思上，striae 和中医的"腠理"并不对等，而且在形式上，striae 是单数形式，语言运用上不够严谨。本句详细解释大偻病的成因，虽然译文略显繁琐，缺失原文的凝练之美，但是整体上语言流畅，表达朴素，更容易帮助读者了解该病的病因，对中医临床起到指导作用，实现了翻译目的。

二、原因分析

(一) 原文解读

吴氏父子所译英文版《黄帝内经》成书于 20 世纪 90 年代。当时已有众多白话文版本可供参考，加之吴氏父子以汉语为母语，对原文理解比较准确，因此他们对原文的解读总体上是到位的。吴氏父子均为中医师，长期从事中医临床工作，有助于他们从不同的视角对《黄帝内经》进行解读。与其他版本不同的是，吴氏父子的译本并不注重从语言的角度解读原文，而是将关注点放在中医医理和临床操作的传播上。古汉语具有高度凝练、一词多义、外延宽泛、词性和词义模糊、通假字使用较多等特点，但是吴氏父子在这些方面不求甚解，倾向于简化深奥的古文，使用通俗的语言来迎合目标读者，形成了独特的翻译风格。

（二）文化意识

吴氏父子的译本注重展现中医的临床价值，希望国外对中医感兴趣的人士能够将中医应用于医疗实践[1]。他们以传递中医医理和行医方法为主，并不重视语言和文化方面的传递和保留[2]。他们不重视语言形式的统一，为迎合普通读者的理解水平，常使用西医术语解释中医内容。这种做法不利于保持和传递中医的文化特色。由于众多中医流派对《黄帝内经》的解读仍存在争议，为了规避争议，实现译文的应用功能，吴氏父子用简练清晰的语言将自己的理解呈现给读者，避免众多矛盾的说法让读者感到模棱两可。因此，该译本受到非学术研究领域的普通读者欢迎，可读性的提升使中医文化的传播成为可能。虽然吴氏父子在翻译过程中体现的文化意识较弱，但是读者的接受度较高。从这个角度来看，他们的工作对中医知识的推广和中医文化的传播起到了很大的促进作用。

小　结

李照国的学术经历及其译本的出版背景决定了李本独特的翻译风格。李本行文简洁流畅，语言精练准确，最大限度地再现原文的句式结构和音韵之美，保留其文学性，实现其可读性。为实现中医文化对外传播的目标，李本

---

[1]　胡犀利.从纽马克功能理论比较《黄帝内经》的三个英译本[D].北京外国语大学，2014：12.

[2]　黄光惠.《黄帝内经·素问》概念隐喻英译研究[D].福建师范大学，2013：53.

非常重视文化传递，大量使用音译、音译加注的方法翻译隐喻等存在文化缺省的内容，着力保留《素问》的文化特色，助力中医药文化的国际传播。

威斯在困难重重的情况下完成《素问》首部较为完整的英译本。该译本的翻译风格同样与译者的学术背景密切相关。威斯从医史学家的视角解读原著，更注重交际目标的实现，运用归化策略对文化内涵丰富的内容进行语言转换，大量采用意译的方法解释复杂抽象的中医概念，以便增加译文的可读性。威本语言流畅，文字优美，通俗易懂，深受英语国家读者欢迎，具有较强的影响力。

文树德在文化意识的影响下，选择直译结合大量注释的方法进行翻译。译文在语言上字斟句酌，在形式上遵循古汉语的语法和句法，在内容上追本溯源，对未尽其意或存在争议之处添加注释，力求在语言形式和内容上重现原文。尽管对一些隐喻的翻译存在译不达意、语言晦涩的遗憾，但是瑕不掩瑜，文本在西方读者中的接受度较高，在保留原著隐喻特征、传递中医文化方面做出了重要贡献。

吴氏父子选择风格独特的阐释译法翻译《素问》。这是由译者身份、目标读者和翻译目的决定的。身为美籍中医师，吴氏父子将目标读者确定为对中医感兴趣的西方读者，因此译文重内容，轻形式，简化复杂晦涩的中医语言，重视中医临床技能的传播。虽然对一些隐喻的翻译存在语言不严谨之处，但整体上译文的可读性较强，通俗易懂，受到普通中医爱好者的欢迎，有利于中医医理和中医文化在西方的传播。

第九章 《素问》隐喻的英译策略和方法

第一节 《素问》隐喻的英译策略

隐喻是一种普遍存在的思维认知方式，也是一种常见的语言修辞手段。从修辞学角度来看，隐喻由本体、喻体、喻底三部分组成。在《素问》中，本体主要指中医学各方面的内容，包括病理、病象、治则等。与本体相对，喻体是对本体特征有效而形象的描述。受"天人合一"和"取象比类"思想的影响，《素问》常将人体的生理病理状况与人们熟悉的、具体的、容易感知的事物进行类比，利用事物之间的相似性达到认识人体生理病理规律的目的。喻底即本体和喻体之间的相似性。《素问》中的隐喻通过各种相似性构建联系，既表明喻体特征又表明本体功能。

《素问》中的隐喻以"三要素"（本体、喻体、喻底）为基本结构支点，加之传统"取象比类"的思维模式，形成了既具有修辞性又有思维性的语言特色[1]。因此，在隐喻的英译过程中，既要注重译语和源语之间在语言内容上的准确转换，又要注重中医思想和文化的准确传达，力求实现译语和源语在文本形式和功能上的对等。

国内翻译界对"翻译策略"的概念和内涵一直存在争议。熊兵认为，狭义的翻译策略是指为实现特定的翻译目的所依据的原则和所采纳的方案集合，可以概括为归化和异化策略[2]。文旭将隐喻的翻译策略概括为四类：隐喻概念

---

[1] 刘璞莹，陈嘉或，陈骥.《黄帝内经》中隐喻的语言特征及英译策略 [J]. 中国中医基础医学杂志，2018，24（18）：1144.

[2] 熊兵.翻译研究中的概念混淆——以"翻译策略""翻译方法"和"翻译技巧"为例 [J]. 中国翻译，2014，5（3）：84.

域的对等映射、转换喻体、隐喻和喻底结合、舍喻体译喻义[1]。邓恋玫从认知角度提出隐喻翻译的对等策略、转换策略和移植策略[2]。刘璞莹等针对《内经》中的隐喻提出三种翻译策略，分别为类比推理、本体补偿，精确描述、喻体直译，重视文化、喻底意译[3]。

通过对比和分析《素问》的四个译本可以看出，《素问》隐喻的英译主要采用以下四种翻译策略：对等策略、本体补偿策略、舍喻体译喻底策略和隐喻显化策略。

一、对等策略

人类生活的外部环境及其自身生理结构的共性决定了来自不同语言文化背景的人可以对同一事物产生相同或相似的心理认知。基于这些心理认知而建构的隐喻具有共通性。因此，在翻译此类隐喻时，可以在译语中找到相同或相似的隐喻，进行对等翻译。

1. 夏至四十五日，阴气微上，阳气微下。（《素问·脉要精微论》）

李本：During the forty-five days from the Summer Solstice [to the Beginning of Autumn], Yinqi is gradually ascending while Yangqi is gradually descending.

文本：During the 45 days [following] "summer solstice", the yin qi is feeble and ascends and the yang qi is feeble and descends.

吴本：the first Yin generates on summer solstice and on the forty-fifth day after it, the Yin-energy ascends slightly, and the Yang-energy descends slightly.

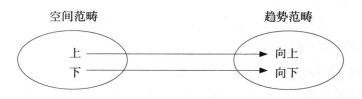

图 9-1　空间隐喻"上 – 下"表示趋势

[1] 文旭，肖开容 . 认知翻译学 [M]. 北京：北京大学出版社，2019：34–37.
[2] 邓恋玫 . 隐喻翻译策略的认知研究 [J]. 湖北开放职业学院学报，2020，33（18）：177–178.
[3] 刘璞莹，陈嘉或，陈骥 .《黄帝内经》中隐喻的语言特征及英译策略 [J]. 中国中医基础医学杂志，2018，24（18）：1144–1145.

"上"和"下"原本属于空间范畴，此处映射到趋势范畴，表示阳气和阴气"向上"或"向下"的运行状态。"上－下"空间隐喻为英汉两种语言共有，因此翻译时可以寻找英语中相同或相似的隐喻，进行对等翻译。李本、文本和吴本均采用此策略，将"上"和"下"对等翻译为 descend 和 ascend，实现隐喻由空间范畴向趋势范畴的映射，准确再现原文信息，完成有效交际，同时成功实现两种文化之间的转换。

2. 复则炎暑流火，湿性燥……（《素问·气交变大论》）

李本：Retaliating [activity leads to] flaming summer–heat, [change of] moisture into dryness...

文本：When it comes to revenge, then there is flaming summerheat [as if there were] fire flowing. That which is of damp nature dries out...

吴本：As the wood energy is restricted causing the crops to become grey and white, its son energy (fire energy) will be retaliating for its mother, the weather will become as hot as fire, all the wet things will become dry...

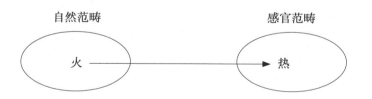

图 9-2　本体隐喻"火"表示感官

此句描述木气受到克制导致子气（火气）来复将会出现的各种状况。句中以"流火"（炎热如火）隐喻木气受到克制时子气（火气）来复的炎热状况。原本属于自然范畴的"火"映射到感官范畴，隐喻为"热"。因此，李本和文本将其译为 heat，吴本译为 hot，都采用对等策略进行翻译，成功表达"火"的隐喻含义。

二、本体补偿策略

中医语言中的一些隐喻是由中国古代哲学等理论类比推理得来，因此具有间接性、抽象性及明显的心理相似性[1]。此类隐喻包括中医学核心概念"精""阴""阳"等。这种本体概念在英文中缺乏对应的概念和语言形式，无法直接进行对等翻译。多数译者采用音译的方法，将其译为Jing、Yin、Yang等。然而，对于没有中医文化背景的读者来说，这样翻译根本无法在头脑中形成相应的心理认知，也就不能实现有效交际。不过，在音译的基础上采用加注的方法，可以为读者提供更多的本体信息，帮助他们更好地理解原文。

1. 故天有精，地有形……（《素问·阴阳应象大论》）

李本：So the heavens has Jing (Essence-Qi) and the earth has forms...

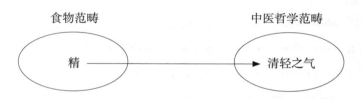

图 9-3　结构隐喻"精"表示中医哲学概念

精，本义为"挑选过的好米，上等细米"，属于食物范畴。句中的"精"指构成宇宙万物的灵气，专指气的精粹部分，即"清轻之气"。对于"精"的翻译，李本采用本体补偿的策略，运用音译加注的方法，译为 Jing (Essence-Qi)。通过音译尽力保留中华文化特色，加注 Essence-Qi（精华之气）以便读者更好地理解"精"的内涵，从而实现有效交际。

2. 余闻天为阳，地为阴。（《素问·阴阳离合论》）

威本：It is said that Heaven was created by Yang (the male principle of light and life), and that the Earth was created by Yin (the female principle of darkness and death).

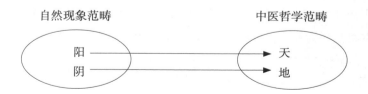

图 9-4　结构隐喻"阴阳"表示中医哲学概念

---

[1] 汤思敏.关联翻译理论指导下的中医隐喻翻译[J].嘉应学院学报（哲学社会科学），2010，28（3）：79.

阴阳最初指太阳的向背，属于自然现象范畴。古人认为，天在上，天气轻清、上浮为阳；地在下，地气重浊、下沉为阴。因此阴阳常被隐喻为"地"和"天"。

威本在翻译"阴""阳"时，采用音译加注的方法，对本体信息进行必要的补充，分别译为 Yang (the male principle of light and life) 和 Yin (the female principle of darkness and death)。此种译法不但可以有效传播中医文化，而且可以加强读者对原文的认识与理解，提高读者对译文的接受度。

三、舍喻体译喻底策略

不同语言和文化的巨大差异决定了来自不同语言文化背景的人可能会对同一事物产生不同的心理认知。作为中医学的奠基之作，《内经》中的许多隐喻带有明显的中医学特色，为汉语所特有，在英文中找不到对应关系。翻译此类隐喻时，一般会舍弃喻体，在译语中寻找恰当的语言形式对喻底进行意译，从而帮助读者实现对原文的认知和理解。

1. 外内相得，无以形先……（《素问·宝命全形论》）

李本：Both the external [manifestations] and the internal [changes] must be taken into consideration, avoiding giving first priority to the external [manifestations]...

威本：But one should rely upon one's combined examinations of the external and the internal circumstances, and one should not rely upon past experience...

吴本：Examine the pulse condition of the patient, be sure the pulse of the exhausted visceral-energy is existing and must not examine the outer appearance of the patient only...

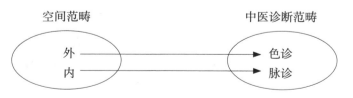

图 9-5 空间隐喻"内－外"表示中医诊断方法

"外内"原本属于空间概念，此处表示中医学的两种诊断方法，"外"指察色，"内"指诊脉。英文中有很多表示"外内"概念的语言表达，如 outside 和 inside、external 和 internal 等，但这些表达均不具有"察色"和"诊脉"这一隐喻含义。英译时，李本、威本和吴本都采用舍喻体译喻底的策略。与李本和威本相比，吴本将"外内"译为 examine the pulse condition of the patient 和 examine the outer appearance of the patient，不但更为准确地再现原文的喻底，而且最大限度地保留喻体"外内"的中医文化内涵。

2. 风客淫气，精乃亡，邪伤肝也。（《素问·生气通天论》）

李本：When wind attacks the body, [it gradually] damages Qi and exhausts Jing (Essence). [This is because of] the impairment of the liver by Xie (Evil).

威本：If the wind enters the body and exhausts man's breath, then his essence will be lost and the evil influences will injure his liver.

文本：When wind settles [in the body] and encroaches upon the [proper] qi, then the essence vanishes, and the evil harms the liver.

吴本：Owning to the wind associates with the liver (liver correspond to the wind and wood), when one is hurt by excessive wind-evil, the essence of life and blood will suffer severe damage. As blood is stored in the liver, the wind-evil will hurt the liver too.

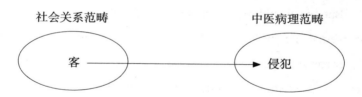

社会关系范畴　　　　　　　　　　中医病理范畴

客　　　　　　　　→　侵犯

图 9-6　社会关系隐喻"客"表示中医病理概念

"客"的本义是"来宾、宾客"，与"主"相对，属于社会关系范畴。句中"客"作动词使用，指风邪侵入人体。"客"在英语中的对应词为 guest，但 guest 并没有"侵入""侵犯"这一隐喻含义。英译时，四个译本都采用舍喻体译喻底的策略，分别译为 attacks the body、enters the body、settles [in the body] 和 hurt。其中，attacks the body 最为到位，不仅形象地表达出外来风邪对人体的侵害，还保留了原文的战争隐喻色彩。

四、隐喻显化策略

翻译时，若能将源语语言文化中建立的隐喻关系最准确最直接最大限度地映射到译语语言文化中，其翻译效果无疑是最佳的 [1]。《内经》隐喻语言形象、精练，在翻译时，可以将那些隐含意义较深、不太明显的隐喻进行显化处理。通过增加 like，as，similar to 等喻词将隐喻转化为明喻，使译文更加生动形象，意思更为清晰，从而更好地向读者传达原文信息。

1. 肺者，<u>相傅之官</u>，治节出焉。（《素问·灵兰秘典论》）

李本：The lung is the organ [similar to] a prime minister and is responsible for Zhijie (management).

文本：The lung is the official functioning as chancellor and mentor. Order and moderation originate in it.

吴本：The lung governs the various vessels and regulates the energy of the whole body, like a prime minister assisting the king to reign the country.

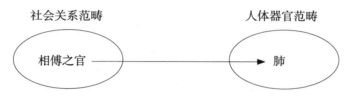

社会关系范畴　　　　　　　　人体器官范畴

相傅之官　　　　　　　　　　肺

图 9-7　社会关系隐喻"相傅之官"表示人体器官

"相傅之官"，即宰相，具有辅佐君主的职能，原属社会关系范畴。此处，以"相傅之官"隐喻肺，把肺比喻成朝廷的宰相，以此说明肺具有辅助心脏的功能。李本、文本和吴本都采用隐喻显化的策略，分别译为 the lung is the organ similar to a prime minister、the lung is the official functioning as chancellor and mentor 和 the lung...like a prime minister。将隐喻转化为明喻，更加凸显本体"肺"和喻体"相傅之官"之间的相似之处，强调肺的生理功能。同时，译文不但易于读者理解和接受，而且可以很好地保留源语特色。

---

[1]　盛洁. 中医语言隐喻分析及其翻译方法研究 [J]. 北方文学，2016（13）：151.

2. 三阳为<u>父</u>……三阴为<u>母</u>……（《素问·阴阳类论》）

李本：Triple-Yang [is equivalent to the position of] father... Triple-Yin [is equivalent to the position of] mother...

吴本：The third Yang is equivalent to the honorable father... the third Yin is equivalent to the mother who is good at breeding...

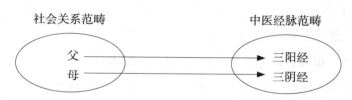

图 9-8　社会关系隐喻"父母"表示中医经脉概念

"父"和"母"本属社会关系范畴。此处将三阳经隐喻为"父"，因为三阳经总领诸经，高尊如父；将三阴经隐喻为"母"，因为三阴经能够滋养诸经，像母亲养育子女一样。李本分别将其译为 triple-Yang [is equivalent to the position of] father 和 triple-Yin [is equivalent to the position of] mother；吴本分别译为 the third Yang is equivalent to the honorable father 和 the third Yin is equivalent to the mother who is good at breeding。两个译本均通过使用短语 be equivalent to 将隐喻转化为明喻，形象准确地表达"三阳"和"三阴"在人体内的作用。译文通俗易懂，有效地传递了信息。

隐喻是《素问》中一种常见的语言现象，体现了中医学独特的思维方式。隐喻构建了中医学的诸多核心概念，如风、水、火、土等，进而从根本上建构中医学经典理论体系，包括阴阳学说、五行学说、藏象学说、精气学说等。因此，在《素问》英译过程中，隐喻翻译的好坏对整个译本的质量起着举足轻重的作用。在隐喻翻译过程中，翻译策略的选择至关重要。只有深刻理解隐喻的本体和喻体特征、找到二者之间的相似性，熟练驾驭源语和译语两种语言，才能找到最佳的翻译策略，最大可能地实现原文文本和译语文本在形式和功能上的对等。

第二节 《素问》隐喻的英译方法

关于隐喻的翻译方法，传统上一般采用描写的方法，公认的有三种：直译法、替换法和意译法[1]。《素问》隐喻的英译策略主要有对等策略、舍喻体译喻底策略、本体补偿策略、隐喻显化策略等，在翻译实践中具体表现为直译法、意译法、直译和意译结合法、音译（加注）法等翻译方法。

一、直译法

《素问》中的很多隐喻来自古人对自然界和社会关系的观察以及生活经验的总结，这种认知方式为不同文化共有，存在相似和共通之处。因此，翻译时可以使用直译法将汉语隐喻植入到译语中，使用译语中的对应词或相似的语言符号进行表达，实现两种语言和文化之间的直接转换。这样，一方面能够使译文在内容和句式上忠实于原文，另一方面又可以保留汉语言的文化特色。直译法主要用于翻译下面五种类型的隐喻。

（一）自然隐喻

自然隐喻是《素问》中最常见的一种本体隐喻。古代医家借助水、火、海、土、风等自然现象隐喻致病因素和病理变化。这些用语描述了自然界客观存在的事物，在其他语言中也能找到对应语，因此翻译时通常采用直译法。

体若燔炭，汗出而散。（《素问·生气通天论》）

李本：[If they] run a fever, their body may feel as hot as a piece of burning coal. [However] the fever disappears after sweating.

威本：Then their body resembles burning charcoal and the (sickness) can be dispersed only through perspiration.

文本：The body resembles burning coal. Sweat flow lets [the internal heat]

[1]　胡壮麟.隐喻翻译的方法与理论 [J].当代修辞学，2019（4）：2.

disperse.

吴本：...and his body will be hot like the burning charcoal. The stagnated heat-evil can only be dispersed by perspiration.

"体若燔炭"形容病人发高热，像炭火烧灼一样，用于隐喻暑邪伤气时身体发热的感受。李本和文本将"炭"译为 coal，威本和吴本将"炭"译为 charcoal。四个译本虽然用词有所差别，但都使用直译法将"体若燔炭"分别译为 as hot as a piece of burning coal/resembles burning charcoal/resembles burning coal/be hot like the burning charcoal。"炭"在中英文化中皆为生活常见之物，因此采用直译法将"燔炭"译为 burning charcoal，不仅语言生动形象，而且行文上也更加忠实于原文，可以有效地实现交际目标。

（二）动物隐喻

动物隐喻在用来表现脉象、病理变化和外候时，有些在原文中出现了喻词，喻体较明显，为不同文化所共有的常见之物。翻译时多采用直译法。

平脾脉来，和柔相离，如鸡践地……（《素问·平人气象论》）

李本：The normal Spleen-Pulse beats smoothly and softly as a chicken putting its claw on the ground...

威本：When man is tranquil and healthy the pulse of the spleen flows softly, coming together and falling apart like a chicken treading the earth...

文本：The arrival of a normal spleen [movement in the] vessels is [as follows]: harmonious, soft, and distanced, resembling chicken stepping on the earth...

吴本：When the coming of the spleen pulse with stomach-energy is mild but adhering with energy, likes a cock's claws falling leisurely on the ground when walking...

"如鸡践地"用于隐喻平脾脉和缓，像鸡足落地一样轻。四个译本均采用直译法，分别译为 as a chicken putting its claw on the ground/like a chicken treading the earth/resembling chicken stepping on the earth/likes a cock's claws falling leisurely on the ground。使用喻词 as/like/resembling/likes（吴本的 likes 为误译，应为 like）对原文隐喻进行显化处理，形象描述出鸡足落地时从容不迫的画面，既帮助读者体会"平脾脉和缓"的脉象特征，又保留原文的隐喻色彩。

（三）植物隐喻

植物隐喻的数量相当可观，主要用来表现病理变化、脉象、外候、大小、尺寸、形状等，部分喻体为不同文化中所共有的常见之物。翻译时多采用直译法。

云物飞动，草木不宁，甚而摇落……（《素问·气交变大论》）

李本：...clouds are flying, things are fluctuating, grasses and trees are unstable. [Under serious condition, grasses and trees] are broken...

文本：[As a result,] cloudy things fly by. Herbs and trees are kept in constant motion. In severe cases, they are shaken and fall down...

吴本：So, the wind energy will be running wildly, causing the clouds flying in the sky, the grasses and woods on earth swaying, and the leaves and branches falling down...

"草木不宁，甚而摇落"描述草木不平静的状态，是自然界的常见现象，用以隐喻"反胁痛而吐甚"的病理变化。李本、文本和吴本分别译为 grasses and trees are unstable. [Under serious condition, grasses and trees] are broken./ Herbs and trees are kept in constant motion. In severe cases, they are shaken and fall down./the grasses and woods on earth swaying, and the leaves and branches falling down. 虽然三个译本在选词上有所差别，但对"草木""不宁""摇落"都采用直译法；同时，三个译本都将"草木不宁，甚而摇落"译为两个分句，结构上与原文保持一致。

（四）容器隐喻

容器隐喻是最典型的本体隐喻之一，用于说明脏腑像容器一样具有贮存、容纳或传化水谷精微的属性和功能，隐喻为致病因素会进入、停留在脏腑之中，病理产物会经由脏腑排出。翻译时常用直译法。

所谓五脏者，藏精气而不泻也……六腑者，传化物而不藏……（《素问·五脏别论》）

李本：The so-called Five Zang-Organs only store up Jingqi (Essence-Qi) and will not discharge it... The so-called Six Fu-Organs only transport and transform food and will not store it up...

威本：The so-called five viscera store up the essences of life and do not dispel them... The six bowels conduct and transform substance and do not store...

文本：As for the so-called five depots, they store the essence qi and do not drain [it]... As for the six palaces, they transmit and transform things, but do not store [them]...

吴本：The function of the five solid organs is to store the essence without discharging... The function of the six hollow organs is to digest, absorb and transport the food...

五脏六腑都具有容器的功能，例如"藏""泻""传"等。对此，四个译本主要采用直译法，将"藏"译为 store up/store，皆有"储藏"之义；将"泻"译为 discharge/dispel/drain，皆有"倾泻"之义；将"传"译为 transport/conduct/transmit，皆有"传送"之义。此译法一方面帮助读者理解"藏""泻"与"精气"，"传"与"物"之间的关联，另一方面也可以最大限度地保留原文的隐喻特色。

（五）空间隐喻

空间隐喻，尤其是"内－外"空间范畴，用来隐喻病邪在体内的运行状态。在说明致病邪气侵犯人体的路径、描述疾病发生的位置、阐释疾病发生的机理时，多采用直译法。

风气藏于皮肤之间，内不得通，外不得泄。（《素问·风论》）

李本：[When attacking the body,] wind tends to stay [in the region] between the skin [and the muscles] and is difficult to penetrate inside or escape to the outside.

文本：When wind qi is stored in the skin, it cannot penetrate into the interior and it cannot flow away to the outside.

吴本：When the wind-evil invades into the skin, it can not be dispersed to the interior, nor can it be diffused to the exterior.

"内""外"本为方位词，用以隐喻风气在身体内外的运行路径。三个译本均采用直译法，李本译为 inside 和 to the outside，文本译为 into the interior 和 to the outside，吴本译为 to the interior 和 to the exterior。三个译本使用副词或介词短语将原文的内 – 外隐喻转化为一种运动趋势，帮助读者更好地理解风气侵入人体皮肤的路径，描述出既不能在内部流通、又无法向外部疏泄的情景，成功实现交际目标。

二、意译法

在《素问》中，很多隐喻的喻体完全脱离字面意思，例如"天地""日月"用于喻指地位、月事等，"内""外"用于表示诊断方法、房事等，官职用于喻指脏器，战争过程用于解释疾病的经过与转归等。对于这类隐喻，一般舍弃喻体的字面意思，对喻底进行意译，以求达到译文内容忠实于原文。意译法主要用于翻译下面五种类型的隐喻。

（一）自然隐喻

"天地""日月"相关的自然隐喻意义非常繁杂。"天""日"经常被用来隐喻至高无上的地位、阳气、人体上部等，而"地""月"则被用于隐喻月经、寿命长久、人体下部等。在这些情况下，"天地""日月"均脱离了字面意思，使用意译法优于直译法。

1.……长而敦敏，成而登天。（《素问·上古天真论》）

李本：...When growing up, he became the Emperor.

威本：...When he became perfect he ascended to Heaven.

文本：...After he had matured, he ascended to heaven.

吴本：...He became an emperor when he grew up.

"天"隐喻至高无上的"天子"，"登天"指登上天子之位。句中"天"与自然界所指的天空毫无联系，翻译时需采用意译法。李本、吴本将"登天"意译为 became the/an emperor，准确理解原文的内涵意义。而威本、文本将"登天"直译为 ascend to heaven，容易造成理解偏差。英语文化中，heaven 常指人死后去的极乐之地，因此 ascend to heaven 容易使读者联想到死亡，导致交际失败。

2.……天癸竭，地道不通，故形坏而无子也。（《素问·上古天真论》）

李本：...and menstruation stops, she becomes physically feeble and is no longer able to conceive a baby.

威本：...Her menstruation is exhausted, and the gates of menstruation are no longer open; her body deteriorates and she is no longer able to bear children.

文本：...The way of the earth is impassable. Hence, the physical appearance is spoilt and [a woman can] no [longer] have children.

吴本：...her menstruation severs as her Taingui being exhausted. Her physique turns old and feeble, and by then, she can no more conceive.

女性的子宫有时被喻为自然界的"（土）地"，句中"地道"用来隐喻"月经"，完全脱离其字面意思，因此翻译时需采用意译法。李本、威本、吴本都使用 menstruation 表达"地道"，明确其内涵意义为"女子月经"，在内容上做到忠实于原文。而文本却将"地道"直译为 the way of the earth，未能传递出其内涵意义，无法有效地实现交际目标。

（二）空间隐喻

由于中西语言和文化的差异，在"内-外"空间隐喻表示范围时，直译容易造成歧义，宜采用意译法。同时，"内-外"空间隐喻用于表示房事以及诊断方法时，带有明显的中医学特色，这一类隐喻是中文所特有的。英语中找不到对应语，因而只能进行意译。

1.……游行天地之间，视听八达之外。（《素问·上古天真论》）

李本：...and roaming around on the earth and in the heavens. So they could see and hear [things and voices] beyond the eight directions.

威 本：...They roamed and travelled all over the universe and could see and hear beyond the eight distant places.

文 本：...They roamed between heaven and earth and their vision as well as their hearing went beyond the eight reaches.

吴本：...They travelled extensively and to hear and see things in distant places.

"八达之外"喻指中古至人游历丰富，见闻广博。"外"虽是一个方位词，但句中不能独立使用，需与"八达"共同构成整体概念。因此，翻译时应采用意译法。吴本将"八达之外"意译为 in distant places，忠实于原文且通俗易懂。相反，李本、威本和文本均采用直译法，将"八达之外"分别译为 beyond the eight directions/beyond the eight distant places/beyond the eight reaches，这三个译文均不达意，未能表达出"八达之外"在句中"遥远的地方"之内涵意义，无法有效地实现交际目标。

2. 名曰肺痹，寒热，得之醉而使<u>内</u>也。（《素问·五脏生成》）

李本：...known as Feibi (Lung–Bi Syndrome). It is caused by cold–heat and sexual intercourse after drinking of alcohol.

威本：The name of the disease is "numbness（痹）of the lungs" and the external evidences are chills and fevers. This disease is caused through toxicity which influences the inner body.

文本：This is called lung block, as well as cold and heat. One gets it when one is drunk and then sends inwards.

吴本：The disease is called lung *bi*–syndrome, which is caused by cold and heat and the conducting sex intercourse after being drunken.

"内"隐喻为房事，完全失去其字面意思，因此宜采用意译法。李本和吴本分别将"内"意译为 sexual intercourse 和 the conducting sex intercourse，准确表明肺痹的致病原因是寒热，并在醉后入房。同时，intercourse 选词精准，既忠实于原文意思，又在形式上保留了原文隐喻。相较而言，威本和文本采用直译法，分别将"内"译为 inner body 和 inwards，未能表达出"内"的内涵意义，容易造成理解偏差，导致交际失败。

（三）植物隐喻

一些植物隐喻用来表现脉象、病理变化等，喻体的内涵意义与其字面意思有很大偏差，直译容易造成词不达意或者引起歧义，因此宜采用意译法。

太虚深玄，气犹<u>麻散</u>……（《素问·六元正纪大论》）

李本：[During this period of time,] the sky looks profound and dark, Qi appears like scattered hemp...

文本：When the Great Void is deep dark, when the [cloud] qi resembles powdered hemp...

吴本：When the sky is high and far with yellowish–dark energy like disorderly fibre...

"气犹麻散"用以隐喻天空中云气隐约不清的景象，"麻"指麻类植物纤维，而非麻类植物本身。李本和文本采用直译法，将"麻散"分别译为 scattered hemp 和 powdered hemp。名词 hemp 指的是用来制绳索、衣料、毒品的一种植物，称为"大麻"。因此李本传递的信息是散落一地的大麻这种植物，而非其纤维，用词不够准确，无法传递"混乱、凌乱不清"之义；文本传递的信息是粉末状的大麻，容易让读者联想到毒品，产生误解。反之，吴本将"麻散"意译为 disorderly fibre，形象地描绘出"气犹麻散"所隐喻的云气混乱、隐约不清的景象。

（四）社会关系隐喻

社会关系隐喻是指利用官职、父母、母子等社会关系概念隐喻人体不同部位之间的关系和变化。这些社会关系或具体或抽象，其中一些是中国文化的特有现象，在不同语境中意思也不尽相同。因此，翻译时宜用意译法。

1. 愿闻十二脏之相使，贵贱何如？（《素问·灵兰秘典论》）

威本：I desire to hear how it is possible that the twelve viscera send each other that which is precious and that which is worthless.

吴本：I would like you to tell me the mutual relations between the twelve viscera in human body and their principal and subordinate status in functions.

"相使"泛指官职，用以隐喻人体内的十二脏器。"贵贱"指职位的高低，用以隐喻十二脏器之间的相互关系。句中"相使""贵贱"完全脱离字面意思，因此宜采用意译法。吴本将"相使""贵贱"分别意译为 the mutual relations between the twelve viscera 和 their principal and subordinate status in functions，准确表达出十二脏之间的相互作用和主从关系。相较而言，威本采用直译法，将"相使"译为 send each other（相互支使、派遣），将"贵贱"译为 precious/worthless，未能忠实传递原文的内涵意义，无法实现有效交际的目标。

2. 鬲肓之上，中有父母。（《素问·刺禁论》）

李本：Over the diaphragm there are parents.

文本：Above the ge-huang, in the middle there are father and mother.

吴本：Above the diaphram, there is the sea of energy which maintains the life.

句中"父母"用以隐喻心、肺二脏，肺主于气，心主于血，共营卫于身，故为父母。"父母"完全失去字面意思，因此宜采用意译法。李本、文本将"父母"分别直译为 parents 和 father and mother。此译法虽然在形式上忠实于原文，但皆未译出喻指对象的具体内容，不能实现有效交际的目标。吴本舍弃"父母"的字面意思，将其意译为 the sea of energy which maintains the life，明确表明"父母"在句中指的是维持机体生命的气海，即心、肺二脏。

（五）战争隐喻

战争隐喻用于阐释抽象而复杂的疾病过程、致病因素、病理变化等，以动词居多。这些动词的意义随着语境而变化，失去其字面意思，翻译时宜采用意译法。例如，"客"用作动词时，兼具"寄居"和"侵害"两层意思。翻译时应该根据语境变化，采用意译法，表达出其内涵意义。

1. 此皆卫气之所留止，邪气之所客也……（《素问·五脏生成》）

李本：These are all the places where Weiqi (Defensive–Qi) maintains and Xieqi (Evil–Qi) stays...

文本：All these are locations where the guard qi [can] come to a halt and where the evil qi [can] settle as visitor...

吴本：All of them are the places for the Wei–energy to stay, and they are also the places for the evil–energy to reside...

"客"为动词，意为"留止"，而非其字面意思"做客"，宜采用意译法。李本、吴本将"客"分别意译为 stay 和 reside，隐喻邪气像人一样客居于某处，是对原文的忠实表达。文本将"客"直译为 settle as a visitor，貌似较为形象地表达出邪气是外来之物，但对译语读者来说，可能很难理解 the evil qi 与 visitor 之间的联系，不利于交际。

2. 风雨之伤人也，先客于皮肤，传入于孙脉。（《素问·调经论》）

李本：[When] wind and rain attack human beings, [they] first invade the skin. [Then they are] transmitted to the fine Collaterals.

文本：When wind and rain harm a person, they first settle in the skin, whence they are transmitted into the tertiary vessels.

吴本：When the wind and rain hurt the body, it invades into the skin first, then enters into the minute collateral.

"客"为动词，隐喻为"外邪寄居并侵犯人体"，句中强调"侵犯"之义，宜采用意译法。李本、吴本都将"客"意译为 invade，表达出风雨由外向内进入皮肤并对皮肤进行侵害这两层意思，保留了原文的战争隐喻。文本将"客"直译为 settle in，表达出"客居"之义，但未能体现出风雨对皮肤的侵害之内涵意义。

三、直译和意译结合法

《素问》中很多隐喻的喻体不明显，或者喻义表达得较为含蓄，仅进行直译可能会导致意思不清或产生误解，此时最好采取直译与意译相结合的方法进行处理。

1. 毒药攻邪，五谷为食，五果为助……（《素问·脏气法时论》）

李本：Duyao (drugs) [can be used] to attack Xie (Evil), the five kinds of grain [can be used] to nourish [the body], the five kinds of fruit [can be used] to assist [the five kinds of grain to nourish the body]...

威本：The poisons and medicines attack the evil influences. The five grains act as nourishment; the five fruits from the trees serve to augment...

文本：Toxic drugs attack the evil. The five grains provide nourishment. The five fruits provide support...

吴本：Poisonous drugs are to expel evils. The five kinds of cereals are to nourish the body, the five kinds of fruits are for supplementing...

"攻"为动词，意为"祛除（邪气）"，"毒药攻邪"指使用药物祛除邪气。"邪"作为中医术语，一般被约定俗成地直译为 evil。"攻"具有明显的战争隐喻特色，李本、威本和文本均将其直译为 attack，保留了原文的隐喻，也表达出"毒药"对"邪"的侵袭之义。但是，从语言角度来看，attack evil 并不搭配。吴本采用直译意译结合法将"攻邪"译为 expel evils。动词 expel 意为"排出（气体或毒素等）"，expel evils 搭配恰当，准确表达出"攻邪"在句中"祛除邪气"之内涵意义，为佳译。

2. 其眚四维，其主败折虎狼……（《素问·五常政大论》）

李本：[...bringing on] calamities to the four directions. [Retaliating activity of

《黄帝内经素问》隐喻英译对比研究

Metal–Qi] mainly impairs [animals like] tiger and wolf...

文本：...Disasters occur at the four ropes. This is responsible for ruin and destruction [caused by] tiger and wolf...

吴本：Its calamities are from the four corner (southeast, northwest, southwest and northeast), and its corruption and injury are like the ferocious damage of the wild beasts of tiger and wolf...

"其主败折虎狼"指农作物的生长受到影响，给人类社会造成极大的破坏，如同虎狼伤人一样。翻译时应将此句当作一个整体，"虎狼"为字面意思，宜采用直译法；"其主败折"指农作物受到破坏，失去字面意思，宜采用意译法。三个译本都将"虎狼"直译为 tiger and wolf，实现了语言和文化的成功转换。李本、文本都采用意译法翻译"其主败折"，但是未能正确理解原句的逻辑关系。吴本将"其主败折"意译为 its corruption and injury are like the ferocious damage of (the wild beasts of tiger and wolf)，对隐喻进行显化处理，指出本体和喻体，准确地传递出原文所蕴含的中医文化。

四、音译（加注）法

《素问》中的部分词语为中医学独有，在现代医学中没有对应语，对于这类具有民族性的词语，翻译时多采用音译法。然而，单纯的音译法虽然保留了汉语言的文化特色，但却很难忠实传递原文的内涵意义，也就无法实现有效交际的目标。因此，翻译时多采用音译加注法，使用汉语拼音进行音译，并在其后附加注释。音译（加注）法主要用于翻译下面四类术语。

（一）阴阳、精气相关术语

许多中医学概念，尤其是与阴阳、精气相关隐喻中的术语，为汉语言所特有，如阴、阳、精、气、邪等，多采用音译法。

1. 天有阴阳，地亦有阴阳。（《素问·天元纪大论》）

李本：[There are] Yin and Yang in both the heavens and the earth.

文本：Heaven has yin and yang; the earth has yin and yang, too.

吴本：There are Yin and Yang in the six kinds of weather in heaven, and there are Yin and Yang in the five elements of earth.

"阴阳"为中医学的特有术语，在现代医学和英语文化中都没有对应语，直译和意译皆不合适。三个译本都采用音译法，将"阴阳"译为 Yin and Yang 或 yin and yang。当前的中医术语英译国际标准一般都采用这一译法。

2. 以长为短，以白为黑，如是则精衰矣。（《素问·脉要精微论》）

李本：[If the eyes] take long as short and white as black, [it is a sign that] Jing (Essence) is declining.

吴本：If one can no more distinguish the length and the black and white, his vital energy has already been exhausted.

"精"指构成宇宙万物的灵气，为中医学的特有术语。翻译时，"精"常被译为 essence/spirit/energy 等，相应地，"精气"被译为 essence qi。例如，吴本一般将"精"或"精气"意译为 vital/refined/healthy energy，但是此译法也常被吴本用于表达"正气"，二者容易相混淆。实际上，随着中医学的对外传播，诸如"精""气"等概念也逐渐被译语读者接受，因此可以将"精"音译为 Jing。同时，"精"在不同语境中具有不同内涵意义，例如"水谷精微"，此种情况下采用音译加注法不失为良策。李本多采用音译加注法翻译此类术语。

（二）容器相关术语

容器隐喻中的部分容器概念为汉语言文化所特有，在英语中没有对应语，例如鬼门、净府、仓廪等，可采用音译（加注）法。

开鬼门，洁净府……（《素问·汤液醪醴论》）

李本：[Besides,] [the therapeutic methods for] opening Guimen (sweat pores) and cleaning the Jingfu (the bladder)...

文本：Open the demon gates and clean the pure palace...

吴本：Then, try to make the patient to perspire thoroughly, and keep his urination unobstructed...

"鬼门"和"净府"为汉语言特有术语，汗孔被喻为"鬼门"，膀胱被喻为"净府"。二者在英语中没有对应语，如果直译为 demon gates 和 pure palace（如文本），从文字层面来看确实保留了原文隐喻，但未能忠实传递原文的内涵意义，不能达到有效交际目的。如果意译为 make the patient to perspire thoroughly 和 keep his urination unobstructed（如吴本），能够达到交际目的，但是完全摒弃了原文的文化内涵，行文也较为繁琐。此种情况下，采用音译法为宜。李本采用音译加注的方法将"鬼门"和"净府"译为 Guimen (sweat pores) 和 Jingfu (the bladder)，音译保留了汉语言的文化特色，注释帮助译语读者理解原文的内涵意义，不失为一种较好的处理方式。

（三）藏象相关术语

一些中医藏象概念为中医学所特有，英语中找不到对应语，例如脏腑、三焦等，多采用音译（加注）法。

三焦者，决渎之官，水道出焉。（《素问·灵兰秘典论》）

李本：Sanjiao (triple energizer) is the organ [similar to] official in charge of dredging and is responsible for regulating the water-passage.

威本：The burning spaces are like the officials who plan the construction of ditches and sluices, and they create waterways.

文本：The triple burner is the official functioning as opener of channels. The paths of water originate in it.

吴本：The triple warmer takes the office of dredging water in the watercourse of the whole body, it takes charge of the activity of the vital energy of the body fluid and the regulation and the dredging of the fluid.

"三焦"是中医藏象术语，是上焦、中焦和下焦的合称，翻译时多被直译为 burning space/triple burner/triple burner 等。以上译法容易引起译语读者的曲解，因为"三焦"不具有 burn（燃烧，烧焦）的意思。李本采用音译加注的方法将"三焦"译为 Sanjiao (triple energizer)，既保留了汉语言特色，又注解了三焦主持诸气、总司人体气化的功能特点，为佳译。

（四）脉象相关术语

脉象是中医学术语，指脉搏的形象与动态，是中医辨证的依据之一，为中医学特有。翻译时多采用音译（加注）法。

女子二七而天癸至，任脉通，太冲脉盛……（《素问·上古天真论》）

李本：At the age of fourteen, Tiangui begins to appear, Renmai (Conception Vessel) and Chongmai (Thoroughfare Vessel) are vigorous in function...

威本：When she reaches her fourteenth year she begins to menstruate and is able to become pregnant and the movement in the great thoroughfare pulse（太冲脉）is strong...

文本：With two times seven, the heaven *gui* arrives, the controlling vessel is passable and the great thoroughfare vessel abounds [with qi]...

吴本：Her Taingui (the substance necessary for the promotion of growth, development and reproductive function of human body) appears at the age of fourteen (2×7). At this-time, her Ren channel begins to put through, and her Chong channel becomes prosperous...

"脉"本义指人体中的血管，常被译为 pulse/vessel/channel。"太冲脉"属奇经八脉之一，是中医核心术语。威本、文本将"太冲脉"意译为 the great thoroughfare pulse 和 the great thoroughfare vessel，表达出其内涵意义，但行文繁琐，不符合术语简洁性的特点，也失去了汉语文化特色。吴本采用音译和意译相结合的方法，将"太冲脉"译为 Chong channel，未能表明其指代的具体内容。李本使用音译加注法将"太冲脉"译为 Chongmai (Thoroughfare Vessel)，不仅明确其具体内容，而且保留脉象术语的汉语言特色，符合术语简洁性和民族性的特点。

需要说明的是，音译（加注）法通常用于翻译具有民族性的词语，这种词语在中医学中所占比例很小。一方面，音译（加注）法有利于中医药的对外传播，帮助译语读者在潜移默化中逐渐接受中医文化特色；但另一方面，音译（加注）法只是无奈之举，除非确实找不到对应语，一般情况下应该慎用音译（加注）法。

小　结

隐喻是《素问》中常用的一种认知手段，借助比喻的手法对古代生命科学进行诠释。《素问》隐喻的英译主要采取对等策略、本体补偿策略、舍喻体译喻底策略和隐喻显化策略等四种翻译策略。《素问》成书年代较为久远，文辞深奥，内涵丰富，增加了翻译的难度。这主要体现在三个方面：

第一，翻译质量在很大程度上取决于对原文的准确诠释。在四位译者中，李照国和吴连胜父子的华人背景使得他们对原文的理解较为充分，因此译文基本忠实于原文。相对而言，文树德和威斯有时对中医术语和喻指对象之间的关系理解不够透彻，导致译文释义不明、译不达意，甚至出现误译。

　　第二，翻译策略与方法需要随着语境的变化而变化。一些表示自然界和人类社会中客观存在的隐喻，为世界各民族文化共有，可以采用对等策略进行直译，例如自然隐喻、动植物隐喻、部分容器隐喻和内外空间隐喻等。但是，绝大多数隐喻的喻体是汉语言文化中特有的，在译语中找不到对应语，例如天地日月相关的隐喻、部分容器隐喻和动植物隐喻、官职隐喻等。有些词语由于语境变化而导致语义多变，例如社会关系隐喻和战争隐喻中的动词等。此种情况下宜采用意译法或直译意译结合法。

　　第三，很多中医核心术语是汉语言文化独有的，例如"阴""阳""精""气"等。这些术语多为名词，使用意译法会导致译文过于冗长，而且形式上与原文相差太大，不符合术语简洁性的特点，因此翻译时多使用音译（加注）法。

后 记

2018年暑期伊始至2022年暮春，历时三年多的时间，书稿终将付梓，不禁感慨万千。本书承蒙教育部人文社会科学研究青年基金项目"基于语料库的《黄帝内经素问》隐喻英译对比研究"（18YJCZH017）的资助，以我的著作《〈黄帝内经素问〉隐喻研究》为基础，从隐喻英译对比研究的角度进行拓展和延伸。三年多来，编委会成员在考查求证上力争精益求精，从最基础的译本收集与整理、文本校对，到语料库建设与维护，再至后期的译本分析、著作撰写等，无不凝聚成员们的汗水和心血。在此，谨向资助机构和编委会成员表示诚挚的谢意。

中医典籍翻译是翻译活动的重要组成部分，在当前"一带一路"国家战略中承担着"讲好中国故事、传播好中国声音"的重要使命。作为"医之始祖"，《黄帝内经》代表着中国传统医学的理论基础及思想精髓，是几千年来我国古代先哲和医家探讨生命科学的智慧结晶。其翻译工作对传承和发展中医药事业、推动中医药文化走向世界发挥着重要作用。自1925年以来，《黄帝内经》的英译工作和相关研究已有近百年时间，国内外已有20多个不同版本的英译本。本书选取《素问》较为典型的四个英译本。由于译者学术背景各不相同，四个译本呈现出迥异的翻译风格，在语言和内容这两方面各有千秋，各有所长。本书对其中的隐喻译文进行对比分析，总结出隐喻英译的策略以及对应的方法，以期为其他典籍的英译提供有益的借鉴。

词无定义，译无定法，对于《素问》这样一部中医经典巨著尤为如此。一个优秀的英译本最终取决于对原文的准确诠释和对翻译技巧的灵活使用。这就要求译者不但要具备强大的英语语言驾驭能力，还需要兼具深厚的汉语言文化知识基础。采众家之所长，集古今之精华，是我们不懈努力的方向。

希望本著作之浅见能够拓展《素问》隐喻英译研究的视角与深度，进一步丰富认知语言学隐喻理论，搭建中医语言与现代语言的沟通平台，为推动中医典籍翻译事业和中医药跨文化传播事业的发展略尽绵薄之力！

陈战

2022 年 4 月于济南